Understanding Dental Insurance

A Guide for Dentists and their Teams

Travis Campbell, DDS

Understanding Dental Insurance

A Guide for Dentists and their Teams

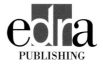

This edition first published 2021

©2021 Edra Publishing US LLC – All rights reserved
Reprinted 2021, 2022

ISBN: 978-1-7351497-5-2
eISBN: 978-1-7351497-7-6

Edra Publishing US LLC
3309 Northlake Boulevard,
Suite 203,
Palm Beach Gardens,
FL, 33403
EIN: 844113980

info@edrapublishing.com
www.edrapublishing.com

Printed by Versa Press, Inc., East Peoria, IL in July 2021

Table of Contents

Introduction

As dentists, when we each got our start in the profession, chances are we graduated from a school which taught us thoroughly how to clinically treat a patient. However, what the school did not teach us was the real-world part of life in dentistry, that is, how to handle patients outside of an institution-based clinic. While in the controlled school environment, we rarely had patients decline care because they did not believe it was needed, it is hard to disagree with dental school instructors that you didn't need that SRP or crown! Despite receiving top-notch dental training, we received minimal training in business skills. And most relevant of all, we were not taught anything about how to deal with the vast and complex arena of dental insurance.

Since graduating from dental school, I have opened multiple dental practices and now speak to and consult with dentists and their teams across the country. The most common misunderstandings, frustrations, and complaints I hear from both in-network and out-of-network offices are about dental insurance and insurance companies. Many of these concerns are legitimate, while others are due to a lack of understanding of what dental insurance is to begin with.

> **NOTE**
> Many, if not most, of the common insurance challenges can be avoided when you understand more about dental insurance.

When an office does not get paid for services that were provided, it can cause a lot of stress and headaches for both the patients and the dental team. The good news is that many, if not most, of the common challenges and problems can be avoided when you and your team really understand how dental insurance is designed, what companies are looking for, and learn how to anticipate, act, and advocate for your patient and your office.

When working with insurance representatives and claims examiners, you are working with people who possess minimal knowledge about the dental industry as a whole. Insurance company employees are typically taught what to do within their specific department and little about the rest of the company. This narrow viewpoint can lead to challenges when a dental team member calls the insurance company to get a question answered and is subsequently given incomplete or sometimes incorrect information. Many of you may have had a patient tell you their insurance customer service representative told them one thing, when just the day before, you talked to the same insurance company and were told the exact opposite. This scenario is a common occurrence experienced by dental offices across the country.

After becoming a practicing dentist, I had the opportunity to work with some excellent team members who knew significantly more than I about how life in the real world worked. However, even with all their practical knowledge of oral hygiene, dental systems, patients, and patient care, the level of insurance knowledge was low across the board. The few individuals who were highly skilled in dental insurance often could not easily teach it to others because their expertise was gained exclusively through years of experience. It was like talking to a great baker who never used a set recipe.

Some of the best bakers in the world tend to craft foods by experience more than recipe. If you have ever watched *Iron Chef*, you know what I mean. These chefs can create dishes on the fly without a recipe—they rely on taste, feel, and experience. The challenge becomes how to take a novice and bring them to that level of skill without undertaking years of similar experience. Other bakers, such as me in the kitchen, can follow a recipe to the letter and make a decent cake. However, that will never get us to the level of mastery to be called an expert. The second something does not go right, we get lost quickly, and the cake is not recoverable.

Just like bakers, most of the dental office professionals I have met who have a good grasp of insurance have been either experiential or cookbook. The cookbook individuals know what they know well but are greatly challenged when claims don't go the way they should. The experiential individuals have a better grasp of the art of insurance but sometimes have a hard time training other people. Both types often fall into the trap of believing a lot of the myths that exist about insurance and insurance companies because their training or experience is incomplete.

Over the course of my own career, any time I had a question about insurance, I usually had to research the answer for myself. It required a significant investment of time because the answers are not always clear cut and certainly not documented anywhere as a whole. There just has been no good single source of dental insurance information in the industry. Even the dental insurance companies can sometimes be poor sources for *correct* information.

Therefore, the goal of this textbook is to serve as that source: to be a training tool for those new to dental insurance, a reference guide to the experienced, as well as an overall resource for everyone on the dental office team. When the team is well trained and knowledgeable about insurance, you can either avoid or quickly overcome most of the challenges that come with handling dental insurance.

KEY TO SUCCESS

At the outset, it is worth emphasizing that obtaining greater insurance expertise in your dental office is about more than just reducing stress, overcoming challenges, and minimizing headaches.

The fact is that the better your office team understands the complexities of and tactics for dealing with insurance claims, the more likely:

1. Your office will be promptly paid for the services you provide;
2. Your patients will receive the maximum benefits from the insurance policies for which they are paying; and
3. Your bottom-line profitability as a business will increase.

Dental insurance has been here for 70 years and is not likely going away. It is a critical source of realizing revenue for your office as well as a way to reduce costs for your patient. If you don't fully understand insurance you might want to ask yourself the following:

- Why would you want to write off any services you legitimately provide to your patients?
- Why would you accept less revenue than you and your team deserve?
- Why would you want your patients to pay more than they need to because of an incomplete understanding of their insurance?

When you think of it that way, gaining expertise in today's world of dental insurance becomes critical toward the ultimate success of your dental practice and its ability to serve the patients.

> **TIP**
>
> Gaining expertise in today's world of dental insurance becomes critical toward the ultimate success and profitability of your dental practice.

My greatest hope is that you and your team will find this guide/reference to be a key resource for navigating the complexities of dental insurance in your practice and achieving your profitability goals.

HOW TO BEST USE THIS GUIDE

This textbook is designed first and foremost to be read through in sequential order, a training primer if you will, as many sections will build upon one another.

Part One serves as an introduction to dental insurance, covering the basic concepts and terminology as well as the ins and outs of the day-to-day use of insurance. Part one is a helpful guide for training someone new to dental insurance.

Part Two is an advanced section that covers the more specific concerns and concepts that can turn an average insurance coordinator into an insurance expert.

Part Three focuses on how to infuse insurance principles into the overall business side of the office.

Part Four discusses the changes that emerged within the insurance industry due to the Covid-19 pandemic.

Part Five is a series of case studies that can help solidify many of the concepts taught in this book and demonstrate practical application. This section can serve as a good tool to test your knowledge, as each case poses real insurance scenarios to think about and answer.

Each chapter in this textbook focuses on a discrete topic so that after training, you can easily refer to specific topics or challenges as needed.

The back of the book contains a Q&A section covering the most common questions and where to reference their answers within the text. This Q&A section can be a great quick-start tool if you are just picking up this guide and have immediate challenges to solve.

This textbook is designed to be a ready resource to both the person who has never worked with dental insurance before, as well as those who have worked for years to supplement their knowledge and dispel the common myths.

COMMON INSURANCE MYTHS

- The rules of the insurance game are intentional.
- The insurance company denied a claim because the patient did not need the service.
- Insurance representatives always give you correct information.
- EOBs (Explanation of Benefits) are always correct and must be followed completely.
- You must file all claims to insurance.
- You cannot offer upgraded services in-network.

The ultimate goal of a highly trained insurance team is to create a process that is smoother for the patient, more profitable for the office, and overall, less stressful to all parties involved. The more we know, the better advocates we can be for our patients and our offices.

Part 1

Understanding Insurance Basics

Chapter 1
What Is the Purpose of Dental Insurance?

Most people make decisions in their life based on what they *want*, sometimes neglecting the things they *need*. Have you ever seen someone buy a luxury item when they needed to fix their car that keeps breaking down? Or have you had a friend who bought a big screen TV, and the same day complained about not having enough money to live?

ADA research shows that patients with dental insurance will visit the dentist far more often and will accept more treatment versus patients without dental insurance.

Dental care often falls into the *need* but not the *want* category. People have a tendency to avoid dentistry even more than other needs they have. The American Dental Association's (ADA) research shows that over half the American population does not go to the dentist within a given year. This fact has stayed constant for decades. Dentistry is highly focused on preventive care, and therefore many people need us before they want us.

Affordability

Since dentistry is one of the least desired items on a person's "need" list, patients rarely set aside a budget specifically for dental treatment. A lack of savings for dentistry generally translates to people saying they cannot afford to go to the dentist, which of course isn't entirely true. They simply cannot see how to afford going to the dentist because they never anticipated that expense and did not reserve funds. (They did save the money for that big screen TV, though.)

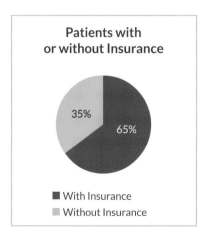

Patients with or without Insurance

35%
65%

■ With Insurance
■ Without Insurance

A large portion of the population does not want to spend their available cash to go to the dentist. Therefore, it is easier in a patient's mind to reserve that money before they even see it. This is where dental insurance comes into the picture. An insurance policy is in part an automatic savings account for patients to build reserve funds in order to receive dental care when needed. Insurance also includes discounted services, as well as sharing of actual costs with the insurance company.

So for the patient, dental insurance provides a structured plan that helps them to afford dental treatment. It is an important tool to plan for the costs of their individual and family health care.

As for the dental office, ADA research shows that patients with dental insurance will visit the dentist far more often and will accept more treatment than patients without dental insurance. An estimated 65% of Americans have dental insurance coverage.

So, as difficult and complex as the dental insurance process can be, it does play a key role in the delivery of dental care.

Who Does the Insurance Company Serve?

When we work with insurance companies on behalf of our patients every day, we would like to think that insurance companies design their forms and procedures to make it easy for the dental office. However, this is not the case at all. Let us look at the primary players in the delivery of dental insurance, and you will begin to appreciate the complexity of the entire system and therefore the priority focus of an insurance company.

Employers. In most cases across the country, it is business employers who contract with an insurance carrier to offer dental insurance packages as a benefit for their employees to purchase. Employers decide how much they are willing to pay for an employee benefit package

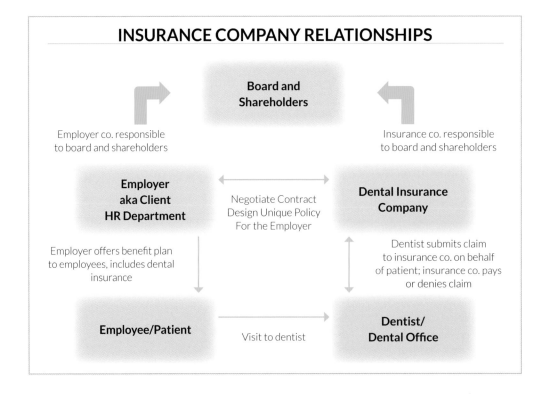

INSURANCE COMPANY RELATIONSHIPS

Board and Shareholders

Employer co. responsible to board and shareholders

Insurance co. responsible to board and shareholders

Employer aka Client HR Department

Negotiate Contract Design Unique Policy For the Employer

Dental Insurance Company

Employer offers benefit plan to employees, includes dental insurance

Dentist submits claim to insurance co. on behalf of patient; insurance co. pays or denies claim

Employee/Patient

Visit to dentist

Dentist/ Dental Office

and therefore what specific benefits will be included in each plan. They review and reassess those benefits every year. The employer is the one who decides each year if a specific insurance company is awarded the contract. Therefore, **the employer is the primary customer**, as they are the ones deciding on procuring insurance benefits for a large number of employees.

Human Resources. It is the human resources (HR) department of most companies who recommend and oversee all employee benefit plans, including dental insurance. The HR department is responsible for evaluating these plans each year and deciding whether to sign up with a specific insurance company.

Therefore, it is this HR department that the insurance company wants to make happy above all else. This is the reason when you hit a major roadblock while working on a claim, you may receive a suggestion to have the patient reach out to their employer's HR department. Most HR departments will have a benefits specialist, who is usually an advocate for their employees and, as a result, can help broker a particularly difficult situation.

Employees (your patients). An insurance policy is legally a contract between the insurance company and the employee policyholder. For a specific monthly fee, the insurance company provides dental benefit coverage to the employee and potentially their family according to the contract provisions. In this regard, the employee policyholder is a customer of the insurance company as well. When a dental office offers to inquire about benefit provisions for a treatment plan or to submit and help to follow up on claims, you are doing so as a service for your patients, not because you have a legal or contractual obligation to do so (in most cases).

> Policies, procedures, and claim forms are designed first and foremost to make it easy for the insurance carrier to handle the high volume of claims they receive from the vast network of providers.

Dental Providers. Dentists and dental offices are considered providers who are contracted with the insurance carrier's network to deliver services. And there are many, many providers that an insurance company does business with. That is why policies, procedures, and claim forms are designed first and foremost to make it easy for the insurance carrier to handle the high volume of claims they receive from the vast network of providers. It helps to explain why working with an insurance company and their forms is not necessarily easy for the single dentist or dental office staff. The dentist is not the customer.

Overall, as you can see, the primary client of the insurance company is the employer in most cases, which means the insurance company will strive to make the employer happy above all else.

TIP

When you have challenges with the insurance company paying what they should on claims, an option to help the patient is through the patient's HR department. HR is who decides whether their employer will retain the contract with a given insurance company each year. HR might have better luck getting the insurance company to pay according to policy. The patient, not the dental office, would need to contact their HR department for assistance.

The insurance carrier sees the dental providers as nothing more than suppliers or vendors. When a business has an ongoing problem with a supplier, they tend to find a new supplier. Keeping this in mind will help you understand the overall dynamics when dealing with dental insurance and the common problems dental offices encounter with insurance companies. One of the most notable challenges is the lengthy average wait time of getting in touch with provider relations or claims departments on the phone in contrast with relatively short patient or employer relations wait times.

How Is Dental Insurance Like or Different from Medical Health Insurance?

Medical health insurance is the insurance most needed and valued by patients and employers. Since dentistry is also part of overall health care, many patients and dentists tend to assume medical and dental insurance are similar. Because of this assumption, many patients (and team members) will mistakenly try to apply rules that work in the medical arena to dental insurance.

> **TIP**
>
> In reality, medical insurance and dental insurance are completely different. It is important to understand the distinctions between the two so you can help educate the patient when they try to mistakenly apply the rules of one to the other.

Medical and dental insurance both cover health-care expenses. This is where the similarities tend to end.

In traditional insurance (medical, home, auto, etc.) the policy will typically have a high deductible and a high or unlimited maximum. This is the true definition of insurance, which is designed to cover the extreme, unexpected outcomes.

Deductibles:

- Medical has a high deductible (often thousands)
- Dental has deductibles below $100

Premiums:

- Medical has high monthly premiums
- Dental has minimal monthly premiums
- "You get what you pay for."

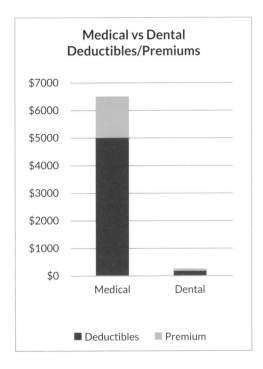

Dental insurance is the exact opposite with low deductibles and low maximums. Instead of paying for the extremes, dental insurance covers costs on the common, expected treatments/services. Medical patients aren't expected to get into a major car accident or develop a severe condition that requires hospitalization, surgery, or extended stays; whereas dental patients are expected to get cavities, need treatment, and see the hygienist twice a year. This alone is a huge distinction with dental coverage as it relates to the total available funds the dental insurance company accumulates. It is also why the cost-to-benefit ratio is so low with dental insurance.

Maximums

Medical generally has no annual maximum (or it is extremely high), but instead works on lifetime maximums. These maximums may be in the hundreds of thousands or millions.

Dental insurance typically has an average annual maximum around $1000–$2000. Lifetime maximums are typically only seen with additional coverage specialty services such as orthodontics and surgery.

This means that patients may never hear the term "maximum" with their medical insurance but may often hit maximum with their dental coverage.

Co-Pays

Medical will typically collect a co-pay on the routine services, such as $15–$50 when you get your routine physical. Medical will then cover 100% of any other treatment or service after the deductible has been met.

Dental insurance does not collect co-pays on routine services and has a large percentage co-pay on other non-routine service (10–50% or more).

Compared to the cost of the treatment, medical starts off higher due to how deductibles work. However, dental costs will quickly ramp up to be higher out-of-pocket cost for the patient due to annual maximums. Patients will often plan to do more medical treatment in a year once they hit their deductible. In contrast, patients may often try to delay dental care once their annual maximum has been reached.

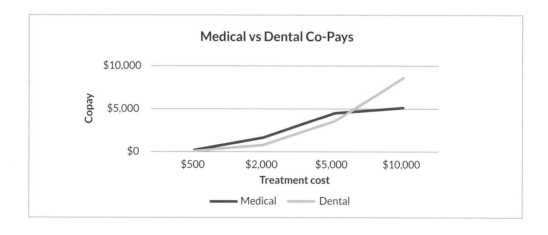

Pre-authorizations/Pre-Determinations

- Medical typically will provide pre-authorizations, or guarantees of payment
- Dental typically only provides pre-determinations, which are *not* guarantees of payment. (See more in Chapter 22)

In actuality, dental insurance is not insurance at all by any other standards, as it does not cover large, unexpected expenses. Dental is more akin to a discount or coupon program with a small treatment assistance benefit attached. This is a challenge because patients tend to assume their dental insurance works similarly to medical. Patients commonly expect to have minimal to no payments for their dental treatment, just like medical. Your team and patients should be aware of these differences so that all involved can have more realistic expectations.

Chapter 2
Basic Dental Anatomy and X-Rays

In order to file insurance correctly, one needs to have a basic understanding of dental anatomy and how teeth are organized. The most commonly used numbering system for teeth is called the Universal Numbering System.

- Primary (baby) teeth are numbered #A – T
- Permanent (adult) teeth are numbered #1 – 32
- The numbering starts on the upper right, most posterior tooth (wisdom tooth)

There are three types of teeth when it comes to filing insurance claims: anterior, premolars, and molars. Anterior teeth include those in the front of the mouth. Molars and premolars are considered posterior teeth in the back of the mouth. It is important to understand when you see a tooth number, which tooth in the mouth this refers to. The location and number (or letter) of the tooth or teeth involved is always documented in a claim to help determine how insurance is billed for treatment. Many services have different coding and pricing depending on the tooth involved.

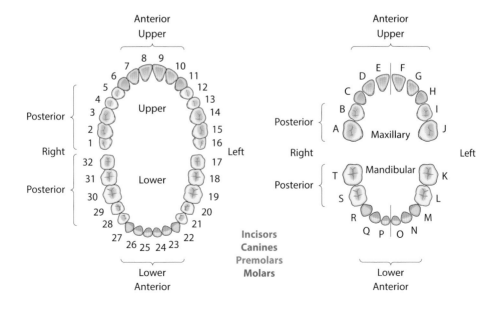

Endodontics codes (root canal services) are identified as anterior, premolar, or molar.

Filling codes are split into groups of either anterior or posterior.

Sealant reimbursement often has the distinction of either molar only or posterior only (includes premolars and molars).

Basic Dental Coding

When there are hundreds of different procedures completed in dental offices every day, offices need a quick way to communicate with the insurance company exactly what was done. This is where dental coding comes in. The American Dental Association (ADA) creates and maintains a list of codes that define most of the common services in dentistry. These codes are designed to use for communication with insurance companies for the purpose of claims reimbursement for procedures undertaken on behalf of their dental policyholders. These codes are used daily in the dental office within your practice management software and are generally referred to as the CDT (Current Dental Terminology).

ADA dental codes are organized by grouping or type of procedure for easier reference. These codes always start with a D and are followed by 4 digits. The first of the four digits corresponds to the category of service. For example, endodontic codes are also referred to as the D3000 codes.

The other three digits correspond to the specific procedure within that category. For example, D3330 is a root canal on a molar tooth. What follows is the ADA table showing a high-level view of the ADA categories. More detailed codes can be found in the coding books from the ADA or Charles Blair.

CDT Codes	Category of Service
D0100–D0999	Diagnostic (exams and x-rays)
D1000–D1999	Preventative (hygiene)
D2000–D2999	Restorative (fillings and crowns)
D3000–D3999	Endodontics (root canals)
D4000–D4999	Periodontics (gum treatments)
D5000–D5899	Removable prosthetics (dentures)
D5900–D5999	Maxillofacial (surgical) prosthetics
D6000–D6199	Implants
D6200–D6999	Fixed prosthetics (bridges)
D7000–D7999	Oral surgery
D8000–D8999	Orthodontics (braces and aligners)
D9000–D9999	Adjunctive

ADA codes are *not* meant to describe every service that can be done in a dental office, only the ones where insurance may provide reimbursement. Later in the book, we will talk about internal coding and how you can apply it to services that will not be covered by insurance (see Chapter 20).

X-Rays

X-rays used in dentistry come in a variety of types. The abbreviations for each of those terms are important to learn as well, as they are more commonly used than the term itself. The common types of x-rays are:

> **TIP**
>
> X-rays are like looking in the mirror; images are flipped. The right side of an x-ray is the left side of the patient, and vice versa. X-rays portray the same view as if you are looking directly at the patient.

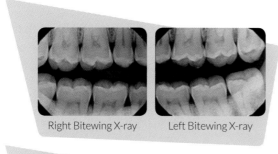

Right Bitewing X-ray   Left Bitewing X-ray

Bitewings (BW) – These show decay occurring between posterior teeth and those under restorations. These are the most common x-rays taken in a general office.

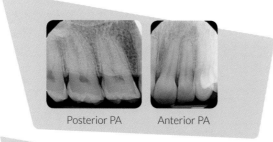

Posterior PA   Anterior PA

Periapicals (PA) – These show the entire length of a tooth and root, often looking for infection or bone loss. These are also used to find decay between anterior teeth.

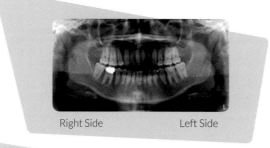

Right Side   Left Side

Panoramic (Pano) – These show the entire jaw and joints. They are most often used when preparing for surgery, dentures, or when there are joint/jaw problems.

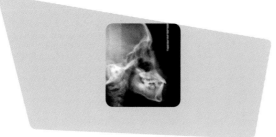

Cephalometric (CEPH) – Shows the profile of a jaw and teeth and is used most often in orthodontics.

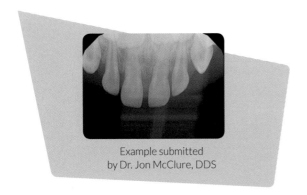

Example submitted
by Dr. Jon McClure, DDS

Occlusal – These are taken on young children to see the development of the anterior teeth when there is no room for BWs and PAs.

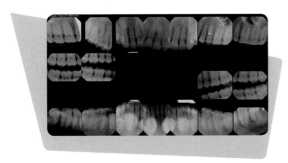

Full-mouth series of x-rays (FMX) – A series of BWs and PAs (14–20) to show the entire mouth. Often used with new adult patients or to see the entire picture of a generalized concern (such as periodontal disease).

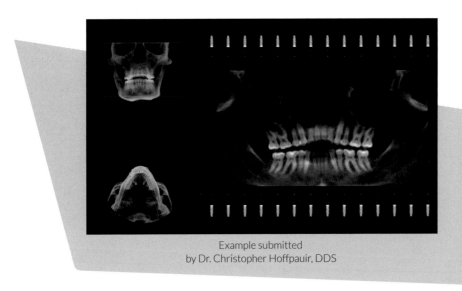

Example submitted
by Dr. Christopher Hoffpauir, DDS

Cone Beam Computed Tomography (CBCT) – 3D rendering of teeth, often showing the same wide view as a Pano does but with better accuracy. It is most often used in specialist endodontic, surgical, and implant cases.

Chapter 3
Types of Insurance

While Preferred Provider Organizations (PPOs) are the most well-known type of dental insurance, there are multiple other types that you will come across working in a dental office. It is important to understand the basics of each so that you know how to handle claims as well as answer patient questions. In general, there are two basic categories of insurance plans in dentistry:

1. Indemnity (traditional insurance)
2. Capitation (managed care)

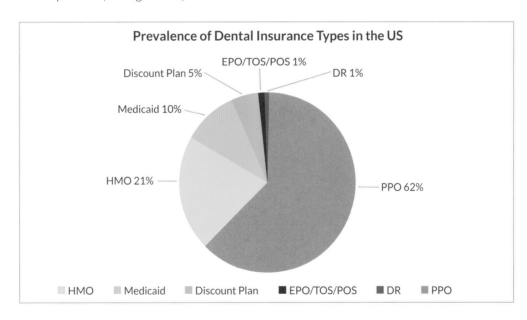

Prevalence of Dental Insurance Types in the US

- EPO/TOS/POS 1%
- DR 1%
- Discount Plan 5%
- Medicaid 10%
- HMO 21%
- PPO 62%

HMO · Medicaid · Discount Plan · EPO/TOS/POS · DR · PPO

INDEMNITY PLAN – "TRADITIONAL INSURANCE"

An indemnity plan is your "traditional" insurance plan, which pays (reimburses) based on dental procedures submitted via a formal claim. Most often they reimburse a percentage of the treatment/service performed. With an indemnity plan, the policyholder can receive dental services from any dentist of their choosing. This is by far the most common type of dental insurance.

Table/Schedule of Allowance (TOA/SOA) Plans

This is an indemnity type plan that pays a flat amount per procedure (instead of a percentage), irrespective of the cost of the procedure. The patient would be responsible for the difference in fees. These plans may or may not have a network arrangement. A common example of this type of plan is Aflac, which reimburses a flat amount when a covered problem occurs. These types of plans are common within medical and uncommon in dentistry.

Preferred Provider Organization (PPO)

The PPO is a type of indemnity plan that is tied to a network of dentists who sign a contract with a specific insurance carrier to provide a set fee schedule and follow a list of rules and guidelines. PPO plans allow reimbursement for both in-network and out-of-network providers. PPOs are the most common type of indemnity plan and the one you will most likely work with every day. Most major insurance carriers offer PPO dental plans, including Aetna, MetLife, and Delta Dental.

Exclusive Provider Organization (EPO)

An EPO is similar to a PPO, except an EPO will not provide reimbursement for out-of-network providers. This severely limits the options for the patient to be able to use their plan benefits. While a PPO plan allows a patient to go anywhere and see any dentist, an EPO restricts them to a specific set of in-network providers if they want to utilize their insurance benefits. Because they are more restrictive, they usually have lower monthly premiums as well. EPO plans are not very common within the dental insurance industry.

CAPITATION PLANS

Capitation plans pay a fixed amount to the dental office each month for each enrolled person assigned to the dental provider, whether or not that person seeks care. The amount is determined by the number of patients assigned to the provider. In exchange for the monthly payment (aka capitation check), the provider agrees to do some procedures for free (typically diagnostic/preventive) and others for a greatly reduced fee.

Health Management Organization (HMO) or Dental Health Management Organization (DHMO)

"HMO" and "DHMO" typically are interchangeable terms. These plans are similar to the EPO in that they will only provide reimbursement for services through an in-network provider. This is where the similarity ends.

While EPO/PPO claims are often reimbursed at a percentage of the office or contract fee, HMO claims are typically paid at a set contract fee instead of a percentage.

EXAMPLE

A PPO plan may pay 50% of the office's crown fee, while an HMO might only pay a flat $200 regardless of the price of the crown.

HMOs typically require some form of co-pay, do not include a deductible, and tend to not have an annual maximum.

Dental services that are not specifically covered by the plan must be paid by the patient, usually at the dentist's normal full office fee.

HMO plans are offered by most of the same major insurance carriers that offer PPO plans. HMO plans often have much lower premiums than PPOs, which makes them attractive to employers. Benefits packages that employers offer to employees often make the HMO plan appear better, in order to nudge the employee to pick the lower cost plan and save the employer money. It is important for dental office team members to understand this so they can correctly advise patients who ask about insurance options.

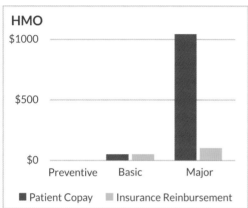

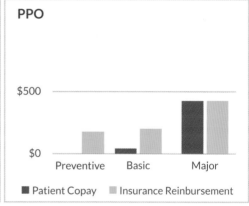

Point of Service Plans (POS)

POS plans are a hybrid of the PPO and HMO. Typically, you still have a network similar to an HMO, where you must designate a primary provider, but there are no capitation checks and therefore no services done for free by the office. Similar to the PPO, POS plans reimburse both in and out of network and have deductibles and co-pays. The difference between an EPO and POS is the POS will cover out-of-network providers and EPOs will not. POS plans are not very common within the dental industry.

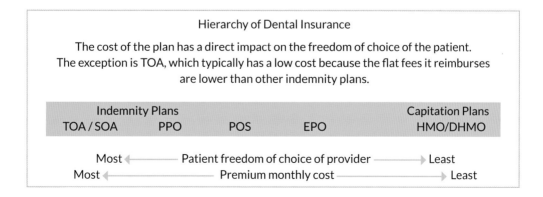

DISCOUNT PLANS

Many of the large dental insurance companies will offer discount plans as a low-cost alternative to a traditional indemnity PPO plan. These are typically the least expensive form of dental benefit a patient can purchase.

Discount plans are not true insurance as there are no claims or reimbursements made from an insurance company. The patient simply pays a monthly premium in order to get access to the network discounts available from a traditional indemnity plan. Then the patient would pay 100% of the network discounted fee directly to the dentist for services rendered.

For the dental office, discount plans are often much easier to manage because there are no claims involved in treatment of patients with these plans. This is basically fee-for-service with a discount. The office is trading a lower fee schedule in order to be listed on the insurance website and to get access to patients who would not otherwise come to the office. Several of the major insurance carriers offer discount plans to patients who do not have benefits from an employer.

SELF-FUNDED PLANS
ERISA (Employee Retirement Income Security Act)

Now that you have seen most of the different types of plans, it is important to understand that insurance plans can be funded in two distinct ways.

- **Traditional insurance** (fully insured) is when an employer pays an insurance company to handle everything related to insurance, including the financial risk.
- **Self-funded plans** are those where the employer takes all financial risk themselves but hires an insurance company to provide networks, call centers, and administrative support.

ERISA is a federal program that oversees the rules governing self-funded plans, so you may often hear self-funded plans being called ERISA plans. Because of their federal status, ERISA plans are not subject to state laws that protect the dental office and patient from certain actions of the insurance company. Common examples of this would be with non-covered services (see Chapter 17) and insurance recoupment laws (see Chapter 21).

How Can You Tell What Plans Are ERISA Plans? – Around 48–49% of dental insurance plans are self-funded plans.

The patient's insurance card may have that data; If you have the patient's insurance card, look for the phrase "administered by," which always means self-funded. The alternative way to find out is to ask upon a breakdown call.

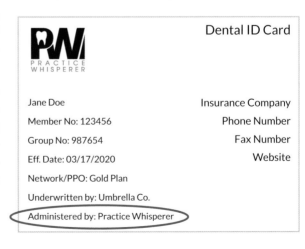

Dental ID Card

Jane Doe

Member No: 123456

Group No: 987654

Eff. Date: 03/17/2020

Network/PPO: Gold Plan

Underwritten by: Umbrella Co.

Administered by: Practice Whisperer

Insurance Company

Phone Number

Fax Number

Website

DIRECT REIMBURSEMENT (DR)

DR plans are self-funded plans that reimburse based on dollars spent instead of type of treatment performed. The patient would typically pay the dentist directly, and the insurance company would reimburse the patient, although occasionally benefits can be assigned directly to the provider. There are no networks to be in or out with DR plans. Some DR plans have minimal or no claims or administrative processing to be done by a dental office or insurance company. DR plans were far more common in the past than they are today.

COBRA

Since most Americans obtain insurance through their employer, when their job ends, their insurance coverage ends as well. COBRA is a way for people to extend their medical and/or dental benefits (up to 18–36 months) beyond their termination date. COBRA is typically more costly to the subscriber because the employer is no longer paying a portion of the premium but can still be less costly than buying the policy as an individual because they are receiving the employer's group rate.

From the dental office perspective, COBRA insurance plans aren't much different than normal, except they can be cancelled at any time by the patient or subscriber. It is a good idea to verify coverage more often on COBRA plans because they are more likely to be cancelled during the year. One may also want to verify status with the patient every visit as well, because they will know more directly whether they still are paying for COBRA coverage.

FEDERAL PLANS

Some insurance plans are federally mandated but locally or individually managed, which include COBRA and ERISA. There is another set of plans that are federally mandated and regionally or federally managed, which include Medicaid, Medicare, and Tricare. The reason these are important to understand separately is because they follow different rules than other non-federal plans. Most importantly, these plans do not follow state laws. Many state laws are designed to protect providers and patients from certain insurance tactics or mistakes. Federally managed plans are not subject to these state laws and protections. (See chapters 17 and 18 for more information on how these federally based plans differ in your day-to-day processing).

MEDICAID/CHIP

The first and most common federal plan in dentistry is Medicaid, which is insurance designed to help low-income and disabled families take care of children's dental care (most common threshold is 138% of the federal poverty level). Most commonly, these plans cover eligible patients 19 and under, often covering 100% of their dental care with no maximum amount of treatment per year. The plan specifics are decided by each state as to what will be covered and what the budget will be, so each state will have a variation of what a plan covers.

Occasionally you may find adult coverage under Medicaid, but the policy or documentation threshold for reimbursement of the treatment is extremely high, making it difficult for the dental office to get paid for treating adult patients.

The main concern of the dental office with these plans is that they are commonly set at the lowest fee schedule. In addition, families covered by these plans can present an office management scheduling dilemma, sometimes lacking reliable means of travel to the office, and may have more life challenges that compete with seeking preventative or general dental care. This tendency can result in a high no-show and cancellation rate. Due to the federal nature of these plans, an office is often disallowed from charging no-show fees or otherwise design incentives to encourage patients to keep their appointments.

CHIP is an offshoot Medicaid plan designed for families that are slightly better off financially (up to 200%–300% of the federal poverty level). CHIP will share fee schedules with Medicaid but include a yearly maximum that will be covered. Many times, you will see CHIP plans with co-payments and premiums the patient is required to pay.

To the dental office, this means that in general, your Medicaid patients will not have to pay anything for dental care, whereas your CHIP patients may have some out-of-pocket costs. Medicaid also allows patients to have dual coverage through private insurance; CHIP does not.

These plans are managed by companies such as DentaQuest and MCNA Dental.

Common Dental Office Question

> **Q: I am not a Medicaid provider; can I still see/treat Medicaid patients?**
> A: Yes, you can see these patients as cash patients. Medicaid will provide no reimbursement at all for services of a non-network provider.

*Note: It is helpful to be sensitive to the fact that the economic level of those who qualify for these plans is quite low. Therefore, they rarely have excess funds available for additional discretionary services to be seen as a cash patient.

TIP

If you were recently (formerly) a Medicaid provider, it would be recommended to obtain a written waiver signed by your Medicaid patient, acknowledging they are aware you are no longer in-network, have the option to go see another Medicaid provider, and understand they have to pay in cash for services going forward.

MEDICARE

Medicare is a federal program of insurance coverage to help patients over 65 with medical care. Dental coverage is not part of Medicare with the exception of hospital-based dental care, such as traumas or procedures required to be done in the hospital. The original Medicare plans have a Part A and Part B.

You may occasionally have patients asking if you take Medicare, and what they are typically asking is if you participate in a dental supplement plan, known as a Medicare Advantage Plan (Part C). These are plans separate from the basic Medicare program and must be purchased separately as additional coverage specifically for dentistry.

The main difference between Medicare and non-Medicare plans is simply what program (or administrator) they run through, which does not affect the dental office much at all. Medicare Advantage Plans are sold and administered by private companies (such as Delta or Humana) and can be anything from HMO to PPO to discount plans.

For the office, there would be no difference whether the patient's plan is a Medicare supplement or a non-Medicare plan.

> **TIP**
>
> When a patient asks you if you accept Medicare:
> You should treat them just like any other patient and ask them what plan they have, along with the details. The patient is unlikely to know what type of plan they have (HMO, PPO, or discount plan); most of them only know that they have a "Medicare" plan.
> Having them provide you with the specific details of the plan off a card or brochure will help.
>
> Many patients have Medicare but did not purchase an additional supplement plan. If they did not purchase additional coverage, they would have no dental plans and would therefore be treated as cash patients.

Typically, there are benefits to the patient for buying a dental policy through Medicare, such as single billing and shared deductibles. This is why you will encounter 65+ patients who do have dental coverage through a Medicare supplemental plan.

TRICARE

Tricare is a federal program for dental care that covers military patients and their families. There are three versions of Tricare based on who is the sponsor (military personnel/subscriber):

Active Duty Dental Program (ADDP)

Active Duty Tricare dental coverage is administered through Delta Dental and United Concordia. This program is specifically designed for active duty military as well as public health services federal employees. This program does not typically cover any service that is considered cosmetic or elective, such as bleaching and veneers. Covered services are paid at 100% by the insurance company, and non-covered services are billed at full fee by the provider to the patient.

A patient may seek treatment through an out-of-network provider but might not be 100% covered if they do so.

Non-Active Duty (Tricare Dental Program – TDP)

This dental coverage is designed for reserve military personnel and families of both active and reserve military. Currently in 2021, TDP is managed by United Concordia. You may occasionally hear the terms CONUS and OCONUS, which stand for the CONtinental United States and Outside the CONtinental United States. CONUS also includes any US territories, unlike what you might expect from the term.

You may come across these patients for their annual exam in preparation for them to go on active duty again, in which case they will need to fill out a D2813 dental exam form. Patients will often bring this form with them, but see the next page for an attached version for reference.

FEDVIP

These plans are for retired service members and their families. FEDVIP plans are managed by several dental companies. The patient has the option of choosing the specific plan, level of coverage, and carrier at time of enrollment (Aetna, Delta, FEP Blue Dental, GEHA, Humana, Metlife, and United Concordia) (see the form on page 25).

TriCare Coverage Table

Coverage percentage depends on the rank of the military person who the plan is sponsored through. The patient or family member will know the rank. See coverage chart below from 2021 for TDP (Non-Active Duty), which are the most likely patients you will encounter:

TDP Cost-Shares (Co-Pays)

	CONUS Pay Grade	
	E1–E4	E5+
Diagnostic	0%	0%
Preventive (including sealants)	0%	0%
Basic restorative	20%	20%
Endodontics	30%	40%
Periodontics	30%	40%
Oral surgery	30%	40%
Miscellaneous services (e.g., occlusal guard)	50%	50%
Other restorative	50%	50%
Implant services	50%	50%
Prosthodontics	50%	50%
Orthodontics	50%	50%

2021 Maximums for TDP patients are as follows:

Annual maximum benefit: $1,500

Coverage year: May 1–April 30

Orthodontic lifetime maximum benefit: $1,750

Accidental annual additional maximum benefit: $1,200

DEPARTMENT OF DEFENSE
ACTIVE DUTY/RESERVE/GUARD/CIVILIAN FORCES DENTAL EXAMINATION

OMB No. 0720-0022
OMB approval expires
Aug 31, 2016

The public reporting burden for this collection of information is estimated to average 3 minutes per response, including the time for reviewing instructions, searching existing data sources, gathering and maintaining the data needed, and completing and reviewing the collection of information. Send comments regarding this burden estimate or any other aspect of this collection of information, including suggestions for reducing the burden, to the Department of Defense, Washington Headquarters Services, Executive Services Directorate, Information Management Division, 4800 Mark Center Drive, Alexandria, VA 22350-3100 (0720-0022). Respondents should be aware that notwithstanding any other provision of law, no person shall be subject to any penalty for failing to comply with a collection of information if it does not display a currently valid OMB control number.
PLEASE DO NOT RETURN YOUR FORM TO THE ABOVE ORGANIZATION.

PRIVACY ACT STATEMENT

AUTHORITY: 10 U.S.C. 136; 10 U.S.C. 1074f; DoD Directives 1404.10, 5101.1, 5136.01, and 6490.02E; DoD Instruction 6025.19; and E.O. 9397 (SSN), as amended.
PRINCIPAL PURPOSE(S): To obtain information in order to record an assessment of an individual's dental health.
ROUTINE USE(S): Information collected may be used and disclosed generally as permitted under 45 CFR Parts 160 and 164, Health Insurance Portability and Accountability Act (HIPAA) Privacy and Security Rules, as implemented by DoD 6025.18-R, the DoD Health Information Privacy Regulation. Information may also be used and disclosed in accordance with 5 U.S.C. 552a(b) of the Privacy Act of 1974, as amended, which incorporates the DoD "Blanket Routine Uses" published at http://dpclo.defense.gov/privacy/SORNs/blanket_routine_uses.html. Information from this system may be shared with other Federal and State agencies and civilian health care providers, as necessary, to provide medical care and treatment and to guide possible referrals.
DISCLOSURE: Voluntary; however, failure to provide the information may result in delays in assessing your dental health needs for military service and/or for possible deployment outside the United States and its territories and possessions.

1. SERVICE MEMBER'S NAME (Last, First, Middle Initial)	2. SOCIAL SECURITY NUMBER	3. BRANCH OF SERVICE

4. UNIT OF ASSIGNMENT	5. UNIT ADDRESS

6. EXAMINATION RESULTS

Dear Doctor,

The individual you are examining is an Active Duty/Guard/Reserve/Civilian member of the United States Armed Forces. This member needs your assessment of his/her dental health for worldwide duty. **Please mark (X) the block** that best describes the condition of the member, using as a suggested minimum a clinical examination with mirror and probe, and bitewing radiographs. **This form is meant to determine fitness for prolonged duty without ready access to dental care and is not intended to address the member's comprehensive dental needs.**

(1) Patient has good oral health and is not expected to require dental treatment or reevaluation for 12 months.

(2) Patient has some oral conditions, but you **do not** expect these conditions to result in dental emergencies within 12 months if not treated (i.e., requires prophylaxis, asymptomatic caries with minimal extension into dentin, edentulous areas not requiring immediate prosthetic treatment).

(3) Patient has oral conditions that you **do** expect to result in dental emergencies within 12 months if not treated. Examples of such conditions are: *(X the applicable block or specify in the space provided)*

(a) **Infections:** Acute oral infections, pulpal or periapical pathology, chronic oral infections, or other pathologic lesions and lesions requiring biopsy or awaiting biopsy report.

(b) **Caries/Restorations:** Dental caries or fractures with moderate or advanced extension into dentin; defective restorations or temporary restorations that patients cannot maintain for 12 months.

(c) **Missing Teeth:** Edentulous areas requiring immediate prosthodontic treatment for adequate mastication, communication, or acceptable esthetics.

(d) **Periodontal Conditions:** Acute gingivitis or pericoronitis, active moderate to advanced periodontitis, periodontal abscess, progressive mucogingival condition, moderate to heavy subgingival calculus, or periodontal manifestations of systemic disease or hormonal disturbances.

(e) **Oral Surgery:** Unerupted, partially erupted, or malposed teeth with historical, clinical, or radiographic signs or symptoms of pathosis that are recommended for removal.

(f) **Other:** Temporomandibular disorders or myofascial pain dysfunction requiring active treatment.

(4) If you selected Block (3) above, please indicate the condition(s) you identified in this patient if they appear above, or briefly describe the condition(s) below:

(5) Were X-rays consulted?		YES		NO	IF YES, DATE X-RAY WAS TAKEN (YYYYMMDD)

7. DENTIST'S NAME (Last, First, Middle Initial)	8. DENTIST'S ADDRESS (Street, City, State, 9-digit ZIP Code)

9. DENTIST'S TELEPHONE NUMBER (Include Area Code)

10. DENTIST'S SIGNATURE/STATE LICENSE NUMBER	11. DATE OF EXAMINATION (YYYYMMDD)

DD FORM 2813, OCT 2013   PREVIOUS EDITION IS OBSOLETE.   Adobe Professional X

Chapter 4
In Network versus Out of Network

Now that you have seen the variety of different dental insurance types, you can start to get a feel for which insurance plans will and will not work for your office.

OUT OF NETWORK (OON)

Being out of network simply means that the dental provider has not signed a contract with a specific insurance company and therefore has not agreed to any network discounts or insurance company rules. The one rule, of course, you must always follow is to not commit insurance fraud per federal law (see Chapter 19).

There are several options you can choose from for how to handle out-of-network cases, the notable difference being how you file claims and manage assignment of benefits (AOB). AOB denotes who receives the reimbursement check from the insurance company, and there are a few different ways you can handle it (see greater detail on AOB in Chapter 10).

- **Patient Pays and Files Claim**. The most traditional approach to managing treatment and claims when you are out of network is to simply not get involved with the patient's insurance carrier. This is typically referred to as being fee for service (FFS). When you provide treatment for a patient, the patient will pay 100% of the cost of that care at the time of service. Your office would then help the patient fill out any insurance claim forms, but the patient would be responsible for mailing and monitoring the claims process. You would not file claims or accept assignment of benefits. This is the simplest way to handle out-of-network insurance cases.
- **Patient Pays, Office Files Claim**. Many patients have a hard time accepting responsibility for the claims process as insurance does not make it simple. As a compromise, many out-of-network offices will collect 100% of the fee but as a service to their patients will file and handle the claims process for the patient, including fight any denials on their behalf. Since the office already collected 100% of the fee, assignment of benefits (reimbursement) would go to the patient. This method can help save your patients a lot of headaches but does add additional time and training needed for the office team in managing insurance claims. This method is also referred to as fee for service (FFS).
- **Office Collects and Files Claim**. The last option is to treat the patient almost like an in-network patient, just without the reduced network discount. Under this method, the

office would collect the estimated patient portion only, file the claim for the patient, and then accept assignment of benefits from the insurance company after the claim has been processed. This is the most patient-friendly option but requires even more knowledge on the part of the office team, especially with estimates and handling claims.

IN NETWORK

Being in-network means signing a contract that you accept the insurance company's rules as well as the network discount that the insurance company sets. The network discount is a reduced fee that the provider agrees to charge as an advertised member of the insurance company's collection of preferred providers. Before signing on as an in-network provider, you will want to clearly understand both the benefits and challenges. (See more in Chapter 16).

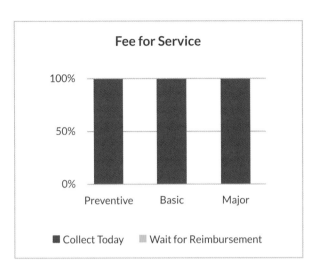

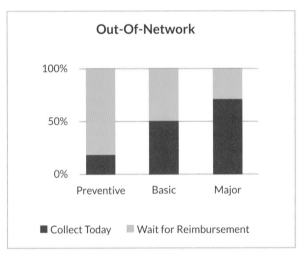

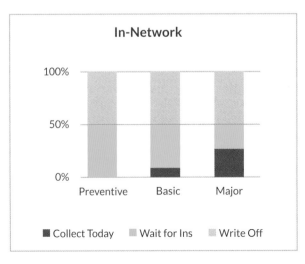

Many dentists want to use high-priced supplies, equipment, and labs. A common misconception is that one can provide high-end materials with in-network pricing. If your preference is high-end-priced options, then being in-network likely is not for you. **It is important to understand that being in-network is not about providing top-price materials at a lower fee.** There are plenty of low-price options that still provide similar quality to not be forced into this pricing mismatch challenge. Being in-network means finding budget options as well as more efficiency to absorb the insurance discounted prices. This makes higher-end materials an upgrade to basic insurance fees.

If you have to accept lower fees and agree to a list of often-onerous rules, why would a dentist ever want to be in-network? There are a few common reasons:

1. **Marketing** – Dental insurance companies save money when patients choose in-network providers and therefore will market or post preferred provider lists of the dentists in a given area who are in-network. Being on this list can help dentists grow their patient population.
2. **Patient Mentality** – A majority of people with insurance have been trained to believe that in-network is the only way to go for a variety of reasons (lower cost, lack of ability to gauge dental quality, and insurance company marketing). In general, unless a patient already has a relationship with your practice, they may well be reluctant to see an out-of-network provider.
3. **Niche** – The more populated an area, the harder it becomes to differentiate yourself from other providers. Keep in mind, most dentists believe they do the best clinical job around, whereas patients have few tools for evaluating quality in dentistry. The more uncommon your practice is in terms of services, customer service, and public perception, the more likely the office can sustain being out of network. (A well-known example is the "denture depots," places that only focus on dentures and extractions.)
4. **Price** – Many dentists decide to go in-network because they feel the patients in their area cannot afford a higher price. The key thing to remember here is that just because you are out of network does not mean you have to be more expensive. Often in medical practices, cash-only clinics typically have lower prices on everything. When a practice does not file or accept insurance, there can be a significant overhead cost savings, which allows lower fees.

Just because you are out of network does not mean you have to be more expensive. You can be out of network and have the same or lower normal prices than the dentist down the street. This allows you to avoid many of the onerous network contract rules and still be more affordable for your patients.

Tips for Offices Choosing to Be Out of Network

1. Understand what patients desire most in a provider/office. While dentists typically believe patients want the highest-quality care, what we often fail to understand is patients have no way to evaluate clinical quality. What patients will often use as their main reasons for going to a dental office are the non-clinical aspects, such as atmosphere, personalities, follow-up and follow-through, and other more emotional aspects of their experience.
2. Know that insurance carriers provide a lot of marketing, so to be out of network, you will likely need to focus heavily on your own marketing to attract patients.
3. Find your niche—you need to answer clearly for the office a few general questions. Why should a patient visit your office over the other dentists in the area? Why should they be willing to spend more money and/or not follow their insurance company's preferred provider list?
4. Focus on customer service and building relationships.

People in general form relationships with their doctors and don't like to change. They usually will stay through minor inconsistencies unless they have a complaint. It is particularly important if you are going to be out of network that you are very conscious of your reputation and referral rating. You need to sustain a top-notch patient experience to maintain patients after you drop their network.

Whether you go to Google, Yelp, Angie's List, and so forth, it pays to research the latest trends and review reasons why patients leave dental offices. Knowing these common complaints can help you avoid these problems, serve patients better, and retain more happy patients. Here are some of the most common reasons found on these review sites why patients left their dental office:

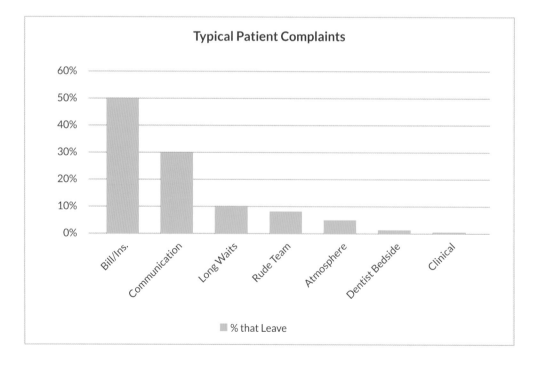

Billing/Insurance Complaints – This is by far the most common complaint with dental offices. People can be quite protective of their money. The usual reason for billing complaints revolves around insurance and estimates that were incorrect and end up with unexpected costs after the treatment is complete. This also becomes a concern when team members cannot articulate clearly why a patient owes money or cannot articulate the value of a service, and the patient then feels something is overpriced.

Unresponsive/Poor Communication – Patients understand that you have other people you are helping, but they do expect when they have a question that someone will provide a prompt response, ideally the same day. If you cannot respond the same day, you should give the patient a reason up front as well as a timetable of when to expect to hear back from you.

Communication can also be an issue when patients feel as if you do not listen to them, do not address their concerns, or do not explain details about their condition and treatment in a way they can understand.

Long Wait Times – This can occur both in trying to make an appointment and in wait time during the appointment. A general rule of thumb for new patients is to schedule a first appointment within a couple of weeks. For emergency situations, many patients want same- or next-day care. Being unable to see an emergency patient quickly is a large reason why patients will leave offices. The dentist who provides care when they are most needed often develops a lot of immediate loyalty.

Rude Team – Teams must manage different personalities and concerns all day, and this can become draining. However, patients all want to be treated professionally and with respect. Sometimes, a visit can start off on the wrong foot as simply as not saying hello when a patient walks into the office. When a patient is already having a poor experience, they will naturally look for more negatives. Make sure you and the team are trained in how to provide the best customer service with a friendly face to all patients, even the difficult ones, from the very beginning of the appointment all the way through the end.

Atmosphere Is Not Welcoming – This feeling could be generated by the tone of team interactions with patients and each other but can also stem from the general appearance of the office. Is the office warm and inviting, or outdated and dingy? Does the look of the office portray the level of service you want to provide? Does the team portray that same level of quality and service as well? Do team members talk to patients as if they are valued, or as if you just want to get them in and out? Do team members talk to each other with respect? All these aspects can affect the atmosphere the patient sees and feels.

Dentist Complaints – Complaints about a dentist are more likely to be about the emotional side, or chair-side manner. Patients cannot often gauge the quality of dental care as long as their procedure does not hurt. What they will focus on is how they feel treated when they are in the office or chair. The most common complaints about the provider directly are that they do not listen, are not interested in patient views, or are more interested in selling services/products than patient care.

Clinical/Post-Op Concerns – When it does come to quality of dental care, typically it's the post-op care that is the focus. If a procedure has a possibility of discomfort after treatment, the patient should be made aware of what might occur and how to respond before you even initiate a procedure, so they understand what is normal. While those who work in dentistry understand that things may not feel perfect immediately post-op, patients typically have the expectation of having no post-op discomfort. When you advise a patient ahead of time a problem might happen, you have helped the patient anticipate the future. When you tell a patient after the fact why something happened, it often sounds like an excuse.

Most post-op concerns can easily be fixed just by educating the patient and then following up with a brief phone call. This is why doctors who call their patients the night after a procedure often maintain a much larger portion of their patients long term.

> **TIP**
>
> Patient Retention Tip: Doctors who call their patients the night after a procedure often maintain a much larger portion of their patients long term.

DISCOUNT PLANS

Discount plans are those where an insurance company gives a patient access to a reduced fee schedule but otherwise does not pay for any care directly. This practice draws some complaints from teams and dentists about why the insurance company should be making money from the office giving a discount.

However, these concerns tend to miss the larger picture of insurance and how it functions. Think of all the many steps required for filing insurance we have just talked about and why medical offices that do not accept insurance can charge lower prices.

Working with insurance involves a lot of challenges. The office must wait to get paid for weeks or months. The claims process can be a huge nightmarish burden, which often becomes one of the main sources of complaints that dentists will ever receive from patients. The office has to deal with denials, disallows, and other aspects of a middleman getting between the decisions of the dentist and their patient over the best course of treatment.

As it turns out, however, the discounted fee can actually be the least onerous avenue for working with insurance companies. Discount plans remove all these frustrations.

- Patients pay you the day they get treatment
- There is no claims process, denials, disallows, etc.
- Estimates become 100% accurate
- Zero need to bill patients after the fact

In an ideal world for a dental office, dropping insurance to become only in-network with discount plans would save a lot of time, effort, and expense.

Chapter 5
Gathering New Patient Information

When working with insurance, you want to ensure you are paid promptly for your services. Therefore, one of the most critical actions you must take before ever treating a patient is to capture accurate information. Details matter! When incorrect information is sent with a claim, you will almost always receive a denial. A denied claim means you now must spend time resubmitting and then waiting for another response. There is also a three-strikes rule. If you strike out three times, the insurance company will no longer process further claims for that service/treatment. Therefore, it is crucial to obtain complete, accurate information from the beginning.

What information do you need to gather from the patient and subscriber?

- Patient's full name and date of birth
- Subscriber name, date of birth, and relationship to the patient
- Mailing address of both the patient and subscriber
- Insurance member ID and group number
- Insurance company name, phone number, address, and payor ID
- Employer name and phone number
- Group name (if different from employer)
- Social Security number

INSURANCE COMPANY INFORMATION

It may seem rather pointless to get this information because there are only so many insurance companies. However, some companies have multiple branches (such as Delta and BCBS) or multiple locations (such as Guardian). If you try to use the incorrect address or phone number, they will be unable to find the patient data or claim you are looking to retrieve.

MAILING ADDRESSES

The mailing address of the subscriber is required by most insurance companies and clearinghouses in order to process the claim. This is partially how the insurance company can keep track of patient locations in order to send out the Estimates of Benefits (EOBs).

MEMBER/SUBSCRIBER ID NUMBER AND GROUP NUMBER

In the early days of dental insurance, a patient's Social Security number was used to identify their policy. Since privacy and security have become more of a concern in the age of identity theft, many companies have switched from SSNs to policy numbers (also called subscriber or member ID numbers) to identify patients.

The group number is assigned to the group that purchased the policy. This group is most often an employer but can also be a marketplace (public) group where people buy individual policies. When you have two patients with the same group number, their benefits will be exactly alike.

What can get confusing is some groups will also have subgroups. This is usually when an employer has multiple layers or options of policy benefits. Subgroups can happen when the employer is large enough to have multiple tiers of employees, or when the employer chooses to offer options to the employees (such as a high-cost and low-cost option).

The benefits will often be different between subgroups but not always. For example, the city may negotiate a single set of benefits for all city employees but separate them out by department, labeled as different subgroups (fire, police, transit, etc.).

EXAMPLE

Example Group number: 12345-678
12345 would be the group number, and 678 would be the subgroup number.

When entering groups into the practice management software, it is recommended to create different insurance policies for each subgroup regardless of whether they are unique or different. This makes it easier in the future for team members, temps, or third-party companies that help with insurance billing to process claims correctly. Subgroups can be a simple matter of copying the group plan into a new group and changing only what is different about that subgroup (if anything).

POLICY NUMBER

You may occasionally hear the term "policy number." The challenge with this term is that it can be used as another name for either the member ID number or the group number depending on the insurance company.

SOCIAL SECURITY NUMBERS (SSN)

In this age of identity theft, patients can offer a little resistance with giving their SSN out. It is important to understand why as an office you still need to capture the SSN when dealing with insurance.

SSNs used to be the primary way insurance companies tracked patients. Although this practice has largely gone away as the primary source, many insurance companies use SSN as the secondary patient identifier. This means that if anything at all is wrong with the claim or data you have for a patient, you can still find the patient with the SSN. If you do not have the SSN, it will make your job working with insurance much more difficult. This is the first reason you should still be collecting SSNs on every patient.

The second reason you need the SSN as an office is an indirect result of working with insurance. When you accept insurance, you are in essence financing the services rendered to the patient until the insurance company reimburses your office. Insurance may not always pay what they should or what you expect, leaving patients with a balance.

If a patient pays this balance as he/she should, there are no problems. However, if you ever must track a patient down or send him/her to collections, you will need several pieces of information, including the SSN. Credit bureaus use the SSN to confirm the identity of the person who owes a debt. While the SSN is not absolutely required, it does make the process much easier.

It is fine if a patient does not want to disclose their SSN, but in the event they do not want to provide it, it is highly recommended *not* to accept assignment of benefits. This means the patient will need to pay the full amount of treatment costs up front and wait for the insurance reimbursement themselves. This is the best way to give the patient the security they want, without becoming a high collection risk later for the office.

> **TIP**
>
> The office should be collecting SSNs from all patients with insurance. This number is often used as a secondary form of identification. It is also used as a way to track down patients by collections agencies.

The next couple of pages have examples of new patient information forms to use or modify.

SAMPLE NEW PATIENT INFORMATION FORM

Patient Name	Home Address	City, State, Zip
Home Phone	Social Security No. Driver's License No.	Birth Date
Cell Phone	Email	Gender (Circle One): Male Female
Work Phone	Marital Status (circle one): Single Married Divorced Other	Contact Preferences (circle all that apply) Email Text Phone

Insurance: ☐ **I have secondary insurance.**

(Please ask us for the secondary insurance form)

Primary Insurance Company	Group #	Member ID
Address	Ph #	Payor ID

Insurance Subscriber Information (if different from patient):

Name	Home Address	City, State, Zip
Home Phone	Social Security No.	Birth Date
Cell Phone	Driver's License No.	Gender (Circle One): Male Female
Work Phone	Email	Relation to Patient:
Employer Name and Ph #	Marital Status (circle one): Single Married Divorced Other	Occupation

Responsible Party (if different from above):

Name:	Birth date:
Social Security No.	Driver's License No.

How did you hear about our office?

Communication and Release

I hereby authorize and request any exam, x-rays, or diagnostic aids deemed necessary to make a thorough diagnosis. I consent to the use of these by the doctor for scientific papers or demonstrations. Upon diagnosis, I authorize the doctor to perform all recommended treatment mutually agreed upon by me and employ such assistance as necessary. I agree to the use of anesthetics, sedatives, and other medications as necessary and understand that using these embody certain risks. I understand that I can ask for a complete recital of any possible complications.

I acknowledge that I have reviewed the Notice of Privacy Policies, can get a copy upon request, and consent to the use of my Personal Health Information for the purposes of health care operations, treatment, and payment activities.

I grant my permission to this office to phone or email me to discuss my account, appointments, or treatment.
I understand if I miss or cancel an appointment with less than 48-hour notice, there will be a failed appointment fee of $50/hour booked, which I agree to pay before any further appointments can be made.

Patient/Parent/Responsible Party (I have read and agree to the above content, terms, and conditions)   Date

SAMPLE FORM FOR SECONDARY INSURANCE

Secondary Insurance:

Secondary Insurance Company	Address
Group #	Ph #
Member ID	Payor ID

Insurance Subscriber Information:

Name	Home Address	City, State, Zip
Home Phone	Social Security No.	Birth Date
Cell Phone	Driver's License No.	Sex (Circle One): Male Female
Work Phone	Email	Relation to Patient:
Employer	Marital Status (circle one): Single Married Divorced Other	Occupation

As a courtesy, I understand this office will file any dental insurance on my behalf. I hereby authorize release of any information needed and also authorize my insurance company to pay directly to this office all benefits accruing under my policy. If the insurance company does not pay, I understand I am responsible for the remaining portion.

I understand secondary insurance can take 2–3 times longer to process, since it requires payment from my primary policy first. I understand in some instances due to my insurance I may have to pay a portion and wait for insurance to reimburse me.

☐ **I have read the above conditions about my insurance and agree to their content.**

_____   _____

Patient/Parent/Guardian Signature (Responsible Party)   Date

Relationship to Patient

FINANCIAL AND INSURANCE POLICY

Our goal is to provide the highest quality of dental care possible and to clearly communicate our financial policy.

I, _____ agree to be responsible for payment of all services rendered to myself and my dependents. I understand payment is due at time of service. I understand any treatment fee will be honored up to 90 days from the date of examination. I understand, in order to collect any debt, my credit history may be checked through use of my Social Security number and any other information given.

I understand that there is a $25 monthly late fee if I do not pay my balance within 30 days of a statement due date. There is a $35.00 processing charge for insufficient funds or returned checks. I agree that in the event my account becomes delinquent due to non-payment and is turned over to an outside collection attorney or agent, I agree to pay all actual and reasonable fees, legal fees, costs, expenses, and court costs incurred in order to collect payments due.

I grant my permission to this office to phone or email me to discuss my account, appointments, or treatment.

As a courtesy to me, I understand this office will file any dental insurance claims on my behalf. I hereby authorize release of all information needed for such claims and also authorize my insurance company to pay directly to this office benefits accruing under my policy. If the insurance company does not pay after 60 days, I agree to pay the full remaining balance.

I understand this office will always do the best to help me maximize my dental benefits; however, ultimate responsibility for payment is mine, and I am obligated and agree to pay this office in accordance with its credit terms and policy.

☐ **I have read the above conditions of treatment and payment and agree to these terms.**

☐ **I do not agree to the terms above and/or do not want to disclose my SSN.** I realize this is my choice and I can still receive treatment here. I do understand this comes with the following changes: (1) all treatment will need to be paid in full at time of service, (2) insurance will reimburse me and not my dentist, (3) I must pay with credit, check, or cash, (4) no payment arrangements will be possible, and (5) often insurance cannot be verified and estimates will be less accurate.

_____   _____

Patient/Parent/Guardian Signature (Responsible Party)   Date

_____

Relationship to Patient

Chapter 6
Verification and Breakdowns

Once you have captured all the correct information from the patient, then you need to obtain all the pertinent information from the insurance company about how it will pay.

First, you will need to verify coverage for the patient to make sure the policy is active and will cover any services rendered. Who do you get the information from? The verification process can vary by insurance company, but most often is through a fax or online portal.

It is important to verify coverage *before* the patient comes to the office; this way you can inform the patient of the latest standing of his/her benefits, along with cost estimates for his/her visit and any future treatment needs. Be sure to contact the insurance company for a status update *before every visit*. If the patient has a job loss or the employer switches insurance carriers, then the patient may lose the dental coverage you currently have on file. This loss of insurance can happen at any point throughout the year.

> **TIP**
>
> If your dental office is accepting assignment of benefits, it is important to verify the patient's coverage before every appointment that you will be submitting a claim to the insurance company for reimbursement. Ideally this verification should be obtained within 48 hours or less before the appointment time.

Next, you will need to gather information from the insurance company on the payment obligations of the patient's policy. This collection of information is called a breakdown. The most common pieces of information to gather are: procedure categories, usual/customary/reasonable (UCR) versus maximum allowable charge (MAC), frequency, maximums, waiting periods, exemptions, deductibles, downgrades (LEAT), and pre-existing conditions. Let's break each of these down:

PROCEDURE CATEGORIES (PREVENTIVE, BASIC, MAJOR)

Insurance companies will itemize how much they cover/pay for services based on categories. This way when getting a breakdown, you only have to ask about the coverage for each category instead for every individual service. However, nothing is ever super simple, each category may differ slightly as to what the specific policy includes within it. Here are the most common category scenarios you will encounter.

Preventive – This category includes services that are considered diagnostic or preventive in nature. These services are typically any dental code in the D0000–D1999 ADA code series, such as exams, x-rays, prophylaxis, sealants, and fluoride. The most common coverage amount for preventive services is 100%.

Basic – This category includes services that are low cost in nature (fillings and extractions). The most common coverage amount is 80%.

Major – These are the more expensive services such as crowns, occlusal guards, implants, and dentures. The most common coverage amount is 50%.

VARIATIONS

Periodontal and endodontic services vary widely, based on policy and generally fall in either the Basic or Major category.

Occasionally wisdom teeth or surgical extractions may be classified as Major by a policy.

Low-cost dental plans may classify periapical x-rays (PAs) as Basic.

Crowns infrequently may be classified as Basic.

It is important to know where these services fall when preparing an estimate for insurance reimbursement.

USUAL, CUSTOMARY, AND REASONABLE (UCR) VS MAXIMUM ALLOWABLE CHARGE (MAC)

Most often insurance companies will reimburse fees at a lower rate than the office's standard fee. Here are the different fees that might exist within an office:

- **Full Fee** – The office's normal fee charged to patients without insurance.
- **UCR** – Stands for Usual, Customary, and Reasonable, which is the average or common fees reimbursed for claims in your geographic area. This term applies primarily to out-of-network providers.
- **In-Network (INN) Contracted Fee** – The discounted fee agreed upon by an in-network contract agreement.
- **MAC** – Stands for Maximum Allowable Charge. It means that reimbursement is capped at a specific fee schedule that is policy based. The reimbursed fee is generally less than the fee that is provided under an in-network plan.

For a single office, UCR rarely changes and is a standard fee schedule used across the insurance company as a whole for a given region. MAC is a fee set according to the specific policy and therefore is different than UCR or the in-network fee. You can often determine UCR for a given company by creating your own blue book (see Chapter 22) and therefore have a good idea immediately how much the insurance company will pay.

If the policy is based on MAC, the fee schedule is going to be different than any other within that insurance company. For example, Cigna may have a UCR crown fee of $900 and an in-network fee of $800, but a specific patient's policy may have a MAC of only $600. This can mean a significant difference in the treatment plan estimates.

Insurance type	UCR OON	In-Network	MAC OON	MAC INN
Office crown fee	$1000	$1000	$1000	$1000
Insurance max fee	$900	$800	$600	$600
% coverage	50%	50%	50%	50%
Insurance pays	$450	$400	$300	$300
Patient pays	$550	$400	$700	$500

The reason behind this difference is what the employer/patient was willing to pay in policy premiums. MAC plans often have lower monthly premiums to the patient. This would be the same as if you bought car insurance. One policy would require more expensive premium payments yet give you full value for a totaled car, while another policy would have cheaper premiums but give you only 50% value of a totaled car. Some people will choose to take the cheaper policy in hopes that they do not get in an accident, while others would choose to have the better coverage. Insurance is all about managing cost vs risk. If you bought the cheaper policy and then ended up in a car accident, it is neither the fault of the insurance company nor the car dealership that you have to pay a lot more to replace that car.

The same is true in dentistry; neither the dentist nor office have control over coverage policies. The more you pay for insurance in premiums, the less your risk will be when something happens that insurance might cover. This is the most important concept to understand when

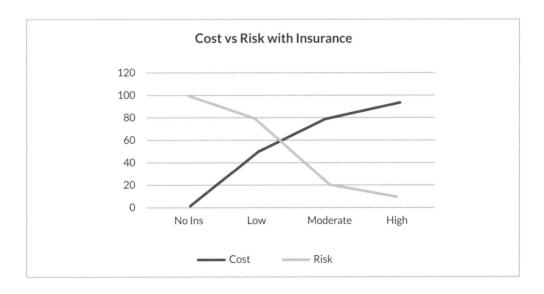

a patient comes in with a policy that does not cover what the patient needs—they (or their employer) likely chose a low-premium option, which comes with minimal benefits.

Notice in the above example that the patient is out of pocket more with the MAC policy regardless of whether they chose an in- or out-of-network provider. It is also important to notice that the in-network provider is still collecting the same total amount ($800). MAC policies do not change the in-network fee schedule, only what the insurance company will reimburse.

FREQUENCY

Many dental treatments come with average expected life spans, such as fillings are 3–5 years and crowns are 5–10 years, or routine necessity, such as a cleaning twice a year. When a dental treatment is performed, insurance companies expect it to hold up for some length of time and therefore will set limits on how often they will pay for that service. Almost every dental code will have a frequency limit, which is determined mostly by the individual policy. Some common examples are:

Exams and Cleanings	Twice per benefit year, or Twice per consecutive 12 months, or Every 6 months, or Every 6 months + 1 day
Bitewing X-Rays	Once or Twice per benefit year, or 1–2 per consecutive 12 months, or Every 6 months, or Every 6 months + 1 day
Pano or FMX	Once every 3–5 years
Fillings	Once per surface every 2–5 years
Crowns	Once per tooth every 5–10 years
Full Mouth Debridement	Once in a lifetime
Scaling and Root Planing (Gum Therapy)	Once per quad every 2–5 years

These frequencies are important to know because if you do the same work inside the frequency time period, there is almost zero chance the insurance company will reimburse for the service. This means the patient would be responsible for the full cost of treatment. What fee the patient is responsible for may vary based on the network contract with the provider as well as your state laws. (See Chapter 17: Non-Covered Services.)

> ### EXAMPLE
>
> If Mrs. Jones comes in for routine care January 1 and has an insurance policy that pays on preventive services every 6 months, then it is important to schedule her after July 1 for her next visit if you want to help her get coverage for her care.

Due to frequencies, one important piece of information to obtain when you call for a new patient breakdown from an insurance carrier is to ask for the history. This will allow you to know whether the patient may have benefits for first-visit services or if the patient would need to pay out of pocket.

> **TIP**
>
> Since policies may vary on preventive care from a loose "twice a year" to a strict "6 months + 1 day," the easiest method is to schedule all patients as if they have the strictest policy. This allows any team member setting next appointments to not have to worry about the patient's insurance when they schedule.

MAXIMUM

Most insurance policies will have a maximum benefit payout for services per year, which is the cumulative total of what they will reimburse for dental services within that time period. This can be based on a calendar year (Jan–Dec) or a fiscal year (e.g., April–March, Oct–Sept, or July–June). The most common policies will have a coverage maximum of $1000–$1500 per patient per year.

Once you exceed the maximum for the policy, you can still provide treatment for the patient, but you should estimate that the patient will pay 100% of the fee.

> **TIP**
>
> Maximums can make your job easier when creating treatment plan estimates for patients with larger treatment plans. Instead of needing to determine coverage for each service, if the patient is going to max out their benefits before all treatment is complete, you can provide just the maximum as the estimate of what insurance will pay.

Lifetime maximums are also common for services like orthodontics. Most often if a policy has orthodontic coverage with a lifetime maximum, the lifetime maximum is separate from the yearly maximum. For example, if the policy has a yearly maximum of $1500 and a lifetime ortho maximum of $2000, the patient can get both general dentistry done as well as orthodontics and receive up to $3500 of combined reimbursement.

It is also highly important to gain information on what remaining benefits exist for the year. While a policy may have $1500 in maximum benefits, that would not help much if the benefits have already been used.

> **NOTE**
>
> Insurance policies may also have an oral surgery maximum as well that is separate, similar to an orthodontic maximum.

DEDUCTIBLES

A deductible is the amount of money that the patient is required to pay first before insurance will cover any treatment. Many times, diagnostic and some preventive services (such as cleanings) are exempt or waived from the deductible. Deductibles are per year and commonly $25, $50, or $100. Once they have been paid during the year, they will not take effect again until the following policy year.

(Fee – deductible) × (% coverage) = insurance reimbursement

Once the deductible is met:

Fee × (% coverage) = insurance reimbursement
Fee – insurance reimbursement = patient co-pay

Deductibles often are not invoked with 100% covered services, such as diagnostic, preventive, and hygiene services.

> **EXAMPLE**
>
> Mrs. Jones has dental insurance and is coming in for her January visit for routine care. She will not have to pay a deductible if she receives only the 100% covered preventive and diagnostic care.
>
> However, if Mrs. Jones has a cavity that needs a filling with 80% coverage, the deductible will need to be paid before insurance will start coverage. Let's say your fee for a filling is $200 with a $50 insurance deductible.
>
> $200 (fee) – $50 (deductible) = $150.
> $150 × 0.8 (80% coverage) = $120
> Insurance will pay $120, and the patient will owe **$80** due to the deductible.
>
> If the patient needs a second filling on another tooth, insurance will now pay 80% of the $200 instead, making the patient's out of pocket cost **$40** ($200 × 80% = $160).
>
> *Note:* the difference between the two payments for this patient is not the $50 deductible. Just adding the cost of the deductible to the normal percentage estimate will not get you an accurate number. See chart below for another visual of this example.

Service	Deductible	Fee	Insurance pays	Patient pays
Exam	No	75	75	0
X-rays	No	100	100	0
Cleaning	No	100	100	0
Filling #1	Yes	200	120	80
Filling #2	Yes	200	160	40

> **TIP**
>
> To calculate a deductible, you must first remove it from the fee before applying the percentage of coverage.

Many family policies will require a family deductible, an amount once anyone in the family satisfies, then the rest of the family does not have to pay it.

> **EXAMPLE**
>
> Let's say Mrs. Jones has a husband and two children, with individual deductibles of $50 and a family deductible of $150.
>
> If Mrs. Jones and her children need treatment, they will each have to pay the $50 deductible. However, if after that Mr. Jones now needs treatment, he would not need to pay a deductible because the family deductible has already been met.

AGE LIMITATION

Like maximums, many policies will have age limits on procedures. These are time periods in which the patient reaching a certain age will no longer be allowed to obtain reimbursement for said service.

Common examples include:

Sealants and fluoride with an age limit between 12–18.

Orthodontics with an age limit between 19–26.

> **EXAMPLE**
>
> Scenario: An 18 year old patient has an insurance policy with a sealant age limit of 16 and an orthodontic age limit of 20. You can provide both services to the patient; however, insurance will reimburse for the orthodontic care but not the sealants due to the age limitation.

> **TIP**
>
> Make sure to ask if the age limit is "through age X" (including) or "up to age X" (not including). This can make a difference if the patient is age X.

WAITING PERIOD

Waiting periods are the time period after which insurance will start paying for dental care. Often waiting periods are added to new policies in order to lower the premium cost of the policy. Waiting periods typically will be based on the service category (preventive, basic, major).

> **EXAMPLE**
>
> A common waiting period on a policy might be:
> Preventive: None
> Basic: 6 months
> Major: 12 months

With a policy like the one above, the patient can come in immediately for preventive and diagnostic care once their policy is active. The patient would have to wait 6 months for basic care if they want coverage (e.g., fillings). The patient would then have to wait a total of 12 months before getting a major service reimbursed (e.g., crown).

You are still allowed to treat the patient within the waiting period timing, the patient will just be responsible for 100% payment without any reimbursement from the insurance company.

> **TIP**
>
> Waiting periods are extremely common with policies that patients purchase individually outside of an employer. If patients ask you about getting insurance on their own, it would be prudent to make them aware of this common trend.

DOWNGRADES AND LEAST EXPENSIVE ALTERNATIVE TREATMENT (LEAT)

Many insurance policies will downgrade reimbursement of certain services. The most common downgrades are with fillings (composite –> amalgam) and crowns (porcelain –> metal). A downgrade means the insurance company will pay less for a service, but the patient is still responsible for the total amount of the service provided.

Let's review a few examples of the common downgrades you will encounter.

Filling Example (80% basic coverage)

Mrs. Jones's composite filling of $200 would normally be covered at 80%, where insurance would pay $160 and the patient would owe $40. However, Mrs. Jones has a downgrade policy meaning the insurance will only pay for the less expensive alternative treatment (LEAT), specifically an amalgam filling. With a downgrade, the insurance company is only going to pay 80% of the cost of an amalgam filling ($140), or $112.

Service	Office fee	Insurance pays	Patient pays
Amalgam filling	140	112	28
Composite filling (normal)	200	160	40
Composite filling (downgrade)	200	112	88

It is important to note that downgrades only change what insurance is going to reimburse. The patient is still responsible for payment of the actual service provided. In this example, Mrs. Jones received a composite filling and owes for a composite filling—insurance is just going to pay a lower amount for the amalgam filling alternative as a downgrade.

Note: Many patients specifically do not want amalgam fillings anymore for a variety of reasons. This trend in dentistry means many offices no longer offer amalgam as an option.

> **TIP**
>
> Downgrades *only* change what insurance is going to reimburse. They do not change what the office needs to collect or what the patient is responsible for.

Crown Example (50% major coverage):

Crowns will commonly be downgraded to either a base metal PFM (D2751) or a gold crown (D2790).

Service	Network fee	Insurance pays	Patient pays
D2790 gold crown	500	250	250
D2751 PFM base metal crown	600	300	300
D2740 porcelain Crown (normal, no downgrade)	700	350	350
D2740 porcelain crown (downgrade base metal)	700	300	400
D2740 porcelain crown (downgrade gold crown)	700	250	450

> **TIP**
>
> If you are unsure whether a policy downgrades, the safest assumption when building the estimate for the treatment plan is that they do. This way if you are wrong, the patient ends up with a credit instead of a balance.

Bridge or Implant Restoration Example (50% major coverage)

Bridges or implant restorations may commonly be downgraded to reimbursement of a partial denture. Typically, a partial is only considered an alternative option if the patient is missing a tooth on both sides of the arch. This is why insurance companies often request a pano or FMX when you do either an implant or bridge; they are looking to see whether a partial denture is a viable alternative option and therefore is subject to a LEAT.

Service	Office fee	Insurance pays	Patient pays
Partial denture	1000	500	500
Bridge (normal)	3000	1500	1500
Bridge (downgrade)	3000	500	2500
Implant (normal)	4000	1500 (max)	2500
Implant (downgrade)	4000	500	3500

An insurance company might also ask for the missing teeth numbers for the same reason. Missing teeth where the gaps that have been closed with orthodontics would not apply to this list.

How Should You Estimate Coverage for Downgraded Services?

First, you should be aware if the patient's policy includes downgraded services. This is an important question to ask when getting a breakdown from the insurance company. When there are downgraded services involved, your office can choose one of two methods for compiling estimates for treatments or dental procedures:

1. Estimate individually.

    Similar to the example tables above, the most accurate way to determine downgrades is to figure out what insurance will pay for the downgraded service and use that alternative service (e.g., amalgam filling) coverage amount instead of a percentage of the service being performed (e.g., composite filling). However, this method can be rather time consuming.

2. Change the percentage of coverage.

    The faster route requires taking time to determine what the percentage difference is between the provided and downgraded service. This way you only have to do the calculation once per insurance company in general.

    In the filling example above, insurance paid $112 on the $200 filling, making it a percentage coverage of 56%. If you use 56% instead of 80% in your coverage table for composites, you will get the same answer.

    The downside of this method is there are a dozen different filling codes based on number of surfaces and whether the filling is in the anterior or posterior section. The percentage difference of each filling type is not going to be the exact same. The best practice if you want to use this type of quick answer is to estimate based on the lowest percentage coverage of any of the different composite codes. This may take a few minutes to calculate them all but will save you time when you create future treatment plans. By using the lowest possible percentage, you set it up so that if there is any inaccuracy on the estimate, it is in the favor of the office. Refunding money is far easier than tracking down a patient to collect on a balance later.

Service	Office fee	Insurance pays	Patient pays
Amalgam filling	140	112	28
Composite filling (normal)	200	160	40
Composite filling (downgrade)	200	112 (56%)	88

PRE-EXISTING CONDITIONS AND MISSING TOOTH CLAUSE

Many people are familiar with pre-existing conditions as used in the medical world. This basically means that if you had a condition before you signed up with the insurance policy, the insurance company would not be responsible for any costs associated with that condition.

In dentistry, there are similar conditions for which insurance will not pay. The most common is the missing tooth clause (MTC). This clause is an exception included on insurance policies that states if the patient was missing a tooth before the policy took effect, then there would be no reimbursement for replacement of that tooth (partial, bridge, or implant).

When getting breakdown information, it is important to ask if there is an MTC exclusion on the policy.

NOTE
Current Events: In June 2020, Louisiana passed a law that prevents dental insurance companies from being able to include a missing tooth clause or other pre-existing condition clause. The ADA is currently advocating for this practice to become a nationwide change. Pre-existing conditions are already being phased out of medical insurance, and we may find in the next few years that MTC and other pre-existing condition clauses will disappear in dentistry as well.
https://www.ada.org/en/publications/ada-news/2020-archive/june/new-louisiana-law-deals-blow-to-downcoding

EXAMPLE

Example 1: You have a patient with a broken #18, a missing #19, and a normal #20 and who wants a bridge. Without an MTC, the insurance company will provide reimbursement for all services (the pontic on #19 and also the abutments on #18 and 20).

If there is an MTC, the insurance company will cover the cost of a crown on #18 because it needed a crown anyway. No reimbursement for #19 due to the MTC. Also, no reimbursement for the abutment on #20 due to the MTC as well as the fact it did not otherwise need a crown.

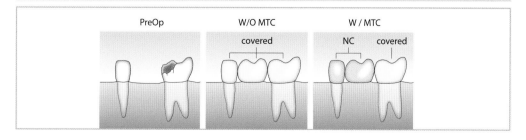

> ### EXAMPLE
>
> Example 2: If you have a patient with an MTC and who is missing #19 from before the policy but also needs #30 removed now, insurance will provide reimbursement for a partial to cover the replacement of #30 after you remove the tooth. The policy would provide no reimbursement at all if you were replacing #19 with a bridge or an implant due to the MTC.

MISCELLANEOUS CLAUSES AND EXEMPTIONS

Many other clauses and exceptions may appear in an insurance policy, all of which are important to understand when gathering information for your patient's breakdown.

Example Progressive Plan	
	Maximum
Year one	$1000
Year two	$1250
Year three	$1500

Progressive plan is one example of such a clause that you might run across. This is a term used for an insurance policy that increases in benefits for every year the subscriber is a part of the plan. Starting with a lower level of benefits helps to keep the initial premium costs of the plan at an affordable level, but eventually it adds higher benefits as a retention incentive. Insurance companies know that many patients and employers change companies often, so this is a potential way for them to help keep their clients long term. Often these progressive benefits can be a positive for both the patient and office.

Exemptions are another type of clause that you may see. An exemption example would be where occlusal guards require either bruxism or osseous surgery to be eligible for reimbursement.

If an insurance policy will cover an occlusal guard only after osseous surgery, but the patient has not had osseous surgery, the patient will need to pay 100% out of pocket for the occlusal guard.

BREAKDOWNS

Now that you have a good basis for the common terms, policies, and exclusions, we can review what a breakdown might look like. Breakdown forms can be one of the most detailed and complex aspects of dealing with insurance. However, if you can read and understand a breakdown form, then it will make your life much easier with insurance as you move forward.

Most offices should customize their breakdown sheet to include only the services you provide. This way you don't need to waste time tracking down information on services you do not offer for your patients. A customized form will also make sure you obtain information on all the services you do provide, which might be different than your colleague's office down the street. See Breakdown Example Form on the following page.

BREAKDOWN EXAMPLE FORM									
Tax ID: NPI:			UCCI number for Dr.				**DATE VERIFIED:** **EFFECTIVE DATE:**		
Service History:	DOB	Exam	Bitewing	FMX/Pano	PX		Fluoride	sealants	SCRP Perio Mnt.
1.									
2.									
3.									
4.									
5.									
6.									

Eligibility Overview   **X-Ray Breakdown**

Ins. Name: **Payor ID:** Ins. Phone: Ins. Address: Subscriber Id: **Group Name:** **Group Number:**	**BW:** D0272 1x12m 2x 12m 1x6m 1xcyr 2xcyr 2x fisc 1x fisc [P B M] D0274 1x12m 2x 12m 1x6m 1xcyr 2xcyr 2x fisc 1x fisc [P B M] **Periapicals:** D0220/D0230 = **FMX** [P B M] **FMX/Pano:** 1x3YRS 1x5YRS Other: ___ [P B M] *Pano & Bitewings filed same day downgrades? [Y] or [N]*

NETWORK: IN or OUT Fee Schedule:
WAITING PERIOD YES or NO if so, For:
Calendar Year or Fiscal year →
Yearly Maximum$ → Remaining Maximum: $
Does Max apply to Diagnostics and Preventive →
Deductible $ → Applies to: Prev Basic Major
(Met) (Not Met)
    Percentages: Preventive: Basic: Major:
    OUT NETWORK BENEFITS: Pays: provider
    or subscriber
Maximum$ Deductible Co-ins
	Doctor Exams
	Comp Exam: (D0150) [P B M] Gives alternate of D0120?
	    Freq: 1x6m 1x 12m 2x12m 2xCYR 2xfisc 1 per DDS
	Periodic Exam:(D0120) [P B M] *anytime or to the day*
	    Freq: None 1x6m 1x12m 2x12m 2xCYR 2x fisc
	Periodontal Exam: (D0180) [P B M] *anytime or to the day*
	    Freq: 1x6m 2x12m 2x CYR 2x fisc or 1 per DDs
	Limited Exam: (D0140) [P B M] *tx same day?*
	    Freq: 1x6m 1x30days 2x12m 2xCYR 3x6mths None
	Pallative Exam:(D9110)[P B M] *Deductible? [Y]or[N]*
	x-rays only Y/N **Freq**: None 1x6m 2x12m 2xCYR 3x 6mths 1xdos

Hygiene Breakdown

Cleanings: (D1120/D1110) 1x6m 2xCYR 2x12m 3xcyr 2X Fisc yr 4xcyr Other: _____ anytime or to the day
Fluoride: (D1206)/ (D1208) [P B] **Age Limit Freq:** 1x6m 1x12m 2x12m 2xcyr 2x fisc 1xcyr
Sealants:(D1351) [P B M] **Deductible:** [Yes] or [No] **Age Limitation Freq:** None 1x24m 1x 36m 1xlife 1x 60M Other:
    Unfilled Perm 1ˢᵗ & 2ⁿᵈ molars/ Bicuspids/Unfilled Posterior {Prim}{Perm} Teeth/ No Tooth restriction
Scaling/Root Planing: (D4341/D4342) [B M] **Freq:** None 1x6m 1x12m 1xcyr 1x24m 1x3yrs [2 Quads] or [4 Quads]
    pocket depth limitation? 2 quads Payable same day with D1110 [Yes]or[No]
Perio PX: (D4910) [P B M] **Freq:** None 1x6m 2x12m 2x cyr 2x fiscal 4xcyr 4x 12m 1x 3m **Share Freq with D1110?**
    [Yes]or[No] 30\ 90 day waiting period after Scaling(D4341/D4342) [Yes]or[No] **Following Active Perio therapy?**
Gingival Inflammation D4346 **[P B M] Freq:**
Arestin: (D4381) [P B M] **Freq: Limitations:**
FMD: (D4355) [P B M]   **Freq: Limitations:**

Restorative TX

Fillings: [B M] **Alternate Benefit of Amalgam?** [Yes] or [No] **If so, applied to?** Molars/All posteriors FREQUENCY: **Root Canals:**(D3310) B M (D3320) B M (D3330) B M **Build Ups:** (B or M) D2954 D2952 D2950 *Bundles with Crown [Y] [N]* **Oral Surgery:** (D7140)B M (D7210) B M (D7220) B M (D7240) B M → *Coordinate with Medical*: **Sedation:** D9239[B M] D9243 [B M] **Notes:** **Crowns:** [B M] **Freq:** 1x5yrs 1x7yr 1x8yrs 1x10yrs other: ___ **Alternate Benefit on Molars?** [Yes]or[No] **Pays:** Prep/Seat **Occ. Adjustment:** D9951[B M]   **Recement Crown:** D2920 [B M] **Bridges:** (D6240/D6750) B or M **Freq:** 1x5yrs 1x 7yrs 1x8yrs 1x10yrs other: ___ **Dentures/partials:** (5100,5120,5130,5140) [B M] **Freq:** 1x5yrs 1x7yrs 1x8yrs 1x10yrs other: ___ **Missing Tooth Clause on policy?** *(prior ext)* [Yes]or[No] (applies to 6010,6058,6057, or crowns?) **Night Guard:** (D9944) B or M **Freq:** None 1x12mth 1x24m 1x 3yrs 1x 5yrs 1xlife **Bruxism only?** [Yes]or[No] **Applied to:** Dental Max or Ortho D9610: D7953 *qualified implant only? Y or N* D9310 Tx same day Y/n D6010/D6057 D6058 D4274 D4260/D4261 D4249 D4266/D4267 Pre-D Pre-D Pre-D Pre-D Pre-D Pre-D Pre-D Pre-D

Orthodontic Coverage: Yes or No
Age Limit Life Time Max: Pays at Deductible: Auto Pay: Y or N Monthly /Quarterly Initial Payment=

Chapter 7
Estimates

After you have verified the patient has active insurance coverage, and you have a detailed breakdown of their benefits, then you have what you need to be able to develop an estimate for any treatment needs the patient may have. The two ways to create an estimate are either through your practice management software (e.g., Dentrix, Open Dental, Eaglesoft) or through a separate Word file or program.

Dentrix Treatment Plan Example

.: TREATMENT CASE Treatment Plan

DATE	VISIT	TH	SURF	CODE	DESCRIPTION	FEE	DelPrem
04/16/2020	1			D1206	Topical fluoride varnish	60.00	30.00
04/16/2020	1			TC301	Periogard/Sock-it Gel	24.00	24.00
04/16/2020	1	LL		D4341	Perio scale&root pln-4+per quad	327.00	198.00
04/16/2020	1	LR		D4341	Perio scale&root pln-4+per quad	327.00	198.00
04/16/2020	1	UL		D4341	Perio scale&root pln-4+per quad	327.00	198.00
04/16/2020	1	UR		D4341	Perio scale&root pln-4+per quad	327.00	198.00
					Visit 1 Totals:	1392.00	846.00
04/16/2020	2	3	MO	D2392	Resin composite-2s, posterior	289.00	156.00
04/16/2020	2	4	DO	D2392	Resin composite-2s, posterior	289.00	156.00
					Visit 2 Totals:	578.00	312.00
04/16/2020	3			D0220	Intraoral-periapical 1st film	39.00	17.00
04/16/2020	3			D0220	Intraoral-periapical 1st film	39.00	17.00
04/16/2020	3	14		02000	Seat Crown	0.00	0.00
04/16/2020	3	14		D2740	Crown-porcelain/ceramic substr	1286.00	922.00
04/16/2020	3	14		D2950	Core buildup, include any pins	298.00	177.00
					Visit 3 Totals:	1662.00	1133.00
04/16/2020	4			D0180	Comprehensive perio evaluation	143.00	70.00
04/16/2020	4			D1206	Topical fluoride varnish	60.00	30.00
04/16/2020	4			D4910	Periodontal maintenance	181.00	96.00
					Visit 4 Totals:	384.00	196.00
04/16/2020	5			D9944	Occlusal guard- hard, full	695.00	464.00
					Visit 5 Totals:	695.00	464.00

.: INSURANCE PROVIDER(S) ::		:: TOTALS ::	
Primary	Secondary	Fee	DelPrem
Delta Dental Premiere		4711.00	2951.00

In the previous Dentrix Treatment Plan example, the patient has been diagnosed as needing some periodontal treatment, fillings, crown, and an occlusal guard on their treatment plan.

The full office fee for this treatment plan is $4711.

After applying the patient's Delta Dental Premier insurance network discounts, that fee is reduced to $2951.

In this example we found out with the breakdown that the patient has an annual $1000 maximum, $0 of which have been used so far. This makes it an easy calculation that the patient's out-of-pocket cost will be $1951 since the individual reimbursements would add up to far more than $1000.

The pros about using the computer-based treatment plans are they can be generated much faster and have most of the information you as a team member would need to finalize the estimate.

The con with a treatment plan like this is it contains a lot of numbers and technical terms, which can become quickly confusing or even overwhelming if shared with the patient.

Patients who become confused often decline accepting treatment for that reason alone. Itemizing the treatment plan can even result in the patient starting to question or even decline parts of the plan to be able to lower the overall cost. This can ultimately cause future challenges for patients as they may not fully understand the consequences of removing items from the treatment plan.

EXAMPLE

Example 1: A patient who needs a buildup on a tooth due to lack of height will often have to deal with reoccurring issues of the crown coming out if the buildup is not completed.

Example 2: A denture patient who does not get alveoloplasty might have to deal with constant denture sores because the bone is not smooth underneath the gum tissue.

Word File Treatment Plan Example

An alternative option is to develop a first draft of the treatment plan using the automated software but then create a more patient-friendly version of the treatment plan outside of the dental software. This patient plan version is based on the same data from the previous computer-generated Dentrix plan; however, it is simplified into a basic Word document (see next page).

Using a Word File instead of a practice management treatment plan	
Pros	Cons
• Easier for the patient to read/understand • No itemizations to incentivize patients to remove treatment elements • Includes financing options on the same page	• Does not include as much detail and may generate more questions from certain outlier patients • Takes a little more time to put together

Whatever method you choose to utilize for developing and presenting treatment plans, it is important to understand them fully and be able to explain them easily to patients. It is also important to be as accurate as possible.

Where there are any estimates you are not confident of, it is recommended that you illustrate the higher cost to the patient. If you use the lower amount, you may overestimate insurance coverage, and as a result you will need to contact the patient later to ask for more money and likely end up with an unhappy patient. If you incorporate the higher cost, you will potentially underestimate the amount of insurance coverage, and may have to refund the patient money or leave the overage as a credit on their account but likely still have a happy patient.

In general, people do not like unexpected bills after the fact. Refunds aren't usually a concern.

EXAMPLE

Which would you rather tell a patient?
"Mrs. Jones, unfortunately, insurance did not pay as much as estimated. You are going to owe another $100."
Or
"Mrs. Jones, great news, insurance paid more than estimated. You have a $100 credit on your account!"

DENTAL TREATMENT PLAN (EXAMPLE)

Patient: Joe Smith   Date: Sept 1, 2021
Treatment Needs: Periodontal therapy, fillings, crown, and night guard

Total Treatment Fee: **$2951**
Insurance allowance: $1000

_____ Pre-payment-in-full discount option: $_1755_
_____ Care credit payment option (48 months): $__0__down and $_46_ /month
_____ In-office payment option (6 months): $_976_down and $_162_ /month

I understand if insurance does not pay for any reason that I am responsible for the full amount.

I acknowledge I have read and understand the treatments recommended along with the associated fees and payment options presented and have received a copy today. I understand the estimated fees in this treatment plan are valid for 90 days but may change after that time. I understand these fees do NOT include general dentistry treatment on other areas or teeth.

_____   _____
Patient signature   Date

_____   _____
Treatment coordinator signature   Date

DENTAL TREATMENT PLAN (BLANK)

Patient: _____   Date: _____

Treatment Needs:

Total Treatment Fee: $

Insurance allowance: $

_____Pre-payment-in-full discount option: $_____
_____Care credit payment option (48 months): $_____down and $_____ /month
_____In-office payment option (6 months): $_____down and $_____ /month

I understand if insurance does not pay for any reason that I am responsible for the full amount.

I acknowledge I have read and understand the treatments recommended along with the associated fees and payment options presented and have received a copy today. I understand the estimated fees in this treatment plan are valid for 90 days but may change after that time. I understand these fees do NOT include general dentistry treatment on other areas or teeth.

_____   _____

Patient signature   Date

_____   _____

Treatment coordinator signature   Date

Chapter 8
Claims Process

Once you have a breakdown from the insurance company, presented an estimate to the patient, and delivered treatment; the next step is to file a claim on behalf of the patient with the insurance company for reimbursement. The office can file these claims through snail mail, fax, or electronically. Electronic processing is the most efficient and fastest. We will focus on the paper claims first to highlight the important parts of the claims forms and what you need to know to file correctly, whether electronically or on paper.

PAPER CLAIMS

The ADA maintains and updates the standard insurance claims forms used throughout the country. The most recent two versions are those from 2012 and 2019. Many insurance companies will no longer accept claim forms from before 2012 as they are unable to be computer processed. 2019 was an editorial change only and does not affect how the computer processes the claim.

> **TIP**
>
> Use current ADA forms for every claim. Use of ADA forms has nothing to do with membership. ADA forms are the common, accepted form of communication with an insurance company. Many insurance companies are no longer accepting claim forms from before 2012.

With paper claims, the insurance company is going to scan the claim to load all the data automatically into its claim system. If anything is in an incorrect location or missing, it will automatically send back a denial. So, when filling out these forms, completeness and attention to detail matters. This scanning process is why some insurance companies may still accept a 2012 form because everything remains in the same location for the scanner and computer. Ideally, it is best to use the most recent form to avoid any issues with getting reimbursement. These claim forms can be found for free on the ADA website or on many insurance company websites.

TIP

Most insurance companies process claims through computers. Keep in mind that paper forms will be scanned and converted to electronic. The ideal paper form is printed and typed from a computer for clarity. If you do have to fill out a form manually, it is crucial to use the cleanest handwriting possible. If a computer cannot read your writing, then your claim will be delayed because it has to run through a human processor (who may also have a hard time reading it).

ADA American Dental Association® **Dental Claim Form**

HEADER INFORMATION

1. Type of Transaction (Mark all applicable boxes)

☐ Statement of Actual Services ☐ Request for Predetermination/Preauthorization

☐ EPSDT / Title XIX

2. Predetermination/Preauthorization Number

DENTAL BENEFIT PLAN INFORMATION

3. Company/Plan Name, Address, City, State, Zip Code

OTHER COVERAGE (Mark applicable box and complete items 5-11. If none, leave blank.)

4. Dental? ☐ Medical? ☐ (If both, complete 5-11 for dental only.)

5. Name of Policyholder/Subscriber in #4 (Last, First, Middle Initial, Suffix)

6. Date of Birth (MM/DD/CCYY)

7. Gender ☐ M ☐ F ☐ U

8. Policyholder/Subscriber ID (Assigned by Plan)

9. Plan/Group Number

10. Patient's Relationship to Person named in #5 ☐ Self ☐ Spouse ☐ Dependent ☐ Other

11. Other Insurance Company/Dental Benefit Plan Name, Address, City, State, Zip Code

POLICYHOLDER/SUBSCRIBER INFORMATION (Assigned by Plan Named in #3)

12. Policyholder/Subscriber Name (Last, First, Middle Initial, Suffix), Address, City, State, Zip Code

13. Date of Birth (MM/DD/CCYY)

14. Gender ☐ M ☐ F ☐ U

15. Policyholder/Subscriber ID (Assigned by Plan)

16. Plan/Group Number

17. Employer Name

PATIENT INFORMATION

18. Relationship to Policyholder/Subscriber in #12 Above ☐ Self ☐ Spouse ☐ Dependent Child ☐ Other

19. Reserved For Future Use

20. Name (Last, First, Middle Initial, Suffix), Address, City, State, Zip Code

21. Date of Birth (MM/DD/CCYY)

22. Gender ☐ M ☐ F ☐ U

23. Patient ID/Account # (Assigned by Dentist)

RECORD OF SERVICES PROVIDED

	24. Procedure Date (MM/DD/CCYY)	25. Area of Oral Cavity	26. Tooth System	27. Tooth Number(s) or Letter(s)	28. Tooth Surface	29. Procedure Code	29a. Diag. Pointer	29b. Qty.	30. Description	31. Fee
1										
2										
3										
4										
5										
6										
7										
8										
9										
10										

33. Missing Teeth Information (Place an "X" on each missing tooth.)

1 2 3 4 5 6 7 8 9 10 11 12 13 14 15 16

32 31 30 29 28 27 26 25 24 23 22 21 20 19 18 17

35. Remarks

34. Diagnosis Code List Qualifier ☐ (ICD-10 = AB)

34a. Diagnosis Code(s) A _____ C _____

(Primary diagnosis in "A") B _____ D _____

31a. Other Fee(s)

32. Total Fee

AUTHORIZATIONS

36. I have been informed of the treatment plan and associated fees. I agree to be responsible for all charges for dental services and materials not paid by my dental benefit plan, unless prohibited by law, or the treating dentist or dental practice has a contractual agreement with my plan prohibiting all or a portion of such charges. To the extent permitted by law, I consent to your use and disclosure of my protected health information to carry out payment activities in connection with this claim.

X _____

Patient/Guardian Signature   Date

37. I hereby authorize and direct payment of the dental benefits otherwise payable to me, directly to the below named dentist or dental entity.

X _____

Subscriber Signature   Date

ANCILLARY CLAIM/TREATMENT INFORMATION

38. Place of Treatment (e.g. 11=office; 22=O/P Hospital) (Use "Place of Service Codes for Professional Claims")

39. Enclosures (Y or N)

40. Is Treatment for Orthodontics? ☐ No (Skip 41-42) ☐ Yes (Complete 41-42)

41. Date Appliance Placed (MM/DD/CCYY)

42. Months of Treatment

43. Replacement of Prosthesis ☐ No ☐ Yes (Complete 44)

44. Date of Prior Placement (MM/DD/CCYY)

45. Treatment Resulting from ☐ Occupational illness/injury ☐ Auto accident ☐ Other accident

46. Date of Accident (MM/DD/CCYY)

47. Auto Accident State

BILLING DENTIST OR DENTAL ENTITY (Leave blank if dentist or dental entity is not submitting claim on behalf of the patient or insured/subscriber.)

48. Name, Address, City, State, Zip Code

49. NPI

50. License Number

51. SSN or TIN

52. Phone Number ( ) -

52a. Additional Provider ID

TREATING DENTIST AND TREATMENT LOCATION INFORMATION

53. I hereby certify that the procedures as indicated by date are in progress (for procedures that require multiple visits) or have been completed.

X _____

Signed (Treating Dentist)   Date

54. NPI

55. License Number

56. Address, City, State, Zip Code

56a. Provider Specialty Code

57. Phone Number ( ) -

58. Additional Provider ID

To reorder call 800.947.4746 or go online at ADAcatalog.org

ADA Claim Form 2019

The most recent update of the ADA Claim Form is 2019, shown on the previous page.

Sections of this form are often either Fixed ⟨F⟩ or Variable ⟨V⟩ meaning that the information does not change or changes based on the office and dentist providing the service, respectively.

We will start first with the fixed sections where the information will likely be consistent for all claims you send from a given office: Authorizations, Billing Dentist or Dental Entity, and Treating Dentist and Treatment Location Information.

For each section, some information to look for and understand:

- Common errors on the form
- Reasons for claim denial
- Tips and tricks
- How insurance companies use the section
- How a dental office uses the section

Completing a Claim Form — Fixed Information

Authorizations – This section captures the patient's consent for the office to do two things:

1. File the claim on their behalf, and
2. Accept assignment of benefits (reimbursement)

The first signature (#36) must be completed in order for the office to file the claim. The second signature (#37) is only needed if the office has agreed to wait for insurance reimbursement rather than require the patient's payment in full up front. Both of these sections are often sent with "signature on file," meaning that the patient signed a different form (new patient paperwork) to allow you to send all claims on the patient's behalf. The second section, #37, pertains to assignment of benefits (AOB), which is where the reimbursement check will be sent. Fee for Service (FFS) offices will have this section left blank. See more about AOB in Chapter 11.

AUTHORIZATIONS

36. I have been informed of the treatment plan and associated fees. I agree to be responsible for all charges for dental services and materials not paid by my dental benefit plan, unless prohibited by law, or the treating dentist or dental practice has a contractual agreement with my plan prohibiting all or a portion of such charges. To the extent permitted by law, I consent to your use and disclosure of my protected health information to carry out payment activities in connection with this claim.

X _____

Patient/Guardian Signature   Date

37. I hereby authorize and direct payment of the dental benefits otherwise payable to me, directly to the below named dentist or dental entity.

X _____

Subscriber Signature   Date

Billing Dentist or Dental Entity – The next section down is the office billing information. This section is blank if being submitted by the patient.

BILLING DENTIST OR DENTAL ENTITY (Leave blank if dentist or dental entity is not submitting claim on behalf of the patient or insured/subscriber.)			TREATING DENTIST AND TREATMENT LOCATION INFORMATION	
48. Name, Address, City, State, Zip Code			53. I hereby certify that the procedures as indicated by date are in progress (for procedures that require multiple visits) or have been completed.	
			X_____	
			Signed (Treating Dentist)	Date
			54. NPI	55. License Number
			56. Address, City, State, Zip Code	56a. Provider Specialty Code
49. NPI	50. License Number	51. SSN or TIN		
52. Phone Number ( ) -	52a. Additional Provider ID		57. Phone Number ( ) -	58. Additional Provider ID

©2019 American Dental Association
J430 (Same as ADA Dental Claim Form – J431, J432, J433, J434, J430D)

To reorder call 800.947.4746
or go online at ADAcatalog.org

#49. NPI (National Provider Identifier): Every provider in the country has a unique NPI number; think of it like a Social Security number for doctors. NPI Type 1 refers to individual providers. Type 2 NPI numbers are organizational providers—those belonging to a corporation, group practice, or other legal entity.

This section of the form can have either Type 1 or 2 NPI numbers.

#50. License Number—if the dentist is the billing provider, enter their license number (which will be the same as #55. If a separate billing entity, leave this section blank.

Treating Dentist and Treatment Location Information – This is for the specific provider who performed the treatment and will always need to be filled out.

Within a single dentist office, this section and the prior section, "Billing Dentist or Dental Entity," will have almost identical information. The sections are separated for the case of an office with multiple providers or a different owner than the provider.

#54. is the individual NPI number only.

#56a. The Provider Specialty Code: HIPAA classification code for which type of dental specialty (General Practice and the 9 recognized ADA specialties.) For the common question whether a dentist might get paid more by being a specialist: yes, and this section must be filled out for that to be possible.

Dentist	122300000X
General Practice	1223G0001X
Dental Public Health	1223D0001X
Endodontics	1223E0200X
Orthodontics	1223X0400X
Pediatric	1223P0221X
Periodontics	1223G0001X
Prosthodontics	1223P0700X
Oral and Maxillofacial Pathology	1223P0106X
Oral and Maxillofacial Radiology	1223D0708X
Oral and Maxillofacial Surgery	1223S0112X

#58. Additional Provider ID (aka Legacy ID, or LID): This is not the SSN, TIN, or NPI. Most offices will not need to fill this out. LIDs are often assigned to different entities (e.g., federal government and third-party payers).

The remainder of the ADA claim form will change for each claim.

Completing a Claim Form - Variable Information

Header and Dental Benefit Information

ADA American Dental Association® **Dental Claim Form**

HEADER INFORMATION

1. Type of Transaction (Mark all applicable boxes)

☐ Statement of Actual Services   ☐ Request for Predetermination/Preauthorization

☐ EPSDT / Title XIX

2. Predetermination/Preauthorization Number

DENTAL BENEFIT PLAN INFORMATION

3. Company/Plan Name, Address, City, State, Zip Code

Here you will designate whether the claim is for a completed service, a pre-determination, or EPSDT (Early and Periodic Screening, Diagnostic, and Treatment), which is a Medicaid program to cover medically necessary services for treatment of identified physical, dental, developmental, and mental health conditions.

If you have a prior pre-determination or pre-authorization, you will enter the reference number at #2.

Insurance information will be placed in #3; this is the section that needs to be visible through the window of an envelope when using snail mail.

Other Coverage (Secondary Insurance)

This is the section to use for Coordination of Benefits (COB). If the patient has other dental or medical coverage, you insert that information here. If you are unaware of any other coverage, leave this section blank. See more on COB and secondary insurance in Chapter 9.

OTHER COVERAGE (Mark applicable box and complete items 5-11. If none, leave blank.)

4. Dental? ☐   Medical? ☐   (If both, complete 5-11 for dental only.)

5. Name of Policyholder/Subscriber in #4 (Last, First, Middle Initial, Suffix)

6. Date of Birth (MM/DD/CCYY)   7. Gender ☐M ☐F ☐U   8. Policyholder/Subscriber ID (Assigned by Plan)

9. Plan/Group Number   10. Patient's Relationship to Person named in #5 ☐ Self ☐ Spouse ☐ Dependent ☐ Other

11. Other Insurance Company/Dental Benefit Plan Name, Address, City, State, Zip Code

Policyholder/Subscriber and Patient Information

This is the main documentation for clarifying who the individual is receiving the treatment (the patient) as well as whomever holds the insurance policy (policyholder/subscriber). This is why it is important to capture all of the pertinent information discussed in Chapter 5, because without it completed accurately, the claim will be automatically rejected.

POLICYHOLDER/SUBSCRIBER INFORMATION (Assigned by Plan Named in #3)		
12. Policyholder/Subscriber Name (Last, First, Middle Initial, Suffix), Address, City, State, Zip Code		
13. Date of Birth (MM/DD/CCYY)	14. Gender ☐ M ☐ F ☐ U	15. Policyholder/Subscriber ID (Assigned by Plan)
16. Plan/Group Number	17. Employer Name	
PATIENT INFORMATION		
18. Relationship to Policyholder/Subscriber in #12 Above ☐ Self ☐ Spouse ☐ Dependent Child ☐ Other		19. Reserved For Future Use
20. Name (Last, First, Middle Initial, Suffix), Address, City, State, Zip Code		
21. Date of Birth (MM/DD/CCYY)	22. Gender ☐ M ☐ F ☐ U	23. Patient ID/Account # (Assigned by Dentist)

#23 Patient ID is your internal method to track which specific patient this claim belongs to. The insurance company ignores this section.

> **TIP**
>
> It is incredibly important to verify the patient has coverage if the office is going to wait for AOB. If you do not, it may take weeks to find out the claim is rejected because submitted information is incorrect.

Treatment/Record of Services Provided

This section is where you enter the information for the services provided such as #27–29 Tooth number/letter, surface involved, and the ADA procedure code.

#24 Procedure Date – This is always the date of service, not the date of the claim. Leave this blank for a pre-determination.

RECORD OF SERVICES PROVIDED

	24. Procedure Date (MM/DD/CCYY)	25. Area of Oral Cavity	26. Tooth System	27. Tooth Number(s) or Letter(s)	28. Tooth Surface	29. Procedure Code	29a. Diag. Pointer	29b. Qty.	30. Description	31. Fee
1										
2										
3										
4										
5										
6										
7										
8										
9										
10										

33. Missing Teeth Information (Place an "X" on each missing tooth.)	34. Diagnosis Code List Qualifier (ICD-10 = AB)	31a. Other Fee(s)
1 2 3 4 5 6 7 8 9 10 11 12 13 14 15 16	34a. Diagnosis Code(s) A_____ C_____	
32 31 30 29 28 27 26 25 24 23 22 21 20 19 18 17	(Primary diagnosis in "A") B_____ D_____	32. Total Fee
35. Remarks		

Area of Oral Cavity (#25) refers to the arch or quadrant. You will need to use one of these 2-digit codes to mark these:

00	Entire Mouth
01	Maxillary Arch
02	Mandibular Arch
10	Upper Right Quadrant (UR)
20	Upper Left Quadrant (UL)
30	Lower Left Quadrant (LL)
40	Lower Right Quadrant (LR)

#26 Tooth System refers to the numbering system you are using. Most dental providers in the US will use the universal system (JP). Orthodontic providers typically will use the international standard system (JO). Review chapter 2 for more information on dental anatomy and tooth numbering.

JP – Universal Tooth Designation System (#1–32 and #A–T).

JO – International Standards Organization (Quads 1–4 and Teeth 1–8).

Common Question for Tooth Numbering

Q: Do I put the number of the tooth or the number for the current location of the tooth?

A: You should always report the number of the **actual tooth involved in the treatment**, no matter where it is located in the mouth. Location can change when a tooth is missing and another tooth moves to fill the space. This makes sure that the insurance company does not deny a service that was previously completed.

Example: the patient lost #18 early in life, and the wisdom tooth #17 grew into the location that #18 used to occupy. You would still need to refer to the wisdom tooth as #17 because insurance might have a history of #18 missing and therefore would not pay for any services involving that tooth.

What if There Are More Procedures Than Lines 1–10 Will Hold?

You will need to fill out a second claim form to house the additional procedures. Each claim will be processed separately, so complete information with signature is required on both.

> **TIP**
>
> Electronic claims often have this same length restriction as most insurance companies do not like processing more than ten procedures at once because there are too many potential sources of errors.

Supernumerary Teeth

When you have extra teeth in the mouth, their numbering is based on the tooth they are matching and add 50 for a permanent tooth or S for a primary tooth. For example, an extra UL wisdom tooth #16 would be numbered #66. A supernumerary #C would be labelled #CS.

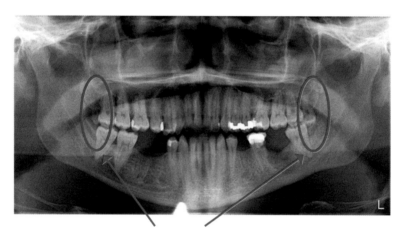

Example Pano of extra wisdom teeth #51 and #66

> **TIP**
>
> Extra (supernumerary) teeth are numbered by adding:
>
> - 50 for permanent teeth
> - S for primary teeth
>
> For example, an extra UL wisdom tooth #16 would be numbered #66. A supernumerary #C would be labelled #CS.

#30 Description – Abbreviation of the code's nomenclature (e.g., two-surface composite filling).

#31 Fee – Always report the *full* fee of the office, not the insurance discounted fee. This is the fee the dentist would usually charge a patient regardless of insurance coverage. (Chapter 19)

#33 – Missing Teeth Information: X out the tooth numbers that are missing for implants, bridges, and partials. Insurance companies often want this information for the entire mouth before approving a claim.

#34/34a. Diagnosis Codes – These are minimally used in dentistry but may be necessary with claims involving medical concerns, state regulation (Medicaid), or insurance contractual requirements.

#35 – Remarks: This is the section where you enter any additional information helpful to understanding the case, such as billing or treatment modifications, secondary claims, and so forth. This is an important section, which we will be referring to a number of times throughout this guide.

ELECTRONIC CLAIMS AND ATTACHMENTS

The previous section reviewed what information is necessary for completing dental claims. Now we can look at the most common way to file claims today, which is electronically, or E-Claims. Here are the basics of how a claim gets processed.

When you submit a claim electronically from your practice management software, the insurance company's software may or may not be able to "read" that information. That is because there are around 50 practice management software platforms in dentistry, and only a few of them are alike in how they package information. Each of the dozens of insurance companies also have their own software that reads information uniquely as well. Getting these all to communicate well together can be a challenge.

For this reason, when you submit a claim electronically, it first goes to a clearinghouse.

> **TIP**
>
> Clearinghouses are data-processing companies that will translate the claim data you sent into one that each insurance company will accept.

The clearinghouse will also screen and detect many of the most common errors with claims submission and inform you almost immediately via their software. The claim will not be forwarded to the insurance company until you correct the error. **Be sure to monitor your clearinghouse software daily to see what claims might need more information or modification before they actually get transmitted to the insurance company**. This can be a huge benefit to the office, as you only get three tries to submit a claim for a specific service.

With many claims, the provider might need to attach additional information (photos, x-rays, perio charts, other documentation, etc.) to communicate with the insurance company, gain approval, and receive reimbursement. Companies such as NEA (National Electronic Attachment) provide attachment services for electronic claims. This step is typically handled within your practice management software, which uses your attachment service to send it out with the claim electronically.

Chapter 9
Managing Secondary Insurance

You may occasionally encounter patients who are covered by two insurance plans. Dual coverage can result in fewer out-of-pocket costs for the patient but does tend to create more confusion and paperwork for the office. This section will help you understand how to most efficiently manage dual coverage.

When a patient is covered under two dental insurance policies, one policy will be responsible for paying first, which is called primary. The other policy will pay after the primary has processed and is therefore called secondary.

Common Examples:

Federal Policies (such as Medicaid) will always be secondary.

Two Jobs — If a patient has policies through two separate, current employers, typically, the plan that has been in effect the longest is primary. If one plan is from a retired job position, that plan will be secondary.

Spouses — If both have policies through their employer, and each include spousal coverage, typically the patient's policy is primary, and the additional spousal coverage will be secondary.

Children — Policies will generally go by the birthday rule. Whichever of the parents has a birthday earlier in the calendar year (month and day) will be the primary policy. These rules may be superseded by court order, establishing the child's responsible party.

> **EXAMPLE**
>
> If the father's birth date is 9/10/75 and the mother's birth date is 2/16/76, then the mother's coverage is primary.

When submitting claims, you must wait for the claim from the primary policy to process and pay first. Then you attach the EOB from the primary coverage insurer to the claim you submit to the secondary insurance carrier.

TIP

When dealing with claims for children of separated parents, it is important to ask the *parent* which insurance company will be primary versus secondary because the answer may be court ordered instead of by the common birthday rule.

TIP

If the patient is unaware of which policy is primary versus secondary, then a suggested route is to go by effective date: whichever policy became active earlier within a calendar year.

What Should You Submit on Secondary Claims?

- ID numbers for both covered enrollees
- Patient's relationship to each enrollee
- Birth date for the patient and each enrollee
- If parents are divorced, the parent with whom the child lives
- A copy of the court-ordered decree (if different than birthday rule)
- **Explanation of Benefits (EOB) from the primary carrier**

Divorce and Remarriage

The following are general guidelines for which policies may be considered priority with blended or separated families. These guidelines may be superseded by court order establishing the child's responsible party.

1. Natural parent with custody
2. Stepparent with custody
3. Natural parent without custody
4. Stepparent without custody

What if Dual Coverage Changes?

If a patient loses dual coverage, please write "patient no longer covered by another plan" on the primary claim form or in a comments section to help ensure correct payment and updating of insurance company records.

What Will Each Plan Pay?

Primary and secondary benefits will typically work together through a concept known as "coordination of benefits."

Coordination of benefits (COB) is a common procedure where the secondary policy will pay a portion of the remainder of the balance after primary pays. This is coordinated so that the combination of payment does not go above a dentist's normal (submitted) fee. This is one of several reasons why it is important to always file claims with your office's full fee. Most commonly, the secondary insurance will pay the patient's portion up to the amount they would have paid as primary.

TIP

It is crucial to always submit the office's full fee on insurance claims.

It is important to note that only group policies will have any coordination of benefit coverage. If a patient buys an individual policy outside of an employer or group, there will be no COB.

TYPES OF COORDINATION OF BENEFITS

Many factors determine how COB is handled: state laws, carrier processing policies, contract laws, fully insured versus self-funded plans, and types of COB. The different types of COB that plans may use are as follows:

Traditional - Traditional COB allows the policyholder to receive up to 100% of the procedure fee from a combination of the primary and secondary plans. This is the simplest to understand of the different types of COB.

EXAMPLE

Traditional Example: Both insurances will normally pay 80% of a $100 filling.
Primary Coverage: $100 × 80% = $80
Secondary Coverage: $100 × 80% = $80. However, only $20 remains. Total coverage is $20.

Maintenance of Benefits (MOB) - MOB reduces covered charges by the amount the primary plan has paid and then applies the plan deductible and co-insurance criteria. Consequently, the plan pays less than it would under a traditional COB arrangement, and the insured patient is typically left with some cost sharing.

EXAMPLE

MOB example 1: Both insurances will normally pay 80% of a $100 filling after they have met the deductible. Primary will pay $80, and secondary will pay $16 (80% of the remaining $20).

  Primary coverage: $100 × 80% = $80
  Secondary coverage: remaining $20 × 80% = $16
  Patient out of pocket cost: $4

MOB example 2: Both insurances will normally pay 80% of a $100 filling, yet secondary has not met the deductible. Primary will pay $80, and secondary will pay $0 since the potential benefits are less than the deductible.

  Primary coverage: $100 × 80% = $80
  Secondary coverage: remaining $20 × 80% = $16
  Deductible $50.
  Patient co-pay: $20 ($16 of which will be applied to the deductible, leaving $34 remaining to be covered before insurance reimbursement will begin.)

Carve Out - Carve out is a coordination method that first calculates the normal plan benefits that would be paid and then reduces this amount by the amount paid by the primary plan. This means that secondary will only provide reimbursement if the policy has higher coverage than primary.

EXAMPLE

Carve Out Example 1:
Primary insurance normally pays 50% of an $800 crown, and secondary normally pays 50% of a $1000 crown. Deductibles have been met. Primary will pay $400, and secondary will pay $100 (normal $500 minus the $400 primary paid).

Primary Coverage: $800 × 50% = $400
Secondary Coverage: $1000 × 50% = $500
Carve Out: $500 – $400 = $100
Patient Co-Pay = $300 ($800 – $400 – $100)

Carve Out Example 2:
Both insurances will normally pay 80% of a $100 filling and have met the deductible. Primary will pay $80, and secondary will pay $0.

Primary Coverage: $100 × 80% = $80
Secondary Coverage: $100 × 80% = $80
Carve Out: $80 – $80 = $0
Patient Co-Pay = $20 ($100 – $80 – $0)

Non-Duplication of Benefits – This refers to a provision or clause in some insurance policies stating that the secondary plan will not pay any benefits if the primary plan paid the same or more than what the secondary plan allows for that dentist. This clause is often found in ERISA-based, self-funded plans (see Chapter 3). The ADA opposes nonduplication provisions and at least one state, California, has enacted legislation prohibiting such provisions.

EXAMPLE

You submit a crown for $1000, and primary paid $500 for that crown; then secondary would only pay if the policy states it would have covered more than $500.

If secondary's policy states it would pay $600 for a crown as primary, then you can expect reimbursement of the $100 difference.

If secondary's policy states it would pay $450 for a crown as primary, then you can expect no reimbursement.

While non-duplication policies do not help the patient as much, they do make the dental office's task of estimating much easier. With non-duplication of benefits clauses, the office just needs to estimate which of the two insurance policies has the highest reimbursement; the patient will owe the remaining balance.

Medicaid/Medicare Coordination

By federal law, Medicaid and Medicare are typically secondary to any other benefit plan.

Affordable Care Act (ACA) and COB

The ACA had almost no effect on COB, contrary to industry myths. COB and claims submission are handled the same now as before ACA took effect.

Current ADA Policy on Coordination of Benefits

The American Dental Association is not a government or regulatory agency, so it does not set laws. However, it is the only entity that develops ADA codes, and it usually serves as a guide for state and federal lawmakers who create the laws. The ADA recommends the following with COB:

When a patient has coverage under two or more group dental plans, the following rules should apply:

1. The coverage from those plans should be coordinated so that the patient receives the maximum allowable benefit from each plan.
2. The aggregate benefit should be more than that offered by any of the plans individually, allowing duplication of benefits up to the full fee for the dental services received (traditional COB method).

For patients and team members who do not understand secondary coverage, the common assumption is that COB is handled as traditional. This poses challenges as every other type of COB reimburses less than 'traditional'.

What if Primary Is Maxed Out?

You should still submit primary claims if the patient is maxed out because you will need the primary EOB denial in order to process the secondary claim.

What Fee Is the Patient Responsible to Pay?

This question often leads to a lot of debate. There is no consistent rule or law across the country. The National Association of Insurance Commissioners (NAIC) has drafted a model of how coordination of benefits should be handled, and the ADA has recommended using this model for uniformity nationwide.

Each state governs how COB runs, and not every state has adopted the NAIC model. Some states, such as Rhode Island, have their own laws on COB that don't match up exactly to the NAIC guidelines. For the purposes of this chapter and simplicity, we will use the NAIC guidelines. You can find these guidelines at:

> http://www.naic.org/store/free/MDL-120.pdf

If you are in-network with either or both insurance plans, the patient is held responsible for the *lowest* of either network's fee.

The common office confusion here is what happens if you get paid more than the lowest fee.

The office is allowed to collect up to the full office fee when the reimbursements come from multiple insurance companies. It is only the patient who is not responsible for any amount above the lower network fee.

TIP

It is important to note that deductibles are PER POLICY. This means that a patient with two insurance policies will need to pay BOTH deductibles. This is a common misconception by patients. Secondary insurance will also require its own deductible to be satisfied before it starts reimbursing services.

The following pages have some examples to help highlight this often-misunderstood section:

NOTE

Please note in all the following scenarios that the patient never ends up with a credit. It would be inappropriate to EVER assign money from an insurance company back to a patient. Any amount paid over the in-network fee is money that belongs to the dental office, NOT the patient. Even in example #3 where the insurance payments exceeded the full office fee the extra money belongs back to the secondary insurance company. Patients can only ever be refunded money that the patient paid and only up to the amount they paid.

SCENARIO 1 - Payment above lowest fee schedule

Your patient has Delta as primary insurance with a crown fee of $1000, 50% coverage.

The patient also has Aetna as secondary insurance with a crown fee of $800, 50% coverage. Secondary COB policy is traditional.

The provider is in-network with both and has a $1200 crown fee.

Delta (primary) processes the claim as it always will. The office gets reimbursed $500 for the crown.

Aetna now receives the secondary claim, with the primary claim EOB showing reimbursement of $500. Aetna reimburses $400.

The office collected a total of $900.

Since the lowest discounted fee of the patient's two policies is $800, the patient owes nothing for the crown. The patient gets the best pricing benefit from either insurance.

The office keeps the total of the $900 because the amount is lower than the normal full fee.

	Primary Coverage
Office fee	$1200
Insurance fee	$1000
Coverage percentage	50%
Insurance reimbursement	$500

	Secondary Coverage
Office fee	$1200
Insurance fee	$800
Coverage percentage	50%
Insurance reimbursement	$400

Office full fee	$1200
Lowest network fee	$800
Primary reimbursement	**$500**
Secondary reimbursement	**$400**
Total insurance reimbursement	$900
Patient co-pay	$0
Office action	Keep all funds

SCENARIO 2 – Payment above highest fee schedule

Now let's switch scenarios and say the Delta plan provides 80% coverage and Aetna provides 50% coverage.

Your patient has Delta as primary insurance with a crown fee of $1000, 80% coverage.

The patient also has Aetna as secondary insurance with a crown fee of $800, 50% coverage. Secondary COB policy is traditional.

The provider is in-network with both and has a $1200 crown fee.

Delta primary reimburses $800.

Aetna secondary reimburses $400.

The office collected up to full fee ($1200) and gets to keep the money.

	Primary Coverage
Office fee	$1200
Insurance fee	$1000
Coverage percentage	80%
Insurance reimbursement	$800

	Secondary Coverage
Office fee	$1200
Insurance fee	$800
Coverage percentage	50%
Insurance reimbursement	$400

Office full fee	$1200
Lowest network fee	$800
Primary reimbursement	$800
Secondary reimbursement	$400
Total insurance reimbursement	$1200
Patient co-pay	$0
Office action	Keep all funds

*This is one of the main reasons an office should always file full fees on insurance claims. If the office only filed the in-network fee of $1000, Aetna would only have reimbursed $200.

SCENARIO 3 – Payment above office full fee

Both insurance companies have 80% coverage.

Your patient has Delta as primary insurance with a crown fee of $1000, 80% coverage.

The patient also has Aetna as secondary insurance with a crown fee of $800, 80% coverage. Secondary COB policy is traditional.

The provider is in-network with both and has a $1200 crown fee.

Delta primary reimburses $800.

Aetna secondary reimburses $640.

The office collected a total of $1440. Since this amount is above the $1200 full fee, it would be a mistake on the part of the secondary insurance company. Eventually Aetna will realize this mistake and request their overpayment back. This money does not belong to the patient or the office.

	Primary Coverage
Office fee	$1200
Insurance fee	$1000
Coverage percentage	80%
Insurance reimbursement	$800

	Secondary Coverage
Office fee	$1200
Insurance fee	$800
Coverage percentage	80%
Insurance reimbursement	$640

Office full fee	$1200
Lowest network fee	$800
Primary reimbursement	$800
Secondary reimbursement	$640
Total insurance reimbursement	$1440
Patient co-pay	$0
Office action	See below

The office has a couple of options here:

1. Adjust off the extra amount on the ledger (it does not belong to the patient as a credit) and be prepared for the insurance company to submit a request for the overpayment in the future.
2. Immediately refund the secondary insurance company any amount over full fee, in this case $240. This is easiest to manage by requesting that the insurance company first submit an overpayment request to the office. Do not just send the money back, you could encounter issues on the insurance company's side.

SCENARIO 4 – Payment below lowest fee schedule

Your patient has Delta as primary insurance with a crown fee of $1000, 50% coverage.

The patient also has Aetna as secondary insurance with a crown fee of $800, 25% coverage. Secondary COB policy is traditional.

The provider is in-network with both and has a $1200 crown fee.

Delta primary reimburses $500.

Aetna secondary reimburses $200.

The office collected $700 from insurance. The patient will owe the $100 difference of the lowest network fee schedule as their co-pay.

	Primary Coverage
Office fee	$1200
Insurance fee	$1000
Coverage percentage	50%
Insurance reimbursement	$500

	Secondary Coverage
Office fee	$1200
Insurance fee	$800
Coverage percentage	25%
Insurance reimbursement	$200

Office full fee	$1200
Lowest network fee	$800
Primary reimbursement	$500
Secondary reimbursement	$200
Total insurance reimbursement	$700
Patient co-pay	$100
Office action	Bill patient co-pay of $100

How Should You Estimate Secondary Insurance?

There is no set rule or requirement on how an office handles secondary insurance. Many offices have a policy that the patient will be responsible for payment of a service in full after 30 or 60 days regardless of insurance.

Secondary insurance benefits may take months to process since you must wait for the primary carrier to pay first. There is also an entire subset of COB rules within individual policies that determine how much secondary insurance will pay, making them much more complicated to estimate ahead of time.

The best practice for managing patient questions with secondary insurance is to estimate as if the patient only had primary coverage and collect from the patient as if they had only one insurance policy. Any secondary benefit can either be:

1. Refunded to the patient directly; or
2. Complete the claim form with the assignment of benefits (AOB) to the patient (see next chapter).

> **TIP**
>
> Any money refunded to a patient should go directly to the original form of payment (such as the exact credit card used).

Following this method avoids any surprise bills for the patient after treatment. Patients are often understandably upset if they owe more money than expected after the fact. However, refunding excess money is simple and does not tend to engender the same negative responses from patients.

What if We Still Do Want to Try to Create an Estimate for Secondary?

First thing you will need to know estimating secondary is how that policy coordinates benefits. You will need to ask during a breakdown call what type of COB the policy goes by. You will also need to know all the details of the breakdown, like you would for primary. You can use the examples in this chapter to come up with your estimate based on the breakdown data.

Chapter 10
Explanation of Benefits, Assignment of Benefits

Assignment of benefits (AOB) is most simply a term stating to whom the reimbursement check from the insurance company is paid. Most insurance companies will allow AOB to go to either the patient or the dental office no matter your network status. (Delta Dental is the notable exception, as they will often *only* send AOB to patients of out-of-network providers.) Filling out point #37 on the ADA claim form will send AOB to the office (see Chapter 8 for more details on where to find this on the claim form). In most cases, "signature on file" will suffice, meaning that the patient signed another document, allowing the office to submit claims on their behalf.

AUTHORIZATIONS

36. I have been informed of the treatment plan and associated fees. I agree to be responsible for all charges for dental services and materials not paid by my dental benefit plan, unless prohibited by law, or the treating dentist or dental practice has a contractual agreement with my plan prohibiting all or a portion of such charges. To the extent permitted by law, I consent to your use and disclosure of my protected health information to carry out payment activities in connection with this claim.

X _____
Patient/Guardian Signature   Date

37. I hereby authorize and direct payment of the dental benefits otherwise payable to me, directly to the below named dentist or dental entity.

X _____
Subscriber Signature   Date

Once a claim has been reviewed and approved for payment, both the dental office and the policyholder will receive a notice from the insurance company explaining in detail what treatment was approved, what amount was reimbursed, and what amount may still be owed by the patient. This is the explanation of benefits (EOB) statement. The EOB always goes to both provider and patient, regardless of where the AOB was sent.

If you work in the front part of a dental office, you will likely be looking at EOBs often. This is the main form of a communication you will have with the insurance companies. Every claim that gets submitted by the dental office will result in an EOB being sent back. It is incredibly important to understand how to read EOBs. You need to learn both what they are trying to tell you and what they aren't trying to tell you (myths). EOBs can have errors in them; the computer system and people at an insurance company are not infallible. Learning how to understand insurance companies and EOBs can prevent tens or hundreds of thousands of dollars every year to be missed.

This understanding is not always easy. Unlike claims forms, EOBs are not standardized by the ADA. Each insurance company has a different layout for their EOBs. It is important to learn how to read these and understand what information they are trying to convey back to you. Let's look at a few different companies' EOBs so you can become familiar with what information you should gather from them.

♥**aetna** P.O. BOX 981106
EL PASO TX 79998-1106
USA

Explanation Of Benefits

Please Retain for Future Reference

Payment Address:

Printed:	9/21/2020
Page:	2 of 2

PIN:
TIN:
Check Number:
Check Amount: $257.40

Provider Address:

Get paid faster – sign up for EFT today!
With electronic funds transfer (EFT), we deposit your payments directly to your account. No more trips to the bank! Sign up through EnrollHub® at **https://solutions.caqh.org**. Or get a paper enrollment form. Medical providers go to **www.aetnaeft.com**. Dental providers go to **www.aetnadentaleft.com**.

Patient Name:
Claim ID: Redc: 08/31/20   Member ID   Patient Account
Member:
Group Name: Group Number:
Product: **Aetna Dental® PPO**   Network ID:
Aetna Life Insurance Company   **Network Status: In-Network**

SERVICE DATES	SERVICE CODE	ALTERNATE BENEFIT CODE	TOOTH NUM.	SURFACE	NUM. SVCS	SUBMITTED CHARGES	NEGOTIATED AMOUNT	COPAY AMOUNT	NOT PAYABLE	SEE REMARKS	DEDUCTIBLE	CO INSURANCE	PATIENT RESP	PAYABLE AMOUNT
08/22/20	D4341		LLQ		1.0	143.00						14.30	14.30	128.70
08/22/20	D4341		ULQ		1.0	143.00						14.30	14.30	128.70
TOTALS						286.00						28.60	28.60	257.40

ISSUED AMT: $257.40

For questions regarding this claim or if you with a review of this decision:
    P.O. BOX 14094 LEXINGTON, KY 40512-4094   *Total Patient Responsibility:* $28.60
    CALL (800) 451-7715 FOR ASSISTANCE
Note: All inquiries should reference the ID number above for your prompt response.   *Claim Payment:* $257.40
                                                                                              $257.40
            Total Payment to:

When reading EOBs there are a few things to look for first:

1. Date of service and patient information – You will want to use this information to track back to the patient and assign the EOB to the correct account for the correct treatment.
2. Services provided and location/tooth number – Next, double check that the services in the EOB match up with what services were provided on that date and confirm nothing was missed.
3. Submitted charges – Next, match the fees assigned here and check for any errors. Full office fees should always show up in this location no matter your network status.
4. Patient responsibility (co-insurance/co-pay) and payable amounts (reimbursement) – Finally, this is the most important number to match to the patient's ledger and account for any differences. See if the patient's amount was already collected or if there is a balance or credit that needs to be communicated and resolved with the patient.

As long as everything matches up the way you expect, you can post the EOB and move on. However, the EOB may show something different than expected. When this happens, you need to understand how to manage the difference. Let's review some of the more common differences.

Anthem.✚

Anthem Blue Cross Life and Health Insurance Company
P.O. Box 1115
Minneapolis, MN 55440-1115

Anthem's Downgrade code is 920. The two composite fillings on #14 and 15 are zeroed out. Instead, two rows are added for the amalgam reimbursement due to the downgrade.

EXPLANATION OF BENEFITS

1-877-567-1804
www.anthem.com/ca

Issue Date: 09/24/2020

EXPLANATION OF BENEFITS
THIS IS NOT A BILL

Provider ID: Provider: Treating Addr: OUT OF
Subscriber ID: Subscriber: Group-Subgrp: NETWORK
Claim: Patient: Patient DOB:

Tooth # Surface	Service Date	Proc Code	Procedure Description	Submitted Amount	Approved Amount	Allowed Amount	Network Savings	Deductible Amount	Cov %	Patient Owes	Plan Payment	*See Notes
14-OBL	09/17/2020	D2393	Resin composite, 3 surfac	0.00	0.00	0.00	0.00	0.00	0	0.00	0.00	920
15-ODL	09/17/2020	D2393	Resin composite, 3 surfac	0.00	0.00	0.00	0.00	0.00	0	0.00	0.00	920
14-OBL	09/17/2020	D2160	Amalgam – 3 surfaces	305.00	305.00	305.00	0.00	50.00	80	101.00	204.00	
15-ODL	09/17/2020	D2160	Amalgam – 3 surfaces	305.00	305.00	305.00	0.00	0.00	80	61.00	244.00	
Totals				610.00	610.00	610.00	0.00	50.00		162.00	448.00	

Appeal Comments	**Current Plan Payment:**	**$448**

Anthem added two amalgam fillings to show the downgraded service payments.

CHECK YOUR UNDERSTANDING

Both fillings were downgraded at the same percentage (80%). Why was the reimbursement different by $40?
Insurance reimbursement for #14: **$204**
Insurance reimbursement for #15: **$244**

CALCULATION FOR #14 FILLING

$305 (Submitted)
−$50 Deductible First
$255 × 80% = **$204**

CALCULATION FOR #15 FILLING

$305 (Submitted)
Deductible already satisfied
$305 × 80% = **$244**

Notes (Downgrades)

In this claim from Anthem, the treatment note 920 is for downgrades. Composite fillings were completed, but the insurance policy downgrades these to amalgam for the purpose of reimbursement. With most insurance company EOBs, you will see the change reflected as services that are zeroed out, and an additional line is added for the downgraded service that was reimbursed instead (as you see here).

> **TIP**
>
> Always remember that downgrades do NOT change the fee the office collects, even in-network. Downgrades only affect the amount the insurance company and therefore patients need to cover of that fee.

> **NOTE**
>
> You may often see a lowered amount than the submitted number in a separate column, such as the "approved amount." This would be because insurance UCR for an amalgam would be lower than the composite. In this specific example EOB, the UCR for an amalgam filling is the same or higher than the submitted composite fee; hence, the fee does not change due to the downgrade.

Another point to see on this claim is the difference in payment between the two fillings: even though both are covered at the same percentage (80%), one was paid at $204 and the other at $244.

This is due to the annual deductible.

Even though the deductible was $50, notice the difference in payment between the two fillings was only $40. This is because the deductible is removed from the filling before the percentage of coverage is applied.

$305 (submitted)

−$50 deductible first

$255

$255 × 80% = $204

> **TIP**
>
> Deductible amounts should be removed from the fee BEFORE you apply the percentage of coverage.

DELTA DENTAL®

Your claim payment

Check Number: Date: September 30, 2020

Summary of claim information

PATIENT NAME	ENROLLE ID NUMBER	DATE OF SERVICE	CLAIM NUMBER	PATIENT PAYS ($)	DELTA DENTAL PAYS ($)
		May 21, 2020		0.00	433.00
		September 23, 2020		85.20	340.80

Claim details

Patient:
Relationship: Spouse
Date of birth: April 3, 1964
Group name:
Group number:

Primary enrollee:
Enrollee ID numbers:

#1 Claim number:

PROCEDURE NUMBER AND TYPE OF SERVICE TOOTH NUMBER AND SURFACE	SUBMITTED FEE ($)	ACCEPTED FEE ($)	MAXIMUM CONTRACT ALLOWANCE ($)	AMOUNT APPLIED TO DEDUCTIBLE ($)	PAID BY ANOTHER PLAN ($)	CONTRACT BENEFIT LEVEL	PATIENT PAYS ($)	DELTA DENTAL PAYS ($)
Date of service: May 21, 2020 Treatment type: Periodontics (D4341) PERIODONTAL SCALING AND ROOT PLANING - 4 OR MORE TEETH PER QUADRANT Tooth: LR	135.00	135.00	135.00	0.00	--	100% Treating provider:	0.00	135.00
Date of service: May 21, 2020 Treatment type: Periodontics (D4341) PERIODONTAL SCALING AND ROOT PLANING - 4 OR MORE TEETH PER QUADRANT Tooth: UR	275.00	146.00	146.00	0.00	--	100% Treating provider:	0.00	146.00
Date of service: May 21, 2020 Treatment type: Oral & Maxillofacial Surgery (D7210) SURGICAL REMOVAL, ERUPTED TOOTH; FLAP ELEVATION, REMOVAL OF BONE AND/OR SECTION Tooth: 04	310.00	152.00	152.00	0.00	--	100% Treating provider:	0.00	152.00
Claim total for	720.00	433.00	433.00	0.00	0.00			433.00

What Is Wrong in This EOB?

A common misconception in dental offices is with what fees should be billed out to the insurance company. Each insurance company has a negotiated in-network fee. However, that in-network fee should never be submitted or shown on a claim. The first reason is that you are bound by the network contract that the dentist signed to ALWAYS submit your full office fee on claims.

The second reason is shown above. This office accidently and incorrectly sent out the network fee they had in their system to the insurance company. Do you see the problem?

Insurance will only reimburse up to the fee submitted, no matter the network negotiated rate. The network rate for this office was $146, and yet one quad of Scaling and Root Planing was only reimbursed at $135 because that was the fee submitted.

NOTE
The office lost money due to multiple errors in this claim submission.

The next step for this office to do is to correct the fee in the system for this treatment code for this insurance company. Then, you should find out why this fee was incorrectly entered and submitted to avoid repeating this same problem. Most likely these are manual entry problems, as the fee is often hardcoded into the software and cannot typically be different for the same code on the claim.

Cigna Dental
Cigna Health and Life Insurance Company

Page 3 of 3
54542225

Explanation of dental payment

THIS IS NOT A BILL

Your payment summary

Enclosed is payment to
Amount: $174.20
Payment date: SEP 24, 2020
Payment number

Claim details

PATIENT NAME: PATIENT'S RELATIONSHIP TO SUBSCRIBER subscriber SUBSCRIBER NAME: PATIENT ID:
HEALTH CARE PROFESSIONAL NAME: HEALTHCARE PROFESSIONAL ID:PROVIDER NETWORK STATUS network
GROUP NAME   GROUP #:   DOCUMENT #:   CLAIMANT #: 01   CLAIM #: 007   PAYMENT #: 001
RECEIVED DATE: Sept 15, 2020   PROCESSED DATE: Sept 18, 2020

AMOUNT YOU CHARGED ($)	YOUR CONTRACTED AMOUNT ($)	AMOUNT ELIGIBLE FOR COVERAG BY THE PLAN ($)	PATIENT COPAY/ DEDUCTIBLE ($)	REMAINING BALANCE ($)	PATIENT COINSURANCE ($)	THE PLAN COVERED (%)	($)
For service on May 21, 2020: D4341* for Tooth#/Quad/Arch: UR							
144.00	144.00	144.00	0.00	144.00	28.80	80%	115.20
				Amount paid by the plan	$115.20		
				Customer's responsibility	$28.80		

PATIENT NAME: PATIENT'S RELATIONSHIP TO SUBSCRIBER depender SUBSCRIBER NAME: PATIENT ID:
HEALTH CARE PROFESSIONAL NAME: HEALTHCARE PROFESSIONAL ID:PROVIDER NETWORK STATUS network
GROUP NAME   GROUP #:   DOCUMENT #:   CLAIMANT #: 01   CLAIM #: 007   PAYMENT #: 001
RECEIVED DATE: Sept 23, 2020   PROCESSED DATE: Sept 23, 2020

AMOUNT YOU CHARGED ($)	YOUR CONTRACTED AMOUNT ($)	AMOUNT ELIGIBLE FOR COVERAG BY THE PLAN ($)	PATIENT COPAY/ DEDUCTIBLE ($)	REMAINING BALANCE ($)	PATIENT COINSURANCE ($)	THE PLAN COVERED (%)	($)
For service on Sept 21, 2020: D0140* *(see note 15)*							
85.00	59.00	59.00	0.00	59.00	0.00	100%	59.00
				Amount paid by the plan	$59.00		
				Customer's responsibility	$0.00		

Notes
15 - Your plan maximum is now paid at the maximum plan level as specified by your employer's plan design.
Additional remarks

Contracted Amount vs Eligible Amount

A common confusion with EOBs involves these two columns and what the difference is between contracted and eligible amount. In most cases these values will be the same in-network. However, occasionally patients may have a low-end policy that covers less than normal (such as a MAC policy), and the "eligible" column might be less. This difference would not affect what the office gets paid in total, only what the patient might be responsible for out of pocket.

If you are out of network, the "contracted amount" column should show either to be blank or to have the same value as the "amount you charged" column.

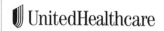

UnitedHealthcare

P.O. Box 30567
Salt Lake City, UT 84130-0567

EXPLANATION
OF DENTAL PLAN
REIMBURSEMENT
THIS IS NOT A BILL

Sheet: Page 3 of 4
Date: Page 3 of 4
Check No:
Check Amt: $315.00

PROVIDER OR MBR NAME AND ID NO; PROVIDER NETWORK STATUS; GROUP NO; CLAIM NO ADA CODE DESCRIPTION	DATE OF SERVICE	TOOTH NO	AMOUNT CLAIMED	AMOUNT ALLOWED	DEDUCT APPLIED	OTHER INS	PATIENT INS	AMOUNT PAID	EOB CODE
ADA CODE D0150 comprehensive oral evaluation – new or established patient	09/21/20	01 32	95.00	82.00	0.00	0.00	0.00	82.00	
ADA CODE D0274 bitewings - four radiographic images	09/21/20	01 32	69.00	64.00	0.00	0.00	0.00	64.00	
ADA CODE D0220 intraoral - periapical first radiographic image	09/21/20	01 32	30.00	28.00	0.00	0.00	0.00	28.00	
ADA CODE D0230 intraoral – periapical each additional radiographic image	09/21/20	01 32	25.00	23.00	0.00	0.00	0.00	23.00	
ADA CODE D0230 intraoral – periapical each additional radiographic image	09/21/20	01 32	25.00	23.00	0.00	0.00	0.00	23.00	
ADA CODE D1110 prophylaxis - adult	09/21/20	01 32	105.00	95.00	0.00	0.00	0.00	95.00	
SUB-TOTAL			349.00	315.00	0.00	0.00	0.00	315.00	

Notes:
This benefit reflects your agreement with   PPO – Careington Dental Network

Plan underwritten by UnitedHealthcare Insurance Company

	AMOUNT CLAIMED	AMOUNT ALLOWED	DEDUCT APPLIED	OTHER INS	PATIENT RESP	AMOUNT PAID
TOTAL	349.00	315.00	0.00	0.00	0.00	315.00

Network Leasing

This EOB from UnitedHealthcare is rather straightforward as a hygiene visit with 100% coverage. The unique part about it is this office has its network contract through an umbrella contract, also known as network leasing. This is where the office signed up to be in-network with Careington, and Careington is sharing that network agreement with UnitedHealthcare. This means that even though the insurance company is United Healthcare, the office will be paid according to the Careington fee schedule. See Chapter 16 for more information about network leasing.

STORAGE OF EOBs

Storing EOBs that are sent individually is simple; however, at times your EOBs may come in batches. Below is an example EOB from Delta where two different patients' claims were attached together. This is a common way insurance companies save money, by combining multiple claims in the same EOB, which reduces their paper and shipping costs. This process does create a small challenge for the office in tracking and storing this data.

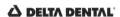
DELTA DENTAL

Delta Dental of Oklahoma	1 of 4
PO Box 548809	
Oklahoma City, OK 73154	**Claim Payment Statement - Dentist**

Forwarding Service Requested

Customer Service Information

Questions? Contact Us
Phone: 405-607-2189
Toll Free: 800-990-7337
E-mail: CustomerService@DeltaDentalOK.org
Online: DeltaDentalOK.org

Reference Info

EFT/Check No.
Check Date: 09/24/20
Paid To:

Date of Issue: 09/24/20

Claim No:
Plan Type: DELTA DENTAL PRO
            PLUS PREMIER   Patient: Provider:
Group No: Patient D.O.B.:   License No:
Group: Rel: SUBSCRIBER   Specialty: GENERAL DENTIST

Date of Service	Tooth Code	Tooth Surface	Submitted Proc Code	Approved Proc Code	Submitted Amount	Approved Amount	Allowed Amount	Provider Adjust.	Patient Deductible	DDOK Co-Ins %	DDOK Pays	Patient Pays	Processing Policies
9/17/20			D0220	D0220	$30.00	$14.00	$14.00	$16.00	$0.00	80%	$11.20	$2.80	
		Claim Totals:			$30.00	$14.00	$14.00	$16.00	$0.00		$11.20	$2.80	

Delta Dental's Total Payment:	$11.20	Other Carrier:	
Total Patient Responsibility to the Dentists:	$2.80	Primary Payment Amount:	$0.00

Claim No:
Plan Type: DELTA DENTAL PRO
            POINT OF SERVICE   Patient: Provider:
Group No: Patient D.O.B.:   License No:
Group: Rel: SPOUSE   Specialty: GENERAL DENTIST

Date of Service	Tooth Code	Tooth Surface	Submitted Proc Code	Approved Proc Code	Submitted Amount	Approved Amount	Allowed Amount	Provider Adjust.	Patient Deductible	DDOK Co-Ins %	DDOK Pays	Patient Pays	Processing Policies
9/15/20	14		D7210	D7210	$310.00	$152.00	$158.00	$50.00	$0.00	50%	$51.00	$101.00	
		Claim Totals:			$310.00	$152.00	$158.00	$50.00	$0.00		$51.00	$101.00	

Delta Dental's Total Payment:	$51.00	Other Carrier:	
Total Patient Responsibility to the Dentists:	$101.00	Primary Payment Amount:	$0.00

Important Notice

Payment for these services is determined in accordance with the specific terms of the patient's dental plan and/or Delta Dental's agreement with your office. This statement is based on individual and /or employment eligibility, and Delta Dental records as of the date of processing.

For questions concerning this statement, please contact Customer Service at 405-607-2189 (OKC Metro) or 800-990-7337 (Toll Free).

There are two common ways to handle multiple claims on the same EOB: individually or in group. Both options have some pros and cons, so you will want to determine which method will work best for your office.

Individual Storage

If you chose to store EOBs individually, this will generally take more time when you process EOBs. You can either physically cut the EOBs and scan them separately or you can find a scanner and software that allow you to trim the EOBs electronically. The upside to individual storage is being able to quickly and easily refer back to the EOB directly through the patient's chart, leading to less confusion if and when a patient question/concern arises about their insurance. This also helps simplify chart audits.

Group Storage

If you chose to store the EOBs in groups, it will take less time to store the information on the front end and more time later if you need to reevaluate an old claim. Some offices choose to store the EOBs in a daily folder. This way if you need to track back to an old EOB, you check what date the EOB was posted (scanned and attached) to the account and check that folder for the EOBs from that day.

No matter which storage option you choose, it is important to save this EOB information. You never know when a patient will have a concern about their current or past coverage, and you won't want to waste time contacting the insurance company again to find this information. It is not uncommon for a patient to question one service or bill on their ledger. Needing to go back several months or years of claims to make sure everything was done correctly can be tedious. The more information you have, the better, when in these patient situations. The EOBs are a helpful resource to show that in general the amount the patient needs to pay is based on what their insurance plan does or does not cover and not due to errors made by the office.

Chapter 11
Avoiding Claims Errors and Denials: The Most Common Mistakes with Insurance

Dental office teams often voice complaints about claims that are denied by insurance companies. Denials can be a constant frustration for the dentist, team, and patients. It is important to understand why denials happen and what you can do about them when they do.

The National Association of Dental Plans (NADP) reports that insurance companies process more than 250 million claims annually. Around 70% of these claims are completed through a computerized process. This means that a human never looks at the claim. Almost all claims that are rejected by the computer are automatic rejections because the claim had submission errors within them, meaning, the office team did not fill the claim out correctly.

Here are the top 10 most common reasons claims are denied by insurance:

1. Lack of information
2. Data entry errors
3. Timing
4. Limitations
5. Incorrect CDT coding
6. Wrong claim form
7. Illegible claims
8. COB issues
9. Not including prior date of placement (delivery)
10. "Dental necessity"

Understanding these points can help you avoid most of the simple, easy-to-fix denials that happen. Let's break them down one at a time.

LACK OF INFORMATION
NADP reports around 50% of claims for basic/major services are returned, either as flat denials or requesting more information. Therefore, it is crucial to make sure all the information on the claim form is complete and accurate before submission. It is also important to attach all the necessary documentation available for many restorative and surgical procedures.

Fillings. In general, fillings tend to be computer-processed without needing more information. Almost every other dentist procedure requires more information to be included with the claim.

Crowns. Crowns are the second most denied procedure. Crowns typically need an x-ray, narrative, and prior crown placement date. The addition of a photo can also help tremendously. See Chapter 23 for more detailed information on what is recommended.

Periodontal Treatment. This is the most frequently denied procedure. Periodontal treatments (surgical and non-surgical) require x-rays, a full periodontal chart, narrative/remark, and inclusion of photos helps greatly. See Chapter 23 for more detailed information.

Extractions and Root Canals. Claims for these procedures always need x-rays, showing the roots, and a narrative/remark. Occasionally root canals also require periodontal charting (insurance will not reimburse for a tooth that has a poor prognosis).

Implants, Bridges, and Partial Dentures. All of these procedures require x-rays, extraction dates, and missing tooth number; bilateral x-rays are often required as well (FMX or Pano).

> **TIP**
>
> All x-rays sent should be less than six months old. Some insurance companies are even requesting same-day x-rays for services, such as crowns and implants.

It is important to know what information and supporting documentation the most stringent insurance companies require for claim approval and payment. This way you can assemble and submit those items of information for every patient. By adopting a high level of standard claim documentation for every patient, the team will avoid being caught unaware. This also helps make the team's job easier, as there is less reason for each team member to know every insurance policy's specific guidelines. Having more available information is better than not enough because it can often be impossible to go back and recreate information that was not generated at the time (such as mid-op photos and x-rays).

DATA ENTRY ERRORS

Often a claim denial or request for more information will say something like, "beneficiary identification incorrect." This means the information on the claim is in error and does not match an existing covered patient in the insurance company's database. These are usually simple errors in name spelling, birth date, tooth number, and so forth. This could also happen when the incorrect insurance company (such as Delta or BCBS, which have multiple companies) or location (such as Guardian, which has multiple locations in the same company) are entered.

> **TIP**
>
> Delta and BCBS are a network of multiple franchises with the same name. Rarely will the franchises within their network talk to each other, so you must make sure you have identified the correct state and contact information.
> Guardian has multiple processing locations and will not transfer data between locations.
> It is important to know which location will process your patient's claim.

This is why it can be vitally important to make sure the team member entering new patient information into a chart is double-checking each item as it is captured. Data entry errors are completely avoidable.

If sending a paper or printed claim, leaving sections blank is rarely an option. Even the "other coverage" section needs to be filled out, even if the patient only has one form of insurance. An empty section means it was missed or ignored. Adding the note "patient has no other coverage" is the correct response for this section if there is no secondary insurance. Electronic claims and clearinghouses will often self-correct any blank spaces.

> ### TIP
>
> If sending a paper or printed claim, leaving sections blank is rarely an option. An empty section is interpreted as it was missed or ignored. Even the "other coverage" section will need a note saying "patient has no other coverage" if the patient only has primary insurance. Electronic claims and clearinghouses will often self-correct any blank spaces for you.

Sending claims to the wrong company is a common-enough problem to be discussed as well. Often patients have medical insurance through one company and dental insurance through another. It is a common mistake for patients to give dental offices their medical insurance information instead of dental. It is also common for a patient to switch insurance companies because the employer changed policies or the patient's employment changed since their last visit. Having old information is a form of data entry error as well.

These problems can easily be solved by verifying coverage on every patient every visit, before their appointment. If you have incorrect information about a patient, you will be unable to verify their coverage. Doing this will allow you to know ahead of time if you have correct information or not. This is also one reason it is still preferable to also capture the patient's Social Security number (SSN) because it can be used as a secondary way to find a patient in the insurance company's system (see Chapter 5 for more details on SSNs).

FILING DEADLINES

The length of time a patient or dental office must file a claim for dental services is regulated by both state laws and policy contract language. Most states and plans have a one-year timeline, but some may be as short as three months.

> ### TIP
>
> Check that claims are sent out daily.
> The deadline to file is different in different states but is a hard limit that insurance companies will not budge with.

It is important to promptly process claims and send them out daily. This will prevent you from missing a claim or forgetting to send one out, thereby missing the deadline for filing.

Q: If we find out a claim was not sent out in time, is there any way to fight it and possibly get reimbursement for our patient?
A: No. These are usually hard limits, and insurance companies will not even process a claim after the time limit is up. It is important to check your system daily to find claims that might not have processed.

LIMITATIONS

Insurance companies are an important vehicle that employers use to be able to offer desirable benefits to their employees. The employer sets the budget, and from that budget, the insurance company designs the terms of a policy that will fit that budget. These terms often come with coverage limits that can range from frequency limitations, yearly or lifetime maximums, service exclusions, and so forth. If the patient needs or obtains treatment outside of the limitations that are set by the insurance company, there is almost no situation in which the insurance company will consider reimbursement. The patient only gets coverage for the services for which the employer is paying.

A common example is with routine cleanings, prophylaxis. If a policy has a limitation of a cleaning every six months, and the patient receives their second cleaning five months and 30 days later, it will be denied with no recourse for consideration.

Waiting periods are another form of limitation. These are commonly set in place to reduce the premium cost of the policy. Waiting periods are time periods where certain procedure categories will not be covered. A common example is a 6–12-month waiting period for major services, meaning the patient will be unable to have a crown reimbursed until the time period has elapsed.

Occasionally policies may even require *pre-determinations* (sometimes called pre-Ds) before certain treatment to be considered for reimbursement. Without them, the insurance company will deny a claim with no way to fight it. Pre-determinations are typically found with more expensive treatments that are not commonly associated with emergencies (e.g., bridges, implants, or dentures).

A breakdown of benefits is important to be able to know these limitations up front, so you can provide the patient the full information they need to make the best decision for their treatment *and* to get the most out of their insurance benefit.

INCORRECT CDT CODING

The ADA updates, modifies, and changes CDT coding yearly. Typically, these changes originate from the most common complaints, challenges, and errors that dentists and insurance companies report. Entering an old or outdated CDT code on a claim form will usually invoke a denial. Occasionally an insurance company may elect to auto-replace the correct, updated coding in its place; however, for most insurance companies, using an old code will simply result in a rejection/denial.

As an example, the most common change in 2017–2021 has been splitting codes to be specifically descriptive of the location of treatment. For example: in 2021, D7960 - frenulectomy (removing a tongue or lip tie) was split into D7961 and D7962 to indicate the difference between a buccal and lingual frenulectomy. The original code D7960 is no longer recognized and will be denied.

The ADA and Charles Blair both offer a revised CDT manual yearly as a reference to the most up-to-date coding options, highlighting the changes that have occurred, helping to prevent mistakes and claim denials.

WRONG CLAIM FORM

Similar to CDT codes that get updated annually, ADA claim forms get updated every few years. Due to the millions of claims processed, it can become nearly impossible for insurance companies to process multiple different versions of claim forms. Therefore, make sure to use the most current ADA form when preparing and submitting your claims. The most current version claim forms can be found free on the ADA website, as well as on many insurance company websites. The most recent ADA forms were updated in 2012 and 2019.

If you get a denial due to the wrong claim form, you can easily resubmit on the correct, up-to-date form.

If you file electronically, this should not be an issue as both practice management software and clearinghouses will keep these updated.

ILLEGIBLE INFORMATION

Paper claims are most often scanned, subsequently shredded, and then processed by a computer. If anything is unclear or faint, it will be denied. If you are still using paper claims, make sure to have clear handwriting, fresh ink, and avoid smudges or extra markings.

LOST X-RAYS AND LOST CLAIMS

One of the largest complaints among team members who handle insurance and claims is when an insurance company reports lost x-rays or claims. This can happen when a team member gets in a rush to send out a claim and misses submitting the attachments correctly. The insurance company could also lose or misplace attachments.

Electronic claims can help reduce or eliminate this problem almost completely. The clearinghouse or attachment service would keep track of this information and have reference numbers should the insurance company misplace an attachment.

COORDINATION OF BENEFITS ISSUES

When filing secondary insurance, one of the most important steps is to attach the primary EOB to the secondary claim. Without the primary information, secondary insurance has no way of knowing what they would be responsible to reimburse.

Always make sure the primary EOB is attached to a secondary claim and add into the re-marks box the phrase "primary EOB attached."

Secondary insurance *also* requires any documentation that primary might have required, in-cluding x-rays, narratives, and photos.

NOT INCLUDING PRIOR DATE OF PLACEMENT

Insurance companies do not want to pay for dental work that fails repeatedly or before its in-tended lifetime. As a result, insurance companies often build in a frequency limitation within their policy to prevent the insurance company from being responsible for either poor quality work or poor home care compliance by the patient. The more costly procedures often have a frequency limitation, and therefore the insurance company will request the prior date of placement to verify whether the restoration met the mark.

These dates are required with crowns, bridges, dentures, and implant restorations. You can include the prior date of placement in the "initial/replacement date" section of the claim.

"DENTAL NECESSITY"

The term "dental necessity" is commonly misunderstood by dental providers and their teams. Medical insurance requires "medical necessity" for almost every treatment provided in order to consider a claim for payment. However, the term does not mean the same thing for dental insurance.

Dental necessity often comes about when a plan policy does not include or exclude a service from the plan. Dental necessity means that an independent dentist will review each listed service to make sure the service had information supporting the need for such service. The National Association of Dental Plans lists the top three reasons for a "dental necessity" de-nial to be rendered:

1. Asymptomatic third molars
2. Periodontal treatment (surgical or non-surgical) with no documentation of bone loss
3. Buildups

Third Molars. With third molars (wisdom teeth), some policies may only cover removal when there is pain, infection, or damage to adjacent teeth. It is important to document the specific reason for removal in order to avoid denial, or to respond if you do receive one of these denials. If the reason for the removal is not one of the listed covered reasons, the pa-tient will be 100% responsible for the cost of treatment.

Periodontal Treatments. The single, most effective way to avoid questions or denials when submitting a claim is to always attach a full periodontal chart that includes pocket depths, recession, bleeding points, mobility, and furcation involvement. The common mistake by clinical teams is only marking the pocket depths and bleeding. See Chapter 23 for a more in-depth review of how to get periodontal services reimbursed.

> **TIP**
>
> The single, most effective way to avoid questions or denials when submitting a periodontal claim is to always attach a full periodontal chart that includes pocket depths, recession, bleeding points, mobility, and furcation involvement.

Buildups. Buildups under crowns can be another major source of claim denial. The simple answer is to provide good photographic and radiographic documentation illustrating the necessity for a restoration to support a crown. See Chapter 23 for an in-depth review on how to get buildups reimbursed.

Typically, the provider or utilization manual you receive from the company will provide you with more specific guidance about what that insurance company will want to review for each service.

Understanding Dental Necessity on an EOB

It would be inappropriate and illegal for an insurance company to hint that a "lack of dental necessity" means that the service was unnecessary. An insurance company is only legally allowed to deny or approve coverage; it is not allowed to approve or deny treatments. It is also illegal according to almost every state board for a dentist to diagnose a patient without a "hands in mouth" exam. Since dental consultants within an insurance company are unable to provide an exam on a patient, it would be illegal for them to conclude or state that a treatment was unnecessary.

> **TIP**
>
> An insurance company is only legally allowed to deny or approve coverage; it is not allowed to approve or deny treatments.

Often these concerns arise due to the language on an EOB. Correct terminology might state that a "service was denied due to coverage limitations based on the documentation presented."

Incorrect terminology might state something such as "Service was not dentally necessary"; while this might be a technically correct statement to those who understand the exact definition of "dental necessity," it is inflammatory and dishonest to say to a patient who would not have that specific knowledge.

"Disallowing" treatment due to dental necessity may or may not be legal. One would need to read their network contract and see the policies that were agreed to.

If you believe that you have a treatment or EOB description that was illegal or inflammatory, it is important to report these to the state or federal department of insurance that would cover the entity in question. Ideally, you also report this to the insurance company with reasoning for the concern so they might correct a mistake they are unaware exists.

Q: If I am out of network and a claim gets denied due to dental necessity, can I still bill the patient?

A: Yes! The insurance company can only determine benefits, not treatment. If you are out of network, there are no rules determining what you bill to a patient.

For an in-network provider, this would depend on the language of your contract and provider manual.

Do Insurance Carriers Purposely Deny Claims?

Denial experiences often lead to speculation that some insurance companies intentionally deny claims. These speculative stories often involve a claims examiner who purportedly splits incoming claims into two stacks: to process and to automatically deny.

The challenge with these types of stories is that insurance companies are under constant scrutiny from state and federal agencies. Any intentional impropriety can lead to severe fines or revocation of the license to offer insurance. Prompt payment laws require insurance to process and pay clean claims on a timely basis. Many employers also have clauses within the contracts with insurance companies stating that premiums will not be paid if the insurance company does not have a reasonable claim processing turnaround time.

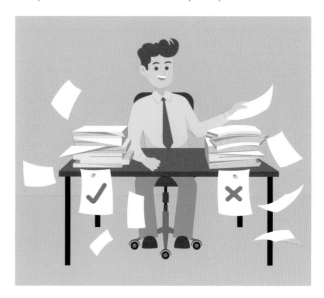

The other challenge with these stories is half of insurance policies now are only administered by the insurance company, whereas the funds come from the employer directly. It serves the insurance company no good to delay claims as they are typically paid per processed claim. In these cases, delayed or denied claims that require resubmission or appeal cost the insurance company time and money that serves them no purpose.

REMARKS SECTION

For services that are commonly denied, placing clarifying remarks or narratives into the claim can be a beneficial in aiding the claim examiner. However, if additional commentary is unnecessary, remarks can cause delays or denials of service. The most common unnecessary remark is "Payment is expected in 30 days." Prompt pay laws take care of this issue without the office needing to state it.

TIP

Do not use the remark "Payment is expected in 30 days," as it is the law, and unnecessary remarks only serve to delay your claim by removing the ability for the computer to automatically adjudicate the claim.

The other major challenge with adding commentary is most claims are processed by a computer (aka auto-adjudicated), meaning no human sees it. Auto-adjudicated claims come back faster and without denials as long as the information is submitted correctly. Claims for preventive procedures and fillings are often processed in this manner. When you include a remark into a claim, it removes it from the computer-driven process and now forces a human to look at it. This extra step brings in unnecessary delays in processing, as well as the potential that the human claims examiner will find something else wrong with the claim and deny it.

Try to leave remarks for only what is absolutely necessary to process a claim. Typically, commentary is more helpful for services that already get processed by hand anyway: periodontal treatments, crowns, bridges, dentures, and implants.

NARRATIVES AND CLINICAL NOTES

Now that you understand *when* you should add narratives, it is important to review *what* constitutes a good narrative. Claims examiners only have the information we give them in a claim. They are not privy to the direct information that the dental team has about the patient and the case. The most common cause for misunderstandings between dental teams and insurance companies is when the dental team *assumes* the claims examiner has all the information they need.

Every insurance company is a little different in its requirements for certain services to be reimbursed. However, in general, insurance companies require the same basic types of narratives. Often these narratives can be confusing because there is a fine line between a great narrative that helps obtain reimbursement and a poor narrative that creates more questions, reduces reimbursement, or even results in denial.

Having templates for narratives can greatly help a team make sure the important information gets documented clearly and effectively. The challenge with narratives is to make sure that they do not become so generic that they no longer become educational for the claims examiner.

First, you have to understand your goal for writing the narrative, which is to convey information to the insurance company clearly enough to enable them to process the claim to benefit your patient, receive timely reimbursement, and ensure your office runs most efficiently with minimal collections concerns.

Don't fall into the trap of just trying to get every claim out immediately with minimal effort. Like any other process, a rushed effort can lead to even more time spent needing to respond to a denied claim and then still doing the work that you could have done with the first claim submission, not to mention what challenges the patient is going to raise when they receive a denial of their claim.

Here are some basic guidelines of what to keep in mind when writing a narrative:

- Keep it simple and brief. Time is valuable to you and the claims examiner
- Use only necessary information
- Use dental language; it is more specific
- Include photos and x-rays when available
- Keep to the facts of why the treatment is necessary
- Don't lie. If something does not add up, the claims examiner will deny before finishing the claim review

Example narrative

Poor example	Good example	Overdone example
Tooth is fractured. Buildup required for retention. Crown prepped to cover cracked/fractured tooth. Patient to return for seating.	#3 fractured tooth: broken ML cusp, internal fractures on D marginal ridge that extend into dentin. Pain to pressure on DL cusp (cracked tooth syndrome). 70% of tooth structure was missing and < 2 mm ferrule. Buildup required to retain the crown.	Pt. is a 65 y/o male who broke their tooth eating a sandwich at lunch. Their ML cusp is broken off and has internal fractures into the distal. Pt. also reports more pain when biting on food after the fracture. Tooth sleuth was used on all teeth in the quadrant and only the DL was involved. This is a common presentation for cracked tooth syndrome. Nitrous was provided because the patient has an intense fear of needles. The patient was given 2 carpules of 2% lidocaine and allowed 15 minutes for anesthetic to kick in. The decay and fractures were removed with round carbide and barrel diamonds to reach to clean, healthy tooth structure past the fractures. Etch was placed for 5 seconds and rinsed for 30 seconds, Scotchbond was placed, scrubbed for 5 seconds, and dried before 10 second curing. The buildup was placed with TiCore to be able to retain a crown. Crown preparation was completed and extended past the damaged tooth structure to provide full-coverage, long-term function. The patient will return for evaluation of the pulpal response in 3 weeks.

In the first example, there is not enough information for a claims examiner to justify the restoration. Remember, at the dental office you have the luxury of seeing the tooth and talking to the patient; the claims examiner does not. Each company has specific guidelines for their claims examiners to be able to approve claims. If that information is not satisfied, the claims examiner (who is often not a dentist) is unable to make a judgment call and therefore has no choice but to deny the claim or send it back with a request for more information.

The good example provides a short but detailed account of why the tooth needed work and what was done to achieve the desired result. It needs to be short enough to be able to fit into the narrative section on the claim, or else it would need to be sent as a separate attachment. But it also needs to be detailed enough to give the reviewer adequate information.

The overdone example is very commonly seen with claims. It provides a lot of unnecessary information, which is going to frustrate the claims examiner, confuse the situation, and possibly lead to denial by itself. It reads more like a clinical note than a narrative. In many cases the first person to evaluate a claim is familiar with dentistry but is not a dentist. The exact nature of the clinical visit is not necessary for the claim. Any confusion in the process will cause the claims examiner to deny the claim or ask for different information.

Chapter 12
Insurance Refund Requests

Insurance companies are large organizations, and as such will occasionally make errors simply resulting from the complexity of their industry. Insurance companies also must deal with their clients, the individual employers, who aren't always prompt with sending them updated information. Insurance companies will routinely conduct financial audits of their systems to find these errors. As a dental office, you may be impacted by such an audit if you receive an insurance refund request.

Insurance companies will occasionally send letters, requesting refunds of benefits already paid on the patient's behalf. Your ability to fight these demands will depend on your state laws as well as the specific insurance company policies. In general, *only in-network offices are subject to comply with refund requests* according to the network contract the provider or office signed.

Refund requests can come in months after treatment is rendered and can be highly detrimental to a dental office team as well as the patients. It is important to understand your state laws and what the insurance company can and cannot do. Insurance companies will often send these letters to all offices, regardless of the laws in place. The letters do not necessarily mean the law forces you to comply with the refund demand, so it is important to understand your state laws.

EXAMPLE

Texas has a 180-day rule. If insurance does not request the refund within 180 days of payment, then the office is not legally bound to comply with the refund request. Each state is different on this timing.

The next few pages will include a detailed reference to the individual state laws. A few general concepts are as follows:

- Most refund requests resulting from fraud, misrepresentation, or inappropriate/abusive billing have no statute of limitations
- Coordination of benefits claims often have a longer time frame to recoup
- Government entities also tend to have a longer time frame to recoup

- If you search the name of the state, with a copy of the state law code, you should be able to find the complete wording of your state law in real time online
- If you do not see details for your state, it means there were no recoupment laws found; therefore, any limitations on recoupment would be based on your network provider contract.

RECOUPMENT LAWS BY STATE

State	Time limit	Other factors	Exemptions	Source law
Alabama	1 year	18 months if related to COB	Fraud	AL 27-1-17
Alaska	No limit			AS 21.54.020
Arkansas	18 months		Fraud	23-63-1802
Arizona	1 year		Fraud	20-3012
California	365 days		Fraud	10133.66.
Colorado	Unique	36 months if COB w/ federal No refunds ever if verification of eligibility within two business days of delivery of services.	Fraud or Misrepresentation	10-16-106.5 10-16-704 (4F)
Connecticut	5 years			SB 764
Delaware				No current law
District of Columbia	6 months	18 months if COB	Fraud or improper coding	31-3133
Florida	12 months	Provider must respond within 40 days. No response = obligated to refund.	Fraud	627-6131
Georgia	1 year			33-20A-62
Hawaii				No current law
Idaho				No current law
Illinois				No current law
Indiana	2 years		Fraud	IC 27-8-5.7-10
Iowa	2 years	No refunds under $25 ever.	Fraud	191-15.33
Kansas				No current law

State	Time limit	Other factors	Exemptions	Source law
Kentucky	24 months		Fraud	304-17A-708
Louisiana	Unique	Same as claims deadline (usually 12 months)		R.S. 22:250.34 B.
Maine	18 months		Fraud	24-A-4303
Maryland		18 months if COB	Fraud	15–1008
Massachusetts	12 months		Fraud or duplicate payment	Section 38, Chapter
Michigan				No current law
Minnesota				No current law
Mississippi				No current law
Missouri	12 months		Fraud or misrepresentation	376.384
Montana	12 months	Max same as claims deadline	Fraud	33-22-150
Nebraska	6 months			TITLE 201, CHAPTER 60, 11.01
Nevada				No current law
New Hampshire	18 months		Fraud	420-J:8-b
New Jersey	18 months		Fraud, COB, inappropriate billing	C.17B:30-48
New Mexico				No current law
New York	2 years		Fraud or abusive billing	S.8417, Spano/A.11996, Bradley
North Carolina	2 years			58-3-225
North Dakota				No current law
Ohio	2 years			3901.38.8
Oklahoma	24 months			36-1250.5
Oregon				No current law
Pennsylvania				No current law
Rhode Island				No current law
South Carolina	180 days			38-94-40
South Dakota				No current law
Tennessee	18 months		Fraud	56-7-110

State	Time limit	Other factors	Exemptions	Source law
Texas	180 days			1301.1051
Utah	12 months	36 months for COB or government programs		31A-26-301.6
Vermont				No current law
Virginia	12 months		Fraud	38.2-3407.15
Washington	1 year	18 months if COB	Fraud	HB 1418
West Virginia	1 year		Fraud	WVC 33-45-2
Wisconsin				No current law
Wyoming				No current law

Why Do These Refund Requests Happen? Did the Insurance Company Lie to Us When Providing Verifications?

There are three common reasons insurance companies send out refund letters.

1. The insurance company system had an error in processing that ended up with an over-payment.
2. The patient was let go from their job prior to the treatment and no longer was covered by the employer's insurance policy.
3. The patient went through a divorce and was no longer on the spouse's policy.

The first reason is fairly self-explanatory. The second may require some background knowledge to understand.

When a patient's employment ends, their paperwork is processed through the human resources (HR) department. HR will at some point send that information to the insurance company, which may be days or weeks later. Most insurance contracts state the employer is only required to pay benefits for current employees each month. Therefore, if an employee is no longer employed on the date of service, then the insurance company policy would no longer be valid. This is one reason it is important to check eligibility within 1–2 days of each patient's dental appointment if working with insurance for reimbursement. This practice will help reduce some of these refund issues.

Once the insurance company receives the information from HR, it may take a couple of weeks to process the termination of the patient's coverage. After that process completes, a different department within the insurance company that conducts audits of accounts throughout the year will find the overpayment issue. The entire journey from termination to discovering the overpayment might be weeks or months.

Meanwhile, at your dental office, the team would have talked to someone at the insurance company to verify coverage. Most likely at the verification stage, the termination process and the entire audit process will not have been completed. Therefore, the insurance company departments that providers and patients deal with would not likely know the patient is no longer covered, and as a result, the office gets confirmation of coverage even though the patient's employment and insurance coverage has ended.

Insurance claims departments may even send out payment before the insurance company is even aware of the new information from the employer HR department.

As an example, here is a basic timeline:

March 1	Patient employment ended.
March 9	Dental team verifies coverage.
March 10	Patient receives treatment in office.
March 31	HR department notifies insurance company about the employment termination.
April 4	Dental office receives reimbursement for treatment.
April 15	Insurance company processes information from HR department.
May 30	Insurance audit agent notices a lack of active insurance coverage during time of treatment.
June 2	Insurance company sends dental office letter to recoup money.

TIP

Recheck benefits later if the patient knows they are losing their job/coverage, or have the patient pay 100% and set AOB to the patient.

These errors have little if anything to do with insurance companies or agents of the company having any deceit in the process. The process of two large corporations working together (employer and insurance company) can at times be slow and cumbersome and lead to timing errors.

The frustration from dental teams, however, is valid. Of all the players in this scenario, the party who *should* be least responsible is the dental office. If the delay occurs somewhere between the HR and insurance departments, logically they should be the ones responsible for any discrepancy. Ultimately, of course, the policy belongs to the patient, and therefore they are responsible for the cost.

Dental offices are subject to these problems because we either do not fight them or because we signed a contract with clauses included in which the provider agreed to become the collection agent for the insurance company.

This is also why out-of-network providers are not required to comply with any refund requests due to insurance or employer errors; there is no contract requiring the provider to act as a collection agent for the insurance company. Of course, by law you still need to respond to the refund request, typically in writing.

ARE REFUND REQUESTS UNFAIR PRACTICES?

In general, it would be correct to state that it is unfair to place the refund burden on the provider. The original problem stems from the employer and insurance company. However, this is one of many clauses you would have signed as part of an in-network contract.

On the insurance company's side, many errors, especially those concerning eligibility, aren't based on fault of the insurance company either. If the employer did not inform the insurance company promptly about employment changes, there is not much the insurance company can do to correct problems before they happen.

What ideally should happen is the insurance company hold a reserve fund when an employer stops using them, which is where any refunds based on eligibility should draw from. Unfortunately for the dental office, this method is not often used. Alternatively, the insurance company should seek excess funds from the patient directly instead of using the dental office as an ill-equipped collection agency.

This is why it is important to use whatever letters and legal means you have to refute refund claims that were due to errors that the dental office has no control over.

> **TIP**
>
> Always appeal! There are multiple scenarios in which an insurance company might back down from their refund request. Often these requests are sent out automatically either in error or because some offices don't even try to appeal. Stand up for the rights of your patient as well as your right to not have to become a collection agency!

On the next page you will find a sample letter to send back to the insurance company to deny a request for an overpayment refund. If you are in a state with recoupment laws, it would also be a good practice to modify the letter to include those laws as applicable. If you need help with this, please visit www.PracticeWhisper.com, and we will be happy to help you craft your specific letter.

> **TIP**
>
> The office can only be held responsible for refund requests if the insurance reimbursement check was submitted to the office. If the office did not accept AOB, then the insurance company legally cannot request that money back from the office.

Understand that the insurance company by law can only request money back from the entity that accepted AOB. If that entity were the patient, then the office would not need to manage the refund request. This is another reason it can be helpful to find ways to have the patient accept AOB (such as pre-payment discounts).

Letter to Insurance to Deny Refund Request

Dear [Recipient],

We are in receipt of a refund request in the amount of $_____ for client _____.

We have reviewed this account thoroughly, and according to our records, the claim has been paid and the account is closed. You will be pleased to know we find no balance due from your company, nor do we find any payment that you are entitled to recoup. We have applied all appropriate contractual adjustments and the patient has been balanced billed for their responsibility, if any.

According to federal law, as a third-party creditor, we cannot be held liable for mistakes on the insurer's part. We obtained the patient insurance information from your office at the time of service, and there was every indication we were entitled to third-party payment from your company.

If you are claiming an overpayment, we received your payment and your explanation(s) of benefits (EOB) in good faith. Based on your payment and explanation of benefits, we did not bill the patient for the portion covered by the insurance. We have provided services in good faith, and the funds received have been exhausted.

If at this date you have uncovered an error relative to timing or amount of coverage, then we believe that any reconciliation of that error and subsequent monies recouped should be between you and the insured (or former insured).

There are several court decisions that bear on this situation. In 1992, the California Court of Appeals held that, if a provider bills in good faith, and the insurance company accidentally pays too much based on the insurance company's own calculation, the company cannot collect a refund from the provider, so long as there was no misrepresentation or fraud on the provider's part in billing (City of Hope Medical Center v. Superior Court of Los Angeles County (1992) 8 Cal.App.4th 633). The discharge for value rule, or the innocent-third-party-creditor rule, has also been applied in an analogous situation. Numerous courts have held that an insurer is not entitled to recover payments erroneously made to an insured's health care provider. See National Benefit Adm'rs, Inc. v. Mississippi Methodist Hosp. & Rehabilitation Ctr., Inc., 748 F. Supp. 459, 464_65 (S.D. Miss. 1990). See also Time Ins. Co. v. Fulton DeKalb Hosp. Auth., 438 S.E.2d 149, 152 (Ga. Ct. App. 1993); St. Mary's Med. Ctr., Inc. v. United Farm Bureau Family Life Ins. Co., 624 N.E.2d 939 (Ind. Ct. App. 1993); Lincoln Nat. Life Ins. Co. v. Brown Schs., Inc., 757 S.W.2d 411 (Tex. Ct. App. 1988).

Similarly, your company, as the insurer, made a payment to discharge a debt owed by the patient, and we are not required to refund the payment based on your calculations, which we received in good faith.

We feel that we have been properly reimbursed for services rendered, and no refund will be issued. If, in the future, you elect to deduct the so-called overpayment from benefits payable on behalf of other beneficiaries of yours to whom we provide services, we will see that our legal counsel ensures that our rights, and the rights of those beneficiaries as supported by the law, are preserved.

Please do not hesitate to call us if you have any questions or need additional information. You can contact us at (xxx)xxx-xxxx.

Chapter 13
Medical/Dental Connection

When you work in dentistry you may occasionally encounter a crossover into medical insurance. There is a strong connection between what happens elsewhere in the human body with what happens in the mouth. Many diseases first show themselves orally and are often detected by a dentist. Dental disease frequently affects a person's overall general health, especially when it involves periodontal disease and infections. Occasionally you may be dealing with dental problems that are caused by medical conditions, and therefore bring medical insurance into the picture (e.g., accidents or traumas).

Myth: Dental Care Is More Expensive Than Medical Care
When the discussion of the medical-dental connection comes up, often there is a myth that surfaces. This myth is that dental care is more expensive than medical care. This myth is be-

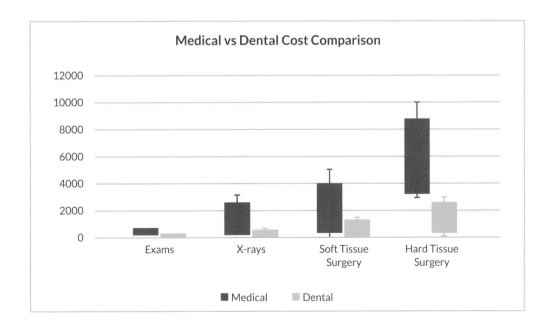

yond false in every way. It is important for dental teams to understand why so they can discuss the topic knowledgeably with patients if they should bring it up.

If you compare exam billings between medical and dental offices, on average, physicians charge and collect more than dentists. When looking at x-rays, dental may be a few dollars for a PA and a couple hundred for a cone beam scan. Comparatively, medical x-rays may range all the way up to multiple thousands of dollars for scans like MRIs. When it comes to dental care, almost every procedure a dentist performs is surgery. Dental surgery costs may range from a couple of hundred for a filling to a couple of thousand for a root canal, implant, or crown. In medicine, most surgeries start in the thousands and can range into the hundreds of thousands. There is almost no case where a comparative procedure in dentistry is more expensive than in medical, and more complex medical surgeries are vastly more expensive than anything in dentistry.

Then why does this myth exist?

The main difference between medicine and dentistry, and the reason for this commonly heard myth, is that medical insurance has no maximum and often pays 100% of medical surgery after the deductible is covered. Medical surgery is far more expensive but comes at a lower out-of-pocket cost due to the way insurance works. This is where this myth arises. Medical insurance is actually insurance in the traditional sense, whereas what is termed "dental insurance", is nothing like traditional insurance. It is more of a fancy discount coupon.

When someone brings up this myth, you have a good opening for educating them about how the two types of insurance differ and the weaknesses of dental insurance.

EXAMPLE

Example team member response:
"I have heard that myth before about dental care being expensive. However, anything you can compare between what physicians and dentists do, we charge less, often far less. The difference is medical has actual insurance, whereas in dentistry "insurance" only barely helps with costs. Dental benefits can be a nice supplement but cannot really be thought of as insurance in the traditional sense."

HOW TO FILE MEDICAL INSURANCE

This is a textbook about dental insurance, so we will only touch briefly on medical insurance.

Occasionally you may find the need to file medical insurance. The patient may have a medical problem that is responsible for their dental concern, and therefore medical insurance may actually cover the treatment. More often, however, you will find some dental plans require you to file with their medical insurance first. This can be common with procedures, such as wisdom teeth removal. You may find dental insurance will only pay after medical insurance has been filed, making dental insurance the secondary policy for coverage of that procedure.

You can then file the dental claim with a copy of the EOB from medical.

There are multiple ways to file medical insurance, but one of the easiest is electronically through a free online service at Availity.com.

You will need to be aware when working with medical insurance of the coding differences. While in dentistry we work with the Current Dental Terminology (CDT) coding, working with medicine, you may occasionally have to work with Current Procedural Terminology (CPT) and International Classification of Diseases (ICD) coding. The ADA and a couple of other entities provide coding crossover books to translate dental procedures into medical codes.

The main difference to remember with medical coding is that medical often requires a diagnosis code modifier. This means you need to file both the treatment *and* the reason for the treatment (modifier) for a claim to be processed.

Another important point working with medical insurance is you won't usually expect the medical insurance carrier to pay the claim. This is because medical insurance typically has a large deductible and does not start reimbursing until after that deductible is covered. This deductible is often in the range of thousands of dollars. When the deductible has not been met, the patient will be required to pay the dental bill. Many patients will not meet their medical deductible each year.

What Happens if Medical Conditions Are the Cause of the Dental Problems?

Here is a common situation that surfaces when working on older patients.

> "My patient is elderly with multiple medical issues and extremely poor oral hygiene. The patient has had multiple fillings completed. A few were on teeth that have had fillings previously about a year ago.
> The dental EOB says the company will not pay and that we are not allowed to collect from the patient! The patient will continue to experience recurrent decay. Normally we would charge the patient with a frequency issue like this, but the EOB specifically says that we can't charge so my front desk just wrote it off. Am I really supposed to keep treating for free?"

This is a great example case on why it is so incredibly important to be an insurance expert. Knowing how insurance works ahead of time will prevent this from ever becoming an issue of doing free work.

Insurance is not wrong, in most cases, with frequency issues. The frequency limitation is set because dental work should last at least a minimum time, and the insurance company should not be held responsible for either poor quality work or poor patent compliance. The challenge is when medical problems interfere and cause dental work to digress more quickly than normal, which is not the dentist's fault either. If a dentist signed a network agreement, then they did sign that quality of work needs to be held to a minimum standard and replacements in a short time period will be no charge to the patient or the insurance company.

What Do You Do with These Cases?

In cases where the patient's medical health is the issue, the *entire* team needs to know how to handle the situation. If you are below the frequency limit and the replacement work is not the dentist's fault, here is how you can proceed:

> *Do not send a dental claim. This will only confuse the situation with how EOBs are worded.

1. Advise the patient this is a *medical* problem, and therefore your dental insurance will no longer assist with payment. If the patient has not met their medical deductible for the year, their medical insurance will not likely pay for treatment either. Even if they have met the deductible, it may be difficult to get medical to pay for a normally dental problem.
2. Request the patient pay up front. This is to make sure the patient is fully aware of the challenges and costs in advance if they choose to have the dentistry redone. It would be unfair to the patient to give them false hope of reimbursement and then hit them with a bill months later.
3. Ideally, have the patient sign a waiver to not submit the claim to dental insurance. See Chapter 18 for more information on HIPAA "Do not bill insurance" release forms.

The patient may elect not to pay and redo the work. This is a possible outcome and the main reason for point #3 above. It should be up to the patient to decide whether they want to keep spending their money for a mouth that may be incapable of staying healthy for long. This situation gives the opportunity for the dentist to have another conversation with the patient about whether to do nothing, or to choose an alternative treatment option that dental insurance might help cover.

Chapter 14
HSA/FSA Usage

Many of your patients may have pre-tax money available to use for medical or dental procedures through a Health Savings Account (HSA) or a Flexible Savings Account (FSA).

FSA is typically managed through an employer and is funds that will disappear if unused at the end of the year.

HSA is typically personally owned and is similar to a bank account. The funds will roll over every year if they are unused.

It is expected for your patients to want to use these funds for their dental treatment. Most of the rules for the usage of FSA and HSA come from the IRS.

Below is a general Q&A from the IRS, slightly edited for clarity in dentistry. If you want the full document you can find it here: https://www.irs.gov/publications/p502

What Are Medical Expenses? (includes dental) – Medical expenses are the costs of diagnosis, cure, mitigation, treatment, or prevention of disease.

Patients can generally include medical expenses they pay for themselves, as well as those they pay for a spouse or dependent either when the services were provided or when they paid for them.

Patients can include only the medical and dental expenses they paid for this year but generally not payments for medical or dental care they will receive in a future year.

Patients can't include medical expenses that were paid by insurance companies or other sources. This is true whether the payments were made directly to them or to the provider of the medical services.

SERVICES THAT ARE ELIGIBLE

Artificial Teeth
Patients can include in medical expenses the amount they pay for artificial teeth (dentures, bridges, implants, etc.).

Dental Treatment

Patients can include in medical expenses the amounts they pay for the prevention and alleviation of dental disease. Preventive treatment includes the services of a dental hygienist or dentist for such procedures as teeth cleaning, the application of sealants, and fluoride treatments to prevent tooth decay. Treatment to alleviate dental disease includes services of a dentist for procedures, such as x-rays, fillings, braces, extractions, dentures, and other dental ailments.

Laboratory Fees

Patients can include in medical expenses the amounts they pay for laboratory fees that are part of medical care.

Medicines

Patients can include in medical expenses the amounts they pay for prescribed medicines and drugs. A prescribed drug is one that requires a prescription by a doctor for its use by an individual. Except for insulin, patients can't include in medical expenses amounts they pay for a drug that isn't prescribed.

SERVICES THAT ARE NOT ELIGIBLE

Cosmetic Surgery

Generally, patients can't include in medical expenses the amount they pay for cosmetic surgery. This includes any procedure that is directed at improving the patient's appearance and doesn't meaningfully promote the proper function of the body or prevent or treat illness or disease. Patients generally can't include in medical expenses the amount they pay for procedures such as face lifts, hair transplants, hair removal (electrolysis), and liposuction.

Patients can include in medical expenses the amount they pay for cosmetic surgery if it is necessary to improve a deformity arising from, or directly related to, a congenital abnormality, a personal injury resulting from an accident or trauma, or a disfiguring disease.

Nonprescription Drugs and Medicines

Except for insulin, patients can't include in medical expenses the amounts they pay for a drug that isn't prescribed. A prescribed drug is one that requires a prescription by a doctor for its use by an individual.

Personal Use Items

Patients can't include in medical expenses the cost of an item ordinarily used for personal, living, or family purposes unless it is used primarily to prevent or alleviate a physical or mental disability or illness. For example, the cost of a toothbrush and toothpaste is a nondeductible personal expense.

Teeth Whitening

Patients can't include in medical expenses amounts paid to whiten teeth.

HSA/FSA CHART

Here is a quick summary list for what can and cannot generally be used for an HSA/FSA:

Eligible	Not eligible	Eligible with letter of medical necessity
• All diagnostics and preventative services • Hygiene and periodontal services • Restorative treatment (fillings, crowns, root canals, etc.) • Extractions • Dentures • TMJ treatments • Prescription medications • Upgrade services that are not cosmetic in nature	• *Cosmetics (veneers/ bonding) • *Bleaching/whitening • Non-prescription medications • Treatment costs covered by insurance	• Ultrasonic toothbrushes • Powered flossers • Medically necessary orthodontics • Periodontal medicaments (e.g., Arestin)

These services can occasionally be covered with either description of medical necessity or other covered treatment on same day.

EXAMPLE

If the patient has bleaching done on the same day as another operative or surgical procedure that requires out-of-pocket costs, the bleaching is likely able to be an HSA/FSA expense. Ideally confirm this with the company that manages the HSA/FSA.

For the brand-name products, such as Sonicare, Waterpik, and Arestin, each company can provide you with letters of medical necessity to allow your patients to use FSA/HSA funds for these devices. Any treatment covered by dental insurance, patients are allowed to use FSA/HSA on patient portions but not on the amount covered by insurance.

What About Botox for Medical Reasons Such as TMJ Problems?

Botox is most commonly used for cosmetic purposes, so alone, Botox would not be eligible for HSA/FSA coverage. However, there are over 20 different applications for Botox, one of which would be to calm down the main clenching muscle, which can be used to help reduce or eliminate TMJ pain. A medical letter of necessity or other documentation may be required. It would be important for the patient to contact their benefit administrator to ensure they have proper documentation for reimbursement.

What Happens if Payment from an FSA or HSA Card Needs to Be Refunded?

You should always refund directly to the card used! Two main reasons why:

1. The cards all charge a fee to the merchant (you). Refunds to the card often remove that fee.
2. With FSA/HSA, the money does not belong to the patient per se to use for anything. They are for approved transactions only. It is fraud to charge the card and refund the money with any other method.

Occasionally you will have patients try to push you to refund them directly. Here is a sample answer you might give them:

"Mrs. Patient,
I would love to be able to provide exactly what you want. But it would be fraudulent for me to refund your FSA/HSA payment in any other way than straight back to your credit card originally used. This is the nature of your card and federal policies governing its use. It has nothing to do with our office, and therefore the decision is not up to us.
I am sorry for any inconvenience, but it is IRS law."

Part 2

Understanding Insurance - Advanced

Introduction

Dealing with insurance can feel very similar to playing a game of chess. On the surface, the game is moderately simple. You have several pieces on the board, each with their own strengths and weaknesses. You move the pieces around the board until one player can conquer the other's king—checkmate. The complexity comes in understanding the relationship between all the pieces and how they must work together seamlessly in order to win against your opponent. The key to becoming a great chess player is being able to think several moves ahead.

The insurance game works in a similar way. At first blush, it seems simple and straightforward. There are different pieces we work with (coding, estimates, claims, narratives, documentation, etc.) in order to achieve a final result—a paid claim.

However, just like in chess, it is actually quite complex. With insurance you must also think a few steps ahead of the insurance company in order to play the game well. You have to know what information to send them that helps you, and what information not to send that can impede your progress later.

"Play the game for more than you can afford to lose—only then will you learn the game."
—Winston Churchill

Winning = achieving two concepts:

1. **maximum benefit for the patient**
2. **maximum reimbursement for the dentist**

If you don't learn all the rules to the insurance game, you are condemning yourself to never fully learning the game at all, and therefore, have a lower chance of maximizing claim reimbursements. Insurance companies thrive when dental offices are ultra-conservative and don't fully understand the process.

This section is designed to help you not only understand the "game" you are playing but also the rules and how to use them so you have the best chance of advocating for your patient's benefit and collecting the funds you are due for their treatment.

While it is a common myth to think the rules are intentional, there is no truth to that thought.

Like many complex businesses, what may feel like "rules" in reality result from a complex arrangement of regulations, corporate structure, and cost-cutting procedures that have evolved over the years within both insurance and dental companies.

Chapter 15
Understanding the Insurance Company

In order to completely understand the insurance game, first you must understand the other major player: the insurance company. Learning how to best navigate through the world of insurance billing, you first need to understand the basics of how the insurance company operates. When you can understand what the insurance company wants and how it functions, you can apply this knowledge to predict how they are likely to respond to anything you send them.

In this section, we will step back and look at the bigger insurance picture and the dynamics that drive the actions and behaviors of the companies we work with, specifically:

- Pressure for profit
- Competition for business/how insurance contracts are sold
- Individual policy election/annual enrollment
- Who is the client of the insurance company?
- Structure of an insurance company/departments/accountabilities
- Working with the claims department
- State department of insurance/insurance commission

Pressure for Profit

Insurance companies are inherently neither good nor bad. They are just a business, like Amazon or any other business. Like Amazon, insurance companies are most often publicly traded companies listed on the New York Stock Exchange. Publicly traded companies are responsible to their shareholders (those who own stock). Their goal as a company is to increase the value of their stock. In order to increase the value of their stock, they must operate as a profitable entity. Their top priority is to maintain a profit to keep their shareholders happy.

Every business on the planet (except for charities) has this same basic goal, to earn profit. Even a dental office needs to show profit, or it will eventually close and be unable to serve its patients.

But for a large, public insurance company, the overarching profit imperative, and constant shareholder scrutiny drives corporations to track progress against metrics and goals. And as a result, they tend to work on a strict quarterly budget and bonus system.

Quarterly Mindset

This constant pressure for results/profit drives a very short-term mindset for most businesses and is certainly true for the insurance business. Thinking long term is not in the nature of most corporations because if you fail this quarter, then your long-term strategies are useless. As a result, they carefully watch results of key metrics through a quarterly budget and bonus system. Each quarter the insurance company needs to show they made a profit. And each department manager in the company is responsible for managing a budget, including the claims department, and will get incentivized to achieve positive results. How does this affect your office?

For example, let's use the first quarter of the year. In March, the insurance company is anticipating the end of the quarter, March 31. Therefore, if they are seeing that they may not be coming under budget, they are going to look for ways to solve this concern, including an increase in denials, delayed claim processing, returns for more information, delays in hiring, and so forth.

Narrow Profit Margins

While you may hear that insurance companies make hundreds of millions in profits, realize that for most carriers the bottom-line result translates to only a 2–3% profit margin. In fact, under the Affordable Care Act's medical loss ratio (MLR) rules, health insurers must spend 80–85% of their premium revenue on medical claims and quality improvements for their clients. No more than 20% of premium revenue can be spent on total administrative costs, including profits and salaries.

In order to show a profit, the insurance company needs to collect more in premiums than they pay out in claims. Simple math:

Profit = premiums collected – claims paid – expenses

So let's focus on that formula for a minute. If the insurance company is struggling to make this formula work, then one side of the equation needs to change. They either need to increase premiums (which we wish they would do), or they need to decrease what they pay out in claims.

Why don't they increase premiums? For the answer to that, one needs to understand how dental insurance is sold.

COMPETITION FOR BUSINESS; HOW DENTAL INSURANCE IS SOLD

Another important dynamic that drives an insurance company's behavior is the manner in which dental insurance is sold. The insurance company does not usually sell a policy directly to an individual. In most cases, dental insurance is first "sold" to an employer who then turns around to offer the insurance to an employee as part of their overall benefits package.

And as you might be aware, medical insurance plans receive a much higher priority and attention than dental plans. Dental insurance is considered a secondary add-on benefit, similar to vision insurance. Therefore, less emphasis is placed on the design and funding of these add-on benefit options.

Designing and Selling the Contract

Because dental insurance is usually part of an employer's overall benefit package for their employees, the insurance contract with the employer must be renegotiated and resold each year. That means the insurance company must present a new or revised contract annually to compete with other insurers for that employer's business. Each year, the insurance carrier selected, the specific array of benefits offered, and the premium pricing to be charged for those benefits are reconsidered, redesigned, and renegotiated. As you can imagine, the competition for business is very fierce. If you've ever wondered why any given dental benefit for one of your patients does not stay the same year to year, even when they are covered by the same insurance company, that is the reason.

As a hypothetical example, we will use American Airlines and Delta Dental.

EXAMPLE

American Airlines has 130,000 employees, and they all want health benefits as part of their employment agreement. American Airlines wants to earn a profit, so they must balance the benefit needs of their employees with the cost to provide those benefits. Therefore, American Airlines is going to negotiate with several insurance companies in order to obtain the best deal for their employees that fits into the budget they can afford (most benefits for lowest premiums). Delta Dental understands that AA has 130K employees and wants to sell a policy to them. But Delta also understands that Metlife, Aetna, Cigna, BCBS all want to have AA's policy too. Therefore, in order to maintain business with AA, Delta must remain competitive in their benefits and premiums to beat out the other insurance companies. Delta has limited ability to increase the premiums they charge unless every other insurance company in the country also increases their premiums too.

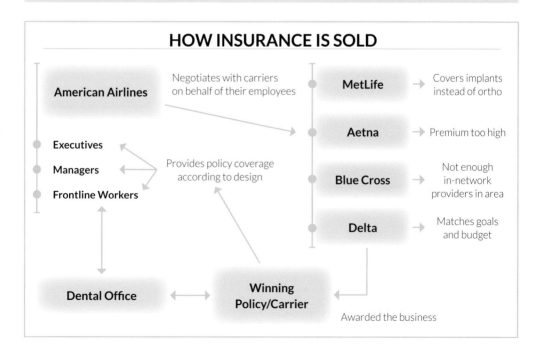

HOW INSURANCE IS SOLD

Selling Dental Insurance to Employees

As we've learned, dental insurance is customarily offered to employees as part of their benefit package. It will be offered to a new employee as soon as they are hired. And if they elect to receive dental benefits, their policy will become effective within the first few weeks, and they will begin paying premiums through payroll deduction.

For all other employees, they will have a chance to review and "re-elect" the various benefits they are interested in once each year during an "open enrollment" period. Open enrollment usually takes place in the fourth quarter of the year. During open enrollment, the insurance carrier selected for the upcoming year will prepare information and brochures to help educate employees about the benefits that will be available in the new year. Employees will have an opportunity to ask questions and review both the benefit changes as well as premium changes, and then decide/declare what they will choose for the next year.

If an employee chooses to purchase (or continue to receive) dental insurance as part of their annual benefit package, the insurance company will be notified, a new insurance card for the year will be issued, and the new benefit plan will commence on January 1 of the new year. Chances are good that the new policy will have a somewhat different mix of benefits and a different premium rate for the new year.

Although their dental insurance plan was procured through their employer, legally, the policy itself is a legal agreement between the employee (your patient) and the insurance company. The employer is merely an intermediary and facilitator.

Why Do Two Patients with the Same Company Have Different Policies?

Very large companies will naturally have a mix of different types of employees. And sometimes because of that mix, the company needs or wants to offer a slightly different set of benefits to each category or tier of employee. As an example, higher levels of managers may be offered one plan/set of benefits, sales employees may be offered another plan/set of benefits, and the remaining employees yet another plan. Employees may also have different options to select for their benefits package each year. This is why you may encounter multiple different policies between patients who work for the same company. Remember this for later, when learning about group numbers. Companies that have multiple policies often have multiple group numbers and subgroup numbers, which confuse many teams who do not realize how insurance is sold.

Now that you understand how dental insurance is sold, you may better understand why benefits may drop over time. Insurance companies would love to charge more premiums! If they did, however, they would likely lose the contract to another insurance company, who is going to come in and generate similar dynamics.

WHO IS THE "CLIENT" OF AN INSURANCE COMPANY?

All businesses in the world work for their clients. As you may glean from the above section about selling dental insurance, the overarching question about "who is the client" of the insurance company is not so clear. The answer to the question is "it depends."

The Employer. At the highest level, the employer company or corporation is the client. It is the employer who decides each year if a particular insurance company will be awarded the dental insurance contract to offer to their employees. If the employer is happy with the performance of the insurance company during the year, then it is very likely the insurance company will be favorably perceived during the annual contract review process. The employer will look at a number of variables in assessing the dental insurance contract, including:

- Percent of employees who opted to take the insurance
- Claims paid out versus budgeted (financial impact on profit)
- HR's experience working with the carrier (positive or negative)
- Employee satisfaction and feedback

The Human Resources (HR) Department. In most companies, it is the human resources department who completes all the leg work to gather proposals from various insurance companies, review and assess the proposals, and prepare a recommendation to the employer's board of directors. Therefore, some might consider the HR department as the primary client of the insurance company. Certainly, HR is a key player in determining whether the insurance company will be awarded the dental insurance contract for the next year or if they will switch to another insurance company. Just how much influence the HR department may have within any employer company will vary widely from company to company.

The Employees. Once an employee elects to sign up for a dental insurance plan, they become a direct client of the insurance company and begin to pay premiums. Of course, the way the insurance company will look at the employee-client will differ somewhat from how the dental office will view that same employee-client-patient. The insurance company will be trying to ensure that the employee-client receives the benefits that have been contracted and paid for, and at the same time to ensure that the dental office where treatment is provided is following the rules and contracts which they are subject to. The insurance company is not really in a position to determine the actual quality of care that a client receives.

The Dental Provider. The dental office, whether in- or out-of-network is not a client. The dentist/dental office is considered a provider, or vendor if you will. And that very fact is why insurance companies do not necessarily design their forms and processes to make it easy for the dental office. Due to the high volume of dental claims that tend to be generated throughout the year, systems and procedures within an insurance company are designed to make it easy for the insurance carrier to process those claims.

Servicing the Client. As we see, the question of "who is the client" is not a simple one. There are several entities that the insurance company views as clients. The largest, most influential clients are the employers who negotiate and purchase large contracts on behalf of their employees. Certainly, the human resource department benefits team would be key clients during contract negotiation as well as ongoing employee education and support. And finally, the employee policyholder/patient become clients when they actually sign up and pay for services rendered.

While many dentists and teams think insurance should be simple and insurance companies should work closely with dental offices to provide great care to patients (which would be amazing), sadly that is not always the reality. Dental teams around the country often observe problems with how they see their patients treated by their insurance company, including one or more of the following dynamics:

- Citing incorrect benefits information
- Not paying for legitimate services rendered
- Limited (or no) coverage for needed treatment

In some cases, what may appear to be poor treatment or service may well stem from the design of the actual contract the employee has purchased. Dental insurance contracts/policies today are not intended to provide full coverage for all potential oral needs of an individual, but are merely to assist, or supplement funding. Therefore, it is important to distinguish the source of the complaint. Is the patient complaint due to a limitation in the policy contract? Their understanding of what their benefit plan covers? Lack of training or experience by the insurance service team member? Or are they a rude/insensitive employee?

To know how best to respond to problem situations or questions raised by patients about treatment, it is helpful to understand how insurance companies are structured to provide support to their various client and provider groups.

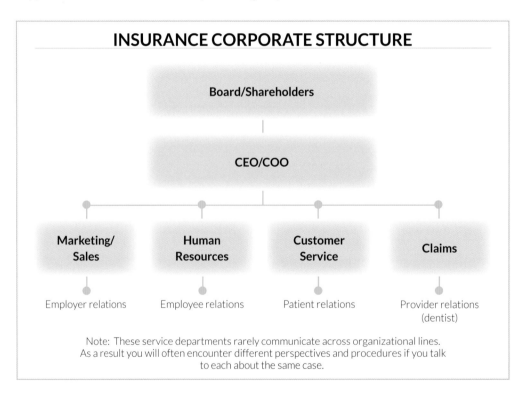

CORPORATE STRUCTURE –
HIERARCHY AND ACCOUNTABILITIES

Most insurance companies are organizations that employ thousands of people. While it is easy to just heap all the blame on the company itself, that is often not the reality of the situation.

If you are a CEO of an insurance company that employs 10,000 people, do you think you are going to know everything that goes on in the company? Of course not! The dentist in your office likely does not know every little thing that goes on in the office. No one person can be everywhere and see everything at once.

The CEO certainly would be responsible for any actions they may have promoted or prioritized for the company to do. Yet most often, the CEO is not the person responsible for the incorrect actions we see on a daily basis. The CEO sets the vision and long-term goals of the company and then delegates what needs to be done to reach those goals to other people, say a vice president. That vice president is likely to delegate tasks to senior managers, who then talk to junior managers, who then work with team leaders, who then set the rules for day-to-day actions within the company. The day-to-day actions are what we as dental professionals tend to see as an end result of that cascade of delegation.

If a team leader decides that they cannot make their budget, they are the ones who decide that they might have to set more stringent rules on how or when claims are approved in order to meet their quarterly goals. The CEO and senior leaders likely have no idea how exactly the daily process is managed to reach each department's goals.

This is why even within the same company, you may get different results from the same question or process. If you end up working with different teams, one team may be doing well and not placing added restrictions on claims, while another team may be struggling and therefore make your life more difficult by throwing wrenches in the process.

Departments

Have you ever had a time where a patient complains that they called their insurance carrier, who told them X, when you know when you called the same company, you were told something completely different?

When this happens, it may well be because you and your patient are dealing with completely separate departments within the company. Here are the primary insurance departments that you may encounter either directly or via your patient:

Provider Relations is the department in an insurance company that you, the dental office, would be contacting if you want to get credentialed or join their network.

Verification/Benefits is the department that handles questions about policies when an office calls for a verification or breakdown.

The **Claims Department** handles questions from dental offices about claims processing or denials. This department often causes the most frustration with offices because it is completely different than the next department that talks to patients.

Member/Patient Relations is the department in an insurance company the patient would be contacting. This group is established to answer questions and address problems that are experienced by their policyholders (your patients).

Those who call insurance companies often will recognize the phrase "Please hit 1 if you are a patient and 2 if you are a dental provider." This is because the phone will get transferred to completely separate departments, depending on which button you push.

All these departments are run by different people. And all these departments have somewhat different rules and regulations within the company.

Most importantly, these departments rarely talk to each other!

Have you ever tried calling a phone company (e.g., AT&T) to resolve an issue? Ever had the frustration of being transferred between multiple departments, where each one says the next department can answer your question, but none actually do?

Large insurance companies can act similarly. What the claims department knows versus what patient relations knows can be quite different. It is even likely in this scenario that no one is lying to you in this process but that the knowledge/training/experience of each person you talk to is different.

If you are a team member for your office, do you know everything your dentist or owner is doing in the background to run the business? Of course not. You are likely trained on your position within the office but may not know every aspect of every other position. The same is true for insurance company employees. Each employee is trained in their position and may have little or no knowledge or training in what employees in other departments are doing.

This is why it is important not to get upset with people on the phone when talking to an insurance company. Most are just doing their jobs the best way possible with the limited knowledge and training they are given. Most are not going to intentionally lie to you. Yelling at someone over the phone is more likely to get them to hang up on you versus encouraging them to help you get what you need out of the conversation.

Now, this does not mean you need to take everything you are told at face value; you shouldn't. We have seen plenty of examples of incorrect information being relayed through an insurance company representative. You just need to be more knowledgeable and better trained than some of the people at the insurance company in order to successfully navigate the game.

WORKING WITH THE CLAIMS DEPARTMENT

Most of your interactions with an insurance carrier will be with the claims department. This department processes a high volume of claims and is usually quite busy. As a result of operating on very thin profit margins and low administrative costs, the claims department is forced to operate as efficiently as possible. Simple claims are fed through automated systems for adjudication. Claims of more medium complexity are given to claims examiners for review. The most complex claims are given to examiners with many years of experience or special training. Rarely are claims examiners also dentists.

Most claims examiners are provided with basic training on what to look for in a claim. And they must review claims covering many different policies/providers. Their goal is to review the claim for:

1. Completeness and clarity of submission
2. Then, ensure the claim is asking for payment for a service clearly covered by the specific policy purchased
3. And only after Nos. 1 and 2, look closely at the need/justification for the service provided to the patient

Claims examiners usually have a high volume of case work, at times even high backlogs, so they review each claim fairly quickly. If information is missing or unclear to them, they will return the claim for more information. And if the information provided does not absolutely conform to what the policy benefits provide, it will be rejected.

Always remember that the customer of the claim examiner is not the dental office. Dentists are providers, not clients or patients. Therefore, the process is not designed to make it easy for the small dental office.

Quarter End Scrutiny

We've discussed the fact that insurance companies, like many businesses, closely track their progress against profit goals, budgets, and key metrics. This is particularly true of the claims department. Remember the profit formula:

Profit = premiums collected − claims paid − expenses

If premiums have not changed and most overhead expenses have not changed, the focus must shift to holding or reducing claims expenses. Therefore, the insurance company may well push their claims departments to reduce costs, particularly as they approach the end of a quarter. What you may notice on the dental office side is near the end of each quarter the number of denied/delayed claims, requests for more information, and so forth, will go up noticeably.

Therefore, if you are nearing the end of a quarter, it can be a good tactic to delay filing your patient claims until the first day of the new quarter. While it is counter-intuitive, you will often get paid faster with fewer hassles by waiting a few days.

TIP

So if you are near the end of a quarter, it can be a good idea to delay filing a claim until the first day of the new quarter.

Does the Claims Department Deny Claims from One Office More Than Another?

Whether intentionally or not, some dental offices do experience a higher rate of claim returns or denials than other offices.

By law, insurance companies need to pay out the contractual benefits on claims for their clients (your patients). If the insurance company can make it more difficult for you to get a claim processed or paid, they know that many offices will give up. In fact, 65% of all dental claims that are denied once never end up being submitted a second time. Do you think the insurance company knows this? Do you think this might give them a reason to question, return for more information, or deny more frequently?

In addition, what can happen over time is that certain dental offices can develop a reputation or will show up on trend reports. If your office regularly submits poor or incomplete claim information, you might begin to stand out, resulting in potentially less rigorous review of your claims and more ready returns/denials. Conversely, offices who are very thorough in their claim documentation and known to fight rejected claims successfully on behalf of their patients will also begin to develop a reputation that can subtly influence the examiner's decision. At the end of a quarter, when claim processing results are not where they need to be and volumes are high, these biases can become even more pronounced and may result in greater denials for your office.

Therefore, it is imperative that your office learn what is expected/preferred by the insurance provider(s) you deal with most frequently. When claims are returned, make note of what is considered missing or problematic, improve the claim documentation, and resubmit. If there is a phone number to call for questions, call it and learn what they prefer to see. And do not ever be afraid to stand by your work, advocate for your patient, and resubmit denied claims (with additional information) if you believe services provided were necessary and within the patient's benefit plan.

It can be incredibly important to also keep track of all this information that you learn about each policy and company, and make sure the entire dental team is trained appropriately to follow the learned guidelines. This can help avoid the office making similar or multiple mistakes.

You will find additional information, recommendations, and examples later in this guide that will help you when resubmitting claims and positioning them for the best chance of approval.

HOW TO HANDLE COMPLAINTS RAISED BY YOUR PATIENTS

It is inevitable that your office will hear complaints on occasion from a patient about their insurance benefits and/or how they are treated by their insurance carrier. It can be easy and convenient for the patient to voice their concerns to the dental team directly while in the office or on the phone even though the team likely has minimal to do with most of these concerns. (with possible exception of a misquoted estimate).

Here are a few types of complaints you may hear and how you might respond:

1. Complaints about policy benefit/coverage. A complaint about benefits may arise when a patient learns their insurance plan does not cover a particular treatment, or if they were confused about a particular benefit. If you are knowledgeable and can clear up a point of confusion, you are performing a great patient service. If you are educated and aware of trends across the common carriers, a legitimate and helpful response might be about the general trend; that is, "That specific treatment is not covered by most carriers." Of course, it would be unprofessional to criticize their insurance carrier.
2. Complaints about rude or unprofessional behavior. While it is tempting to commiserate with a patient, you don't want to criticize any carrier. You never know the other side of the story. Best practice is to suggest they call back to the customer service department of their insurance carrier, ask for a supervisor, and discuss/report what happened. An alternative would be to suggest they contact the benefits coordinator within their HR department and lodge a similar complaint.

The next time your patient has a legitimate concern about their insurance coverage or carrier (or even a non-legitimate concern), the best strategy is to direct them to their employer's

HR department. This is not to push it away from the office necessarily, but to correctly direct the concern where it can be registered by the group who has the most influence over the selection of the insurance carrier and the design of future benefit plans. The HR department has leverage with their insurance carrier, knows who to contact when an employee is experiencing a problem with their insurance, and can address trends/problems on behalf of their employees. This will serve in the best interest of the office, the patient, and all the other patients of the employer. HR has the power to influence a change in a policy contract/employee benefits for the following year.

WHAT ABOUT THE STATE DEPARTMENT OF INSURANCE?

When a dental office encounters a challenge with an insurance company's decision, the generic answer offered by many groups is to just, "Complain to the state department of insurance." Sometimes this tactic works, and sometimes it doesn't. So it is helpful to understand who is the state department of insurance and the insurance commissioner, what is their role in overseeing insurance practices, and when it is effective to engage them into your challenge.

The state department of insurance (SDI) is an organization within each state's finance department. The department of insurance is headed up by an insurance commissioner. The insurance commissioner is either elected or appointed, depending on the state. Insurance commissioners act as advocates for consumer protection, regulators of insurance, and educators who are able to provide consumers with information that pertains to the insurance system within a particular state. While insurance commissioners' duties may vary across states, their roles are generally the same: to act as intermediary figures between individual consumers and insurance companies within the state.

To accomplish their charter, each state grants several powers to insurance commissioners and their offices, including:

- Approval of insurance rates
- Periodic financial examinations of insurers
- Licensing of companies, agencies, agents, and brokers
- Monitoring and regulating claims handling

Once the SDI approves an insurance plan and its associated premium rates for sale within the state, then the insurance company must follow the contract language within that plan. Any subsequent complaints to the insurance commissioner or SDI will hold the insurance company to the patient's policy language. As long as the insurance company is following the language contained in the policy, there is nothing SDI can do; insurance is following its mandate.

Common example: The patient comes to the office with a cracked tooth around an old amalgam filling. The patient is symptomatic to a tooth sleuth. There is no question clinically the patient needs a crown. The patient gets the crown done, feels instantly better even in the temporary, and the crown code gets submitted to insurance with just the PA (which does not show the fracture).

Insurance denies the crown, stating that not enough information was sent to justify reimbursement for the case. This is where many offices will try to invoke SDI. The problem is, SDI can do nothing here because insurance is not the problem. The office documentation was the problem; not enough information was submitted to approve reimbursement based on contract language.

Instead of trying to threaten working with SDI, the office would be better off learning what documentation the specific insurance carrier wants to see and just providing it. This will be much quicker and easier than waiting for the insurance commission to get involved. See Chapter 23 for specifics on getting crowns and buildups reimbursed.

WHEN WOULD YOU WANT TO TRY TO INVOLVE SDI?

If you submit information that the policy states it needs and insurance still denies the claim, this would be a good time to send a letter to the insurance company and carbon copy to SDI. If you provide the written policy language along with this letter, it will work much more effectively.

Do understand that SDI for the insurance company is like the state board for a dentist. They are the last entity that insurance wants to deal with. Think of it in terms of a patient complaining to the state board about your office's dental treatment.

If the office provided medically appropriate, quality treatment, documented the claim correctly, and a poor result happened due to no fault at all of the office, yet the patient filed a complaint with the state board, are you likely to bend to this patient? Or are you more likely to just shake your head and let the patient beat their head against the wall?

This is the exact scenario insurance companies face when they do their job according to the policy contract language and you threaten SDI. It will mean nothing. The insurance company will not want to deal with SDI, but they understand if they followed all protocols, the result of the SDI complaint will be found in their favor.

In the opposite scenario, if the dentist might have made a mistake (missed scanning a consent form, failed to get necessary diagnostics, etc.) and the patient threatens to complain to the board, the dentist is likely to let the patient have whatever they want to go away. There may not have been a specific concern, but the documentation is fuzzy and will create a nightmare with the board that has nothing to do with the clinical case.

Insurance companies are not immune to mistakes (the larger you get, the more errors will happen). Often insurance companies that are shown to have an error will fix it without much hassle. However, if somehow the insurance company did have an error or otherwise did not follow their stated policy, invoking the SDI card may help resolve the problem. Just make sure the problem is with the insurance company and not with the policy itself just having poor reimbursement due to what the employer chose. SDI cannot help if the policy does not cover the treatment in question.

What Other Resources Do You Have for Filing a Complaint?

The SDI/insurance commissioner certainly has strong leverage for brokering complaints on behalf of an insured (your patient). If the complaint, however, is not related to the contract language, then there are other avenues for directing a complaint, including:

Head of the claims department. Writing to a higher level of management will ensure that a complaint is handled by a more knowledgeable, experienced professional. You can direct the letter generically to the "Head of the Claims Department," or you can do a bit of research by calling your normal contact within the company and asking for the name of the individual in charge of claims. It is even more effective to cite the exact name and address for the appropriate individual.

President or CEO of the company. Even greater leverage can be gained by directing a complaint to the insurance company's president or CEO. Same principle applies: you can simply write to "President, _____ Insurance Company," or you can look up the name of the president or CEO and use their specific names. Every insurance company has a group of highly experienced professionals who are trained to respond specifically to complaints to the president, CEO, insurance commissioner, Better Business Bureau, and so forth. Chances are that complaints directed in this manner will be more quickly responded to than those directed to the SDI.

Chapter 16
Insurance Network Contracts

Now that you have a basic idea of how an insurance company works, you need to understand what is involved with signing network contracts. It helps to have a basic understanding of the history of dental insurance.

Dental insurance started becoming popular in the 1950s. Back then, marketing was not done in dentistry, so the insurance network list became one of very few external sources of attracting new patients.

In order to attract a perspective employer client, the insurance company would have to show the value of choosing them versus another company. This means that dental insurance companies need to show they have a wide network of dentists who participate with the plan, or else the plan has no value to the employer and their employees. When dental insurance first started, there were thousands of dental offices that did not participate in an insurance plan. This meant that insurance carriers had to make a lot of concessions to dentists in order to convince them to join the plan. For example: back in 1950, the average maximum coverage for a patient was $1000. To put this in perspective, $1000 in 1950 is worth about $11,000 in 2020. When was the last time you saw an insurance policy with a $11,000 maximum?

The amount of dentistry done per patient was lower in 1950. The cost per person for dental expenses has risen significantly since 1950. The number of providers per patient has also grown significantly over that time. What this has led to is an increase in both total expenditures for dental care as well as the supply of dentists to provide that care.

TREND IN DENTAL BENEFITS

Year	Annual Premium	Maximum Benefit (Average)	Price of a Crown
1950	$33.80	$1,000	$60
1970	$54.40	$1,000	$112
1990	$183		$444
2000	$241		$739
2020	$360	$1,250	$1,400

When you have a lot more providers in an area, the need for dental insurance companies to entice dentists to join their network is much lower. What this means for your office is that if you are in an area with multiple other network providers, the insurance company has minimal or no need for you to sign up. The less need they have for more providers, the less they have to reimburse for services to keep dentists in-network.

Insurance companies and dentist providers have been negotiating since the beginning on what fees are reasonable for the dentist to accept in exchange for the insurance company sending them more patients. In recent years though, most areas of the country have enough providers in-network with each insurance company, so the ability to negotiate with companies as a private dentist is greatly diminished.

BECOMING AN IN-NETWORK PROVIDER

When a dentist or office signs an insurance network contract, it is important to understand the terms you are agreeing to. There are a variety of clauses that tend to be written into a contract, so let's first review the clauses and terms that exist in most network contracts so that you have an idea of what you are signing.

Contract Basics:

1. **Independent Contractor Status**. The dentist is an independent contractor, not an employee of the insurance company. This is mostly for legal and IRS distinction.
2. **Submitting Claims**. This section usually covers the requirement for use of ADA forms, company policy regarding how to fill them out, and procedures on how to submit claims. The content of this section is almost universally standard across the board. For out-of-network offices, contract terms usually must follow the same procedures for reimbursement.
3. **Liability Coverage**. The dentist agrees to maintain a certain minimum level of malpractice insurance.
4. **Hold Harmless**. You also agree that any procedure you conduct on a patient is the liability of the office or dentist, not the insurance company.
5. **Amendments**. Articulates the understanding that the insurance company can amend the contract at any time in the future, with notice (usually 30–60 days). If anything is about to change, they will send you correspondence (typically print) ahead of time to give you the opportunity to accept the change or terminate the contract. This is another reason to make sure you read and understand all the information you receive from the insurance company.
6. **No Balance Billing**. This means the dentist/office will not bill patients for the difference between network fees and your normal office fees.
7. **Non-Disclosure Agreement**. You agree not to share your in-network fee schedule or the insurance company's internal policies with anyone else, another dentist, or insurance company.
8. **Timely Filing**. You agree to file all claims within a timely manner, usually meaning anywhere from 3 to 12 months after completion of a procedure. The specific time frame is dependent upon the contract. Any treatment provided where a claim is delayed or submitted past that point, you agree to neither bill the insurance company nor the patient.

9. **Submit Full Fees**. The provider is required by contract to submit their full, normal fee for all procedures (not the negotiated network fee).

Those are the basics in most contracts that typically cause minimal to no concern. Now let's review the sections that are more likely to cause concern, misunderstandings, and myths.

Refund Demands, Payment Corrections, and Right of Recovery

This is the section that causes issues and can be referenced when insurance companies encounter an error that causes them to demand money back from the dentist/office. If the insurance company finds it overpaid for almost any reason, you are signing that you agree to give that money back to the insurance company (instead of the insurance company getting funds back from the patient).

In this section, the language is typically asking for your agreement to return such a payment by issuing an immediate refund or by deducting the owed money from a payment for another patient. This is what happens when you accept assignment of benefits (for reference, review Chapter 10); you are the one that insurance goes to when money needs to be recovered.

It is also important to note that this section almost always adds in language that a refund demand will "survive the termination of this agreement," which means you agree to comply with refunds for work that was completed while in-network even after you are no longer in-network.

Most state laws place a cap or time limit for these refund demands, often 6–24 months.

Non-Discrimination

The dentist/office agrees to treat all patients the same regardless of differences, but especially differences based on payment source (whether they have insurance or not). This clause means two important things:

1. You cannot perform procedures for your cash patients and refer out those same procedures for your insurance patients. For example, root canals.
2. You cannot have different clinical requirements for your cash patients versus your insurance patients. For example, frequency of exams, x-rays, upgrade fees.

Cost Share/Co-Pay

The dentist/office agrees to make every reasonable effort to collect co-pays for all patients of the insurance company. This means not giving family or employee discounts and not providing insurance-only payments for treatment. The co-pays are the way for the insurance company to make sure the patient has some ownership and skin in the game for any treatment to avoid being overbilled for services the patient may not necessarily agree to otherwise.

This clause, along with the non-discrimination clause, are the anti-fraud stipulations in insurance contracts that often create misunderstandings from providers.

Access to Records

In this section, the dentist/office agrees to provide access to patient records at any time upon request by the insurance company for services performed while they were in-network. This section often survives the termination of the agreement. The difference among insurance companies here is whether you agree to give them access to only network patients of that company or all the patients in the office (regardless of insurance participation). While most companies only want records of their insured patients, some want access to all patient records.

Payment/Fee Arrangements and Non-Covered Services (NCS)

This is one of the most important clauses within an insurance contract to be aware of and read carefully. This section can be what causes an insurance contract to be either mildly annoying or decimating to the office budget. These sections can cause the dentist/office more loss of revenue than the fee schedule discounts.

This section is where the insurance company states the restrictions they have for non-covered services (NCS, services that are not eligible for reimbursement). Most insurance company contracts say nothing about NCS, thereby saying there are no rules, and you can choose with the patient what works best for you and the patient. Other contracts will state the exact terms of what makes an NCS and how to manage it. This is where the rules come into play about what information the patient needs to be given and sign for to get an NCS (Chapter 19).

In rare circumstances, a contract will state that the provider is not allowed to bill patients for an NCS at all (disallow) or they must use network fees (potentially overriding state laws). If the contract states anything like this, it would be prudent for the office to strike out or modify this clause before signing. The insurance company should have no legitimate concern about your charging a patient for a non-covered service, as the NCSs do not affect the insurance company or contractual agreement in any way.

Claims Filing Requirements

This is the section that talks about how and when to file claims. Most contracts only state the method for filing a claim, specifically for covered services. Most often covered service is defined as a service where reimbursement is available according to the policy. These are normal clauses that should cause no concern.

The concern would come into play if one of the two following clauses were written into the contract:

1. You must file a claim for all covered services (including services completed after the maximum benefit has been reached); or
2. You must file a claim for all services, whether covered or not.

This is where a lot of office myths may surface. The myth that an office needs to submit all claims for all services provided to a patient. It is actually extremely rare for a contract to state either one of these above two points. The most common clause by far just says how you must file claims if you want reimbursement for a covered service.

> **EXAMPLE** **MISREAD CLAUSE:**
>
> "Participating providers agree to bill <company> directly for services provided to <company> members at no charge to the patient."
> This clause doesn't mean you have to submit claims. It means you agree to not charge the patient a separate fee to submit the claims.
> Otherwise read:
> "Participating providers agree to bill <company> directly for services provided to <company> members at no charge to the patient (for billing insurance)."

The reason an insurance company may want you to file all claims for covered services (meaning even after maximum is reached) is typically due to frequency limitations. They want to know if you did a crown, even if it was not reimbursed so that it can now have a frequency limit for not being reimbursed again in the future. This concept often upsets providers as they feel like the insurance company should not penalize the patient with frequency limitations on procedures the insurance company did not reimburse.

The challenge for the office is that filing claims costs money and time. There is no legitimate reason for an office to file a claim for a patient who has no chance of being reimbursed (such as after maximum is reached).

The second scenario where an insurance company would want to see all claims for all services, whether covered or not, begs the question as to why the insurance company cares. Non-covered services would never be paid, so frequency limitations are pointless.

The only possible scenario is the insurance company wants to maintain more direct control over the dentist and the treatments being provided for the patient. This does inch into the realm of ethics and legality, however, because it is usually considered illegal for a provider or non-provider to diagnose and treat a patient without a license and physically perform an exam on said patient. While the insurance company might claim that they are not dictating treatment, in reality they know full well that when you control the finances of a treatment, you control the treatment.

This is somewhat similar to what can happen in government. When a governmental body wants to remove a law but does not think they can get the votes to strike it, they remove the budget for that law. No budget to enforce a law typically ends up with a law that is ignored and thereby indirectly removed.

This is why it is important to know what to look for in these clauses and strike out the portions that are on the legally questionable side of the law, that do nothing but harm the patient's ability to receive certain options for treatment.

Non-Covered Services

Starting in 2009, states began enacting laws in dentistry preventing insurance companies from setting fees on procedures that are not covered by the policy. Since then 39 states have enacted a non-covered services legislation to prevent fee capping by insurance on procedures not covered by the plan. (See the next chapter for more details.)

There can also be a few points within the contract which may be ways to circumvent these laws. Some insurance contracts now have clauses basically stating that you agree to not abide by state law and will maintain fee capping on all procedures, covered and non-covered. If you signed a contract with this clause in it, your state laws may not protect you from fee capping.

Legal 101 - Strike Outs

In any contract you are allowed to strike out clauses or lines you do not agree with. The way to do this is use a single line to cross out the section in question, then initial and date it. It is also best to reference the strike out at the end of the document where your final signature is located. This will prevent someone from claiming the changes were made after the contract was in force.

When it comes to the non-covered services, realize this does not affect the insurance company at all. They will not be paying for these services either way. Many insurance companies will not care if you cross certain sections out, this one being the least offensive to the insurance company. If they do push back, then you might want to consider why and whether going in-network with them is a worthwhile venture. Also be sure to keep your own copy of the amended contract.

The other concern that comes into play when filing non-covered services, is often the best way for an office to track and relay information about NCSs to patients is through internal coding (non-ADA codes). This is because the ADA code list is not an exhaustive list of every possible treatment, it is only designed to be a list of all possible codes an insurance company might reimburse. (See Chapter 20 on internal coding.) Insurance company software and processes are not usually capable of correctly processing NCSs, which leads to a lot of patient and provider frustration with EOBs that are in error, confusing, and potentially illegal.

EXAMPLE

CLAUSE TO WATCH FOR AND HOW TO POTENTIALLY AMEND IT:
Base Clause
Dentist agrees to submit complete and accurate claims for all services provided to Enrollees, whether Program Services or not
Amended Clause
Dentist agrees to submit complete and accurate claims for all ~~covered~~ services provided to Enrollees, ~~whether Program Services or not~~ (Initial and Date)

NEGOTIATION VS AFFILIATION (AKA NETWORK LEASING OR SILENT CONTRACTS)

If you work as a dentist in Los Angeles, California, the chance for you to negotiate rates and terms with an insurance company is pretty slim. There are likely 100 dentists within a mile radius of your office, most of whom are already in-network with the insurance company. This is true for a good portion of the urban areas of the country.

This does not mean there isn't a way to get better terms in a dental contract!

Each insurance company has a different fee schedule, which they work with. Different companies use different methods and incentives to get their clients, employers, and patients to sign up. As a result, many insurance companies will choose to network lease or affiliate with another insurance company to share the burden of connecting these groups together.

As a purely hypothetical example, Metlife may affiliate with Cigna to share a fee schedule for the patients who come from that relationship.

In this example, your dental office might join Metlife-Cigna affiliation in one of three different ways:

1. Sign up with Metlife and get auto-affiliation with Cigna
2. Sign up with Cigna and get auto-affiliation with Metlife
3. Sign up with both individually

How you join the affiliation matters because who you sign up with is whose fee schedule you end up using.

	Metlife crown fee	Cigna crown fee
Sign up with both	$650	$800
Sign up with Metlife only	$650	$650
Sign up with Cigna only	$800	$800

Let's use crown fees as an example.

Metlife has a crown fee of $650.

Cigna has a crown fee of $800.

Now let's look at those three ways to join the affiliation:

1. Sign up with Metlife and get auto-affiliation with Cigna; your fee for a crown with both insurance companies is $650.
2. Sign up with Cigna and get auto-affiliation with Metlife; your fee for a crown with both insurance companies is $800.
3. Sign up with both individually; your fee for Metlife patients is $650 and for Cigna patients is $800.

This is how affiliations work in dentistry and why they have become one of the major sources of differences in fee schedules around the country. Knowing which affiliations exist around the country is vital to being able to maintain a higher level of reimbursement with an insurance company.

The challenge is that these affiliation relationships change constantly. Often the only people who can manage the constantly shifting landscape are dental support companies that negotiate with insurance companies every day.

Is Network Leasing Bad for Dentists?

The answer to this question is a little more complex than yes or no because it depends on the situation of the dentist.

Signing up with each individual insurance company can be complex and highly time consuming. If a dentist is new to an office and wants to sign up with multiple insurance companies at once, network leasing can be a great thing. The affiliations will allow you to sign fewer contracts and be marketed/exposed to more patients at the same time.

The savvy office can also use the affiliations to their advantage and sign up with insurance company A who has a higher fee schedule and get affiliated with insurance company B at that higher fee schedule.

There are some challenges with network leasing, so it is helpful to know more about how the process works.

- When you drop a network contract, an insurance company may learn about this drop and send you an offer to network lease directly with a new network offered from that dropped company. Typically, the offer is written to include an automatic yes if you do not respond, which is where the concern comes in. Should you ever drop a network contract, pay attention to your mail and email correspondence coming directly from the insurance company, as they are required to inform you ahead of time, and you can decline being added to the new network.
- "I did not know I was contracted with Company C"—this can occasionally happen with network leasing. Like the example above, the insurance company is required to let you know ahead of time if a network leasing event is taking place. Offices commonly disregard insurance correspondence, which is where the misunderstanding comes in. If you keep track of the communication from the insurance company, you should be able to be informed of or avoid this automatic network inclusion.

One thing to remember about network leasing is why you signed up with an insurance company in the first place. Usually, it is to get access to more potential clients who could increase your office patient pool. Network leasing is just a way for you to expand that patient pool even more, without signing any additional contracts and at the same time benefitting from the same fee that was previously agreed upon.

INSURANCE CONTRACT TRENDS 2020

Here is a summary of the common insurance companies and the main differences among their standard contracts of which a provider should be aware. These contracts do not change very often.

	File claims required	Non-covered services fee capping	COB	Other notes
Aetna	Only covered services	No w/ waiver		
Ameritas	No	Yes, must follow fee schedule for all services. If no fee listed, must be 80% of UCR.		
Careington	Yes	Yes, if fee schedule, 15% (platinum) or 20% (POS/500) discount on non-fee schedule services	Traditional	Specialists 15–20% UCR 90 days to file
DHA	No	Accept or deny capping in contract		
GEHA	No	Cap all services on fee schedule, not off.		
United Concordia	No	No payment = not covered. Fee capping is voluntary on contract		Not location based
Metlife	No			
BCBS	No	No w/ waiver		
Cigna	No	Yes		20% off all non-fee schedule treatment
Delta CA/MD/CO	Yes	No w/ waiver		
Delta Midatlantic (PA, MD, DE, DC, NY, WV)	Same as above			
Delta RI	No	No w/ waiver		6-month file deadline, access to non-Delta patient records
PrimeCare	No	No. Covered = payment		
UniCare	No	No		

Chapter 17
Non-Covered Services (NCS)

In a basic sense, a non-covered service is a dental procedure for which the insurance company will not reimburse any portion of the procedure (pay nothing). It is a procedure excluded from the network contract. The most common example would be teeth bleaching procedures.

However, many states have their own definition of what is considered an NCS from a legal perspective. The most common set of rules is the following:

A covered service is one for which reimbursement is available under the plan outside the following limitations:

- Yearly/lifetime maximum
- Deductible
- Co-pay/coinsurance
- Waiting periods
- Frequency
- Alternative benefit payments
- Downgraded services

This basically means that any procedure insurance would potentially reimburse is considered covered, whereas any procedure that the insurance company will not reimburse in any instance is considered non-covered.

CHECK YOUR UNDERSTANDING

Since Non-covered services are often a point of confusion, here are several examples where insurance will reimburse nothing. See if you can figure out for yourself which ones are covered, and which are non-covered based on the list on the prior page.

1. You have a patient with a crown that needs to be replaced. The original crown was done four years ago, and the policy has a frequency limit of seven years on crowns.
2. Patient has a $1500 maximum and insurance has paid $1500 this year. Patient needs a crown.
3. You made a D2740 (porcelain) crown, insurance downgraded it to a D2790 (gold crown).
4. The patient has a policy with a $100 deductible, and the patient needs an extraction with a network fee of $98.
5. You have an emergency patient come in with pain on a tooth. She just got a job two months ago and her policy has a 6-month waiting period.
6. You have a 29-year-old patient who is getting braces. The policy has an age limitation of 26.

In all of the above examples, insurance reimbursed nothing, but the only scenario where the service is actually non-covered is No. 6. Because age will never go down, there is no circumstance where insurance would consider reimbursement for the service. This is a non-covered service. The rest of the services are considered covered by the most common state law language.

Missing Tooth Clauses and Non-Covered Services

MTCs can become a little complex within the framework of NCS since the procedure would be covered on any other tooth. Like all other NCS, it depends on the language of the state law. Since most states have a defined list of what makes something a covered service if it is not reimbursed, and MTC is not found within that list, an MTC would typically make a service non-covered and therefore subject to no insurance discount. Therefore, services for missing teeth with policies with an MTC are typically considered non-covered services.

EOBs and Non-Covered Services

The challenge with NCS is that many times the insurance contract itself may violate these state laws. The most common example occurs when the EOB shows a coverage table that says the patient only owes the amount if the service was a covered service (the network discounted rate), but then a note with an asterisk (*) at the bottom says something along the lines of:

*Your dentist may charge normal fees in certain states.

Anyone who has worked with patients for a while in the office knows that the patient is not going to read the fine print; they are only going to look at the coverage table. The insurance company will likely claim they are following the law based on the note. The patient is only going to see the coverage table and that you are asking for more money than their insurance company shows they owe. You have a couple of different options in this scenario:

1. Accept the reduced amount. The challenge with this is often you/your dentist will have used labs and materials based on the expected fee they receive. This can lead to paying more for the cost of providing the care than the office is going to be reimbursed.
2. Try to convince the patient about the law and the meaning of the asterisked note. If you have a silver tongue, this might work, but make sure to have all your paperwork in order and be very prepared for a potentially confusing conversation with the patient.
3. Call the insurance company and request a "Corrected EOB" to show the coverage table based on state law. (Some companies will be amenable to this, some will not.)
4. Have the patient sign a HIPAA release form and not send the NCS claim at all (see Chapter 18). This will allow you to avoid the incorrect EOBs completely.
5. Charge the patient an "upgrade" fee and let them keep their network discount on the base service (see Chapter 18). This will allow you to avoid the incorrect EOBs completely.

No matter which option you choose, make sure you understand one important point: **states and the federal government define the laws**. Insurance contracts and terms of service are not law. When the two are in conflict, state/federal law trumps insurance every time.

STATES WITH NON-COVERED SERVICES LEGISLATION

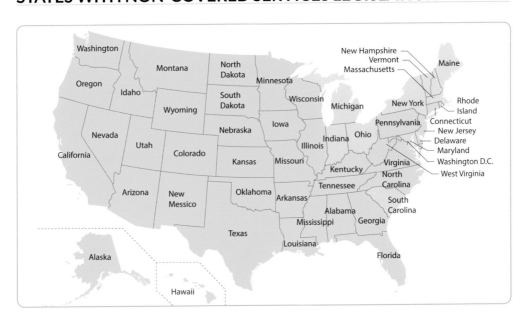

States with Non-Covered Services Legislation (2020)
Alabama, Alaska, Arizona, Arkansas, California, Colorado, Connecticut, Florida, Georgia, Idaho, Illinois, Iowa, Kansas, Kentucky, Louisiana, Maryland, Minnesota, Mississippi, Missouri, Montana, Nebraska, Nevada, New Jersey, New Mexico, North Carolina, North Dakota, Oklahoma, Oregon, Pennsylvania, Rhode Island, South Dakota, Tennessee, Texas, Utah, Virginia, Washington, West Virginia, Wisconsin, Wyoming

Are All Insurance Companies/Contracts Subject to These State Laws?

The simple answer is no.

Realize these laws are created by each individual state. Many insurance policies are state based and therefore subject to these state laws. However, some insurance policies are federal based and therefore not subject to state laws. Here are the following most common policies that are not subject to state law and NCS legislation:

- ERISA (see page 20)
- Medicaid (see page 22)
- TriCare (see page 23)
- GEHA

All of the above are federally based policies and therefore not subject to state law. They might allow you to charge what you want for non-covered services, but they are not legally bound to that. You want to make sure you know when a patient is covered under one of these types of policies and therefore can alert the dentist ahead of treatment to know that they may not be reimbursed if they provide a higher, more costly level of service/care. This may affect the way the patient and dentist determine their treatment plan.

What you can still do with ERISA and GEHA plans is have the patient sign a HIPAA/HITECH release form since HIPAA is a federal law that supersedes almost everything else.

It is not recommended to do this with federally funded plans such as TriCare and Medicaid. The safest route with these plans is to realize the dentist just cannot offer upgraded care, non-covered services (above network capped rates), or "disallowed" procedures (see page 156) on patients with federally funded insurance plans unless you are doing it as a charity.

CURRENT EVENTS

A federal bill is currently sitting in the legislature that might prevent ERISA plans from capping non-covered services for both dental and vision: H.R. 1606 DOC Access Act

Chapter 18
Filing Insurance Claims 102—Advanced

This chapter is going to review the more advanced techniques for handling insurance claims and build upon the lessons learned in Part 1 – Understanding Insurance Basics.

While the basics in Part 1 were about moving through each step, the advanced techniques we will discuss here in Part 2 involve better understanding of the insurance company and how it functions, then applying this knowledge to anticipate pitfalls and pre-emptively addressing them before they happen. This knowledge will also help you more successfully fight claims that do get denied. Please make sure you have already reviewed and understood the information in the prior chapters for the basics of how an insurance company functions internally.

WHY WAS MY CLAIM DENIED? (ADVANCED)

Many dental claim denials that offices receive are not necessarily final, meaning that you can appeal and still get reimbursement for those services. Submission errors are the most common reason that dental office claims are initially denied. In Chapter 11, you can find the most common submission errors which include incorrect info, wrong CDT code, incomplete info, and missing narratives. Within this chapter, we are going to cover what to do when your initial claim was denied and wasn't due to one of the most common errors.

> **MYTH**
>
> The claim was submitted correctly without any errors in data; therefore, the insurance company believes the patient just did not need the service.

This myth has been around a long time, and it is **completely false**. Do realize that most of the time, claims are processed by claims technicians who have minimal training and zero dental experience. These claims are not processed by trained dentists a majority of the time.

How Claims Get Processed

Insurance companies function on very low profit margins and therefore only survive by keeping expenses as low as possible and automating services as much as possible. Claims is one of the largest automated departments in an insurance company. Most often you will find a computer processes claims for the low-cost services where there is nothing up for debate. Preventive and many basic services will be processed by a computer, which is called auto-adjudication.

When you file for preventive services, such as exams, x-rays, and a prophylaxis, a computer processes these claims automatically and generates either payment or denial without any human interaction. If you received a denial on preventive services, it can be due to a submission error or frequency limitation or the insurance company's error.

> **TIP**
>
> Insurance denials can be incorrect due to errors on the insurance company's part; therefore, almost all denials should be reviewed and appealed. Even with frequency issues, there can be errors on the insurance company's side.

Often fillings and extractions will be auto-adjudicated as well.

The more complex, costly services are the ones that are almost always processed by a human claims examiner. These services include buildups, crowns, periodontal treatment, and any replacement of a missing tooth. Almost all major services and some basic services will be human processed (e.g., crowns, buildups, perio treatment). Typically, until a dental office learns to effectively handle insurance claims, they may notice a much higher denial rate for these services.

With human-processed claims you want to make sure you are providing all the information that supports your claim and avoid adding extra information that could possibly cause problems with your claim. Let's dig into the process more deeply.

Who Is the Claims Examiner?

Depending on the type of claim and the step in the process, the one examining your dental claim may be different. Here is a generic way to have an idea who you are dealing with at each step.

Initial (First) Claims

When claims are first submitted to the company, they are scanned into a computer system and are either processed directly by the computer (auto-adjudicated) or forwarded to a human claims examiner. Most claims within a dental insurance company are split off to be auto-adjudicated by a computer. These are the claims for diagnostic, preventative, and often basic restorative work (such as fillings). When these claims are denied, it is almost always due to a processing error on the part of the office or a policy limitation.

The initial claims that get processed by a human are typically sent to junior claims examiners with minimal to no experience in dentistry. Their primary task is to follow a series of checklists to see if the claim you sent matches what needs to be seen by the insurance company policy to process reimbursement. If anything confuses them or does not follow the formula, it will get denied.

Resubmitted Claims (After the First Denial)

When you resubmit a claim a second time for reconsideration, the computer no longer handles these. These claims are always handled by a person and typically are processed by a more senior, experienced claims examiner. While not dentists, these claims examiners have a greater level of experience that will allow them to think slightly out of the box. If you provide the complete information requested and it matches the checklist policy the claims examiner must follow, then your claim should now get approved.

It is important to remember that typically no licensed dentist has seen this claim to this point.

It is worth noting that some insurance companies will process a second electronic claim as a duplicate and automatically deny it. If you see this happening with an insurance company you work with, it would be best to submit the second claim attempt by fax or mail. You can talk to your clearinghouse to find out, as they usually keep track of which insurance companies need specific ways to process second attempt claims.

Third Claim Submission (After the Second Denial)

Only after exhausting the first two steps will a claim ever reach the eyes of a licensed dentist. This is a cost-saving measure by the insurance company, as dentists command a higher salary, and therefore the insurance company will employ very few of them. This is the same reason why a dental office would not want to pay a hygienist or dentist to answer the phones or manage insurance.

This is why the myth about claims being denied because a patient did not need services is so false. Dentists are the only ones who can really make this determination, and they are not involved in the early process of insurance claims.

MYTH-TRUTH

Myth: My claim was denied because the patient did not need the service.
Truth: Dentists are not often involved in the claims process until the very end. Denials have nothing to do with necessity of the service no matter what the EOB might incorrectly state.

At this third try for a claim, the provider office has the right to request that the dentist consultant at the insurance company speak with the provider dentist. Insurance companies often call this a peer-to-peer review.

It is important to understand that the dentist consultant likely had nothing to do with the previous denials. Yelling or getting angry at this dentist will serve no purpose and often will lead to the office having even less of a chance for the claims resolution to end in reimbursement. Dentist consultants can be vital assets to the office as they are the ones who have the ability to recommend overturning the prior denials and leading you to a successful resolution. Attacking them will not embolden them to want to help you at all. This is a situation where you often "win more with honey than vinegar."

This conversation can be your dentist's best way to provide clinical information that is difficult or impossible to relay completely through the normal claims process. It also happens to be your last line of defense for getting the claim approved. **After the third denial, the insurance company will no longer accept further requests for a claim to be reviewed**.

BREAKDOWNS AND ESTIMATES

If you are the one handling breakdowns and estimates in your office, you should realize your number one role is to protect both the office *and* the patients. You protect the patients by providing them the most accurate estimate that you can so they do not incur unexpected expenses. By protecting the patients, you protect the office as well by avoiding complaints that will harm the reputation of the office.

When you call to get a breakdown of benefits, it is extremely important to be detailed and accurate with this information. The benefits agents you are talking to will not care if they make a mistake because there is minimal if any consequence to their being wrong. The consequence of you being inaccurate is the patient will likely come complaining to you later.

A common mistake is asking the wrong questions or assuming the benefits agents are right when all other experience tells you they are not. A great example of this is with company-wide policies, especially those that are not written down anywhere. For example, United Concordia (UC) will likely tell you that they will pay for four quads of SRP if done in the same appointment; however, if you have any experience with UC, you know they rarely will. This makes it rather pointless to ask a benefits agent the question about four quads in a day because you already know the answer. We have had dozens of patients try to fight us on this because they will call patient relations and get the benefit agent's answer that four quads will be covered. When we call after claims are processed, the claims department tells us that four quads are not covered (without rather extreme circumstances). The "unwritten" answer with some companies is what you need to know. You need to know more than the benefits agents so that you can correctly advocate for your patients and help them as much as possible maximize their insurance benefits.

NOTE

Different insurance companies handle treatments such as four quads of SRP in a single visit differently. Delta is an umbrella of dozens of different companies, all which might handle SRPs slightly differently. Some may completely deny no matter what, while some may require a lot more information and documented support (such as sedation, driving long distances, medical restrictions, etc.). The simplest way for a team to handle these is to take the most extreme approach for all companies within the umbrella name. This makes it easier for the entire team to know what to do, such as: "Delta in general does not pay for four quads of SRP on the same visit, so we should always separate them unless absolutely necessary, or the patient is willing to pay more because the insurance company will not."

When you have accurate breakdown information, you are now equipped to give the patient the best estimates possible. Preparing breakdowns and estimates correctly up front will save you a ton of hassle and patient complaints. Most of the estimate side of explanation to a patient is all about their perception of the information you provide (not necessarily the information itself). Your presentation of the details and the words you choose can have a great impact on your success throughout the patient experience.

What Patients Want to Hear from Providers/Offices

Often there is a misconception from both dentists and team members about what patients want or need to hear concerning their treatment, especially when it comes to insurance. In dentistry, we are extremely detail oriented, and therefore it is natural to assume that everyone needs the same information we do.

What we forget is that patients have different personalities and rarely have the same level of background information or training as we do. When we think we are providing great detail and information to the patient, often all we are accomplishing is confusing the patient. A confused patient does not want to move forward with care, and this often triggers multiple questions that many team members complain about receiving.

"Why is my patient asking that? I just answered it three different ways! They must be a crazy person!"

Ever heard or thought something similar?

Many times, the patient is not the problem, we are. We need to realize what the patient really wants and needs to hear in order to make an informed decision. Give enough information to be useful but not so much as to be confusing or overwhelming.

So what do almost all patients in common want/need to hear in order to make an informed decision?

1. What is the problem that needs to be fixed?
2. What is the recommended solution to the problem? (in simple terms, not dental terms)
3. How long will the process take? (hours, days, number of appointments)
4. How much will the solution cost me? (bottom dollar)

There is a small subset of patients who may want more information than this, but not most of them. You can be prepared to answer the questions, but it will save you a ton of time and a lot of patient confusion if you avoid going into too much detail when those details are not requested.

Here is an example of how that treatment presentation may look like for a crown:

"Mrs. Jones, you have a broken tooth on the lower left that is bothering you. The solution is to rebuild the tooth. The process for this will take two visits. The first visit will be 90 minutes; the second visit will be 30 minutes, three weeks later. The cost after insurance for repairing your tooth is estimated to be $500. What works for your schedule to have this taken care of? How would you like to pay?"

This simple explanation is what most patients will respond to best. It takes less than a minute to explain, is in simple terms that the patient uses every day, answers all the basic questions, and there are no points of confusion.

Now let's review several concepts that are common in a dental office that ruin patient clarity.

"Not Covered"

This is a term that should rarely be used in a dental office. The problem with it isn't the word itself but the context it conveys to the patient. Here is what you might well see if you were observing a patient move through a dental office.

- Dentist shows patient the problem
- Patient asks for a solution
- Dentist provides details on the solution
- Patient is very interested in getting the solution
- Treatment coordinator comes in, patient asks how they can get the solution
- Treatment coordinator says the service is not covered, but the patient portion is only $30
- Patient declines the care

What happens often is the patient stops listening after the words "not covered" and now no longer wants the solution or cares about the problem. This one phrase elicits an automatic response that the insurance companies have brainwashed into society: if it is not covered, it is not important. The problem isn't about the $30.

The solution is just to change your terminology to avoid the unconscious response.

"Mrs. Jones, after checking your insurance, your fluoride treatment will be $30."

Or

"Mrs. Jones, your portion after insurance for the fluoride treatment will be $30."

If you are using the phrase "not covered," test this out for yourself for a few weeks and see what happens. You are still being fully honest with Mrs. Jones because you are still telling her what her out-of-pocket portion is, which is the main thing she wants to know. "What will it cost me?"

If the patient asks (most won't) if the service is covered, you can confidently tell them that their insurance does not reimburse for that service (without needing to use the phrase "not covered").

Percentages

Many dental office personnel are trained to use the percentages on breakdowns to create their insurance benefit estimates. This is necessary to learn in order to understand how to estimate, but it is only part of the equation. Realize, however, that patients do not have this background or training. Patients do not understand that the percentage of coverage is often changed by many other factors, such as downgrades or deductibles. Giving patients direct information on percentages is not helpful in most cases. As an example:

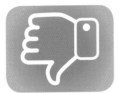

Poor Terminology

Team: "Mrs. Jones, your insurance covers fillings at 80%. Your portion for this $200 filling will be $80."

Patient: "Your math is wrong" (and the patient would be correct, 20% of 200 is $40).

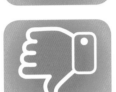

Still Poor Terminology

Team: "Mrs. Jones, your insurance covers fillings at 80%, your insurance has a deductible of $50, and they also downgrade your service, which means they pay less for your filling than normal. Your portion for this $200 filling will be $80."

Patient: (I do not understand half of what you just said, but I am not going to admit it out loud, so instead I am going to ask a dozen questions and then still be confused).

Many offices will use this same example as a reason to go into so much more detail about the coverage, such as downgrades and deductibles. A vast majority of patients do not need or want this information. Refer back to the section about what patients truly want to hear from their doctors and offices. All you do in many cases by giving out too much detailed information is wasting time and confusing the patient.

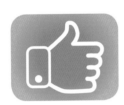

Good Terminology

Team: "Mrs. Jones, the full fee for your filling is $200, however, after insurance, your estimated portion will be $80."

Short, simple, to the point, and answers everything the patient wants/needs to hear.

Itemization

Think of the last time you went to buy groceries and you used the checkout clerks. After they scan every item into the computer, what do they tell you? Do they list off every item with a price, or do they just give you a total price?

If you think about it, most businesses in the world do the same thing. They will give you a total price for the products or service you are purchasing. So why do we think in dentistry that we should be any different? It is a great question because the answer is that we should not be different. The reason most businesses in the world give total prices is they understand that itemization causes a lot of problems from client confusion and frustration to a loss of sales.

When you provide a patient with an itemized list of services included and attach a fee to each one, have you ever noticed that many patients will search down that list and start asking questions about why specific items are needed? This is after the dentist, the assistant, and the treatment coordinator all asked if the patient had any more questions other than financial before you handed them the estimate.

Most Americans are naturally savers. Whether this is instinct, or society taught, the ultimate result is that when you stick an itemized list in front of people, they want to start searching for things to pull out to save money. When you are selling products that have little to do with each other, that isn't much of a problem. However, when you are providing medical/dental care, many items cannot or should not be pulled off that list. The easiest example of this is a buildup and crown. Often the patient has no idea that the buildup is required to support the crown and that doing many crowns without one can cause a lot of problems.

Or have you ever had a patient with a large broken tooth and a few small cavities who tells you they only want to do the fillings because they are cheaper per tooth? The dentist looks at the case and gets frustrated because the broken tooth is likely to get worse far faster than the small cavities. This is the exact reason that perception is everything.

You can avoid these issues a majority of the time when you stop itemizing treatment.

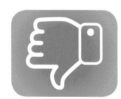

Poor Example:
"Mrs. Jones, your filling will be $100, your crown will be $500, the buildup will be $200, and the sealant will be $50."

Mrs. Jones now has a list of numbers running in her head, she is trying to add them all up, and now is wondering whether all the treatment you recommended for her is necessary.

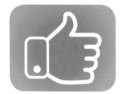

Good Example:
"Mrs. Jones, the total cost to fix your teeth, as Dr. Smith has discussed with you, is $850 after insurance. The process will take two visits. When would you like to schedule the first visit of two hours?"

Short, simple, to the point, and answers everything the patient wants/needs to hear.

HANDLING DISALLOWED SERVICES

One of the most frustrating things to a dental office are services that the insurance company tells you not only are they not paying for it, but the patient is not responsible for paying for the service either. This is what is called a disallowed service.

Dental state boards have condemned disallows as well because they are a violation of state board rules that say in order to come up with a diagnosis one must conduct a clinical exam. And in order to disagree with a doctor's diagnosis, you technically have to come up with a diagnosis of your own. The insurance company cannot do this, nor can dentists who work within an insurance company. This concept is still being fought on a national level to stop. In the meantime, you need to know how to handle disallowed services.

If you are an out-of-network (OON) office, these disallows should not affect you much other than the frustration that the patient has to pay more than they should. To an OON office, disallows are no different than a denial, both result in the insurance company reimbursing nothing. Disallows are not enforceable on an OON office, which should clue you into the illegitimacy of the term.

By saying a procedure should have a value of $0, the insurance company is trying to dictate treatment through money. It is the same as if Congress or the president does not like a law that passed. Instead of repealing the law, they will just give the law a $0 budget, which accomplishes the same task with less effort. This is a violation of everything that medical and dental providers stand for, and you should understand the reason that these should be fought by the office as strongly as possible.

What Are Some Common Disallowed Services?

You will typically find these when you get an EOB back that shows a service with a "covered or allowed amount" of $0 and a patient responsibility amount of $0 as well. You occasionally may see an attached note saying "disallowed," but not every insurance provider is as transparent about the use of this term.

What may be disallowed you can often find if you read the provider manual or claims guidelines.

Here are some common examples:

Perio (Delta): doing four quads of SRP on a single day is often disallowed. This means that if you file four quads same day, they not only won't pay, but they will say the patient shouldn't pay either.

D4212: Gingivectomy to access a restoration is often disallowed the same day as the restoration.

Buildups: often these are noted as disallowed, which is not necessarily true. (See Chapter 23.)

Bone grafts or membranes are occasionally disallowed on the day of a tooth extraction (even though there is no clinical reason to do them separately).

Indirect pulp caps are often disallowed on the same day as the final restoration (any composite or amalgam filling code).

Retainers are disallowed as a separate fee when doing braces. (See Chapter 18: ortho claims.)

What if the Patient Needs These Services, but the Dentist Does Not Want to Work for Free?

Your dentist shouldn't work for free, ever! Do you want to work for free? Of course not.

In some cases, you just need to understand what will likely be tagged as disallowed and reorganize the treatment plan timing to work within the insurance provider's framework. You are not doing this because it is the right thing to do or because insurance is legitimate in disallowing it. You are only doing it because it is the most efficient way to achieve the services for the patient and ensure the patient receives their insurance benefits and the office is appropriately compensated for providing the services.

When Delta Dental (directly) or United Concordia (indirectly) tell you that you cannot do four quads of SRP on the same treatment visit, the easiest answer is to just not do them on a single visit. Split up the treatment into two visits, and you remove most of the problems. The best part of this is if the patient needs other work (e.g., fillings or crowns), then they can get it done at the same time and only have to be numbed once. Turn a lemon into lemonade.

When you know that a gingivectomy to access decay D4212, an indirect pulp cap, or bone graft is disallowed on the same day of service as the restoration/extraction, you can have the patient come back and get numbed twice. Or you can have the patient sign a "HIPAA do not bill insurance form," which prevents insurance from getting involved in the patient's decisions for their own care.

In-Network Frequency Question

> **Q: If a filling we did is under frequency limitation, the insurance company may say the patient share is $0. Do we have to abide by this? Even if the restoration was not the problem?**
>
> A: Not necessarily.
>
> What the insurance company is doing here is making sure that patients are not responsible for poor quality work that does not last. Most dentists who treat patients without insurance and have work fail in a short time period would not charge the patient for replacement. The insurance company is applying this common concept to the claims process.
>
> However, there are times where the works fail due to something outside the dentist's control. A patient could have an accident or injury. The patient could be non-compliant with protective devices such as an occlusal guard. The patient could have habits that are detrimental to the teeth and restorations such as chewing on pens or fingernails or biting on a hard bone. None of these are reasons to provide a free replacement.
>
> There are a couple of ways to handle this. You can provide a narrative on why the work failed that has nothing to do with quality. You then hope the claims examiner understands this and has the ability to send an EOB that says the patient owes the money. Alternatively, you can just not send a claim at all and avoid the insurance system, which may not be designed to understand this concept. EOBs that are incorrect can cause a lot of headaches for the patient, the office, and the insurance company.

HOW TO ALLOW A PATIENT TO DECLINE USE OF INSURANCE

In 2009/2010 the Health Information Technology for Economic and Clinical Health (HI-TECH) Act was passed as an addition to HIPAA. Part of this lengthy act applies to dentistry because it has to do with a patient's rights to specify what information they agree to share with anyone, including insurance companies.

This act states that the patient has the right to restrict a provider (dentist) from submitting information to the insurance company for the purposes of payment (reimbursement) **as long as the patient has paid for the service out of pocket in full**.

In other words, if the patient chooses to restrict you from filing a claim for a service because it would cause the patient to not get the service (disallowed services), then the patient has the legal, federal right to prevent you from filing the claim and the insurance company from getting involved in the payment process.

Simply put: Yes, the patient can sign a form telling you not to file a claim for a service. This is a federal law that supersedes any insurance contracts, in any state.

HITECH ACT

SEC. 13405. RESTRICTIONS ON CERTAIN DISCLOSURES AND SALES OF

HEALTH INFORMATION; ACCOUNTING OF CERTAIN PROTECTED HEALTH INFORMATION DISCLOSURES; ACCESS

TO CERTAIN INFORMATION IN ELECTRONIC FORMAT.

(a) REQUESTED RESTRICTIONS ON CERTAIN DISCLOSURES OF

HEALTH INFORMATION—In the **case that an individual requests** under paragraph (a)(1)(i)(A) of section 164.522 of title 45, Code of Federal Regulations, that **a covered entity restrict the disclosure of the protected health information** of the individual, notwithstanding paragraph (a)(1)(ii) of such section, the **covered entity must comply with the requested restriction** if—

1. except as otherwise required by law, the disclosure is to a health plan for **purposes of carrying out payment** or health care operations (and is not for purposes of carrying out treatment)
2. the protected health information pertains solely to a health care item or service for which the health care provider involved has been **paid out of pocket in full**

Patient – "case that an individual requests"

Dentist/Office – "covered entity"

Does not submit information – "restrict the disclosure of the protected health information"

Dentist/Office must comply – "covered entity must comply with the requested restriction"

If the disclosure is for "purposes of carrying out payment"

As long as the patient has "paid out of pocket in full"

Source:
https://www.hhs.gov/sites/default/files/ocr/privacy/hipaa/understanding/coveredentities/hitechact.pdf

---

How Do You Use This HIPAA/HITECH Law?

When you have patients who need or desire services that are going to be disallowed and therefore the dentist is unable to do them, the patient can sign a single-page form to prevent the insurance company from getting involved at all.

So, if your patients do not want to come back for two visits to do the four quads of SRP for any reason, then they can sign the form and pay the amount in full. Insurance will not get a claim for the SRP, not pay anything towards the SRP, and therefore have no ability to disallow the service being done on the same visit. The same can go for indirect pulp caps, gingivecto-mies, ortho retainers, and so forth.

This will allow your office and dentist to provide the best care that the patient wants without interference in that treatment by the insurance company.

Do realize this is actually no different than if a patient comes to your office with insurance, does not tell you they have insurance, and gets treatment. This scenario may not be common, but it does happen occasionally. The patients who do this mention it is because they are private people, they would rather file insurance themselves, or they just do not trust insurance companies.

But My Insurance Contract Requires I Submit *All* Claims?

This is a common myth in dentistry that has minimal support for the concept. We have read through contracts for the major dental insurance companies that constitute 98% of claims in the country. It is rare for an insurance company to require you to file a claim for any and every service. Most just state how to file claims, or that you cannot charge the patient an extra fee just to file a claim. See Chapter 16 for more details on this myth.

However, let's just say your insurance contract does require you to submit all claims. The HI-TECH federal law overrides any insurance contracts. The patient's privacy rights are more important than any insurance contract. Insurance companies do not and cannot make laws.

To stay safe though, you should always obtain and retain written documentation of the patient revoking the office's requirement to submit the insurance claim. See the next page for this form.

DO NOT BILL TO INSURANCE

Patient HIPAA Restriction Request

Election to Self-Pay for Services

[Section 13405 of Subtitle D of the HITECH Act (42 USC 17935)]

Patient _____

Please do not share the health information specified below to my health insurance company:

Date of service_____

Specific service or test to be restricted: _____
_____

I acknowledge that I understand and agree that:

1. I am covered by a dental discount ("insurance") plan.
2. Despite the above, I do not wish the clinic to submit a claim to the company for services pro-vided to me by the clinic and thereby release the provider from contractual obligations.
3. The dental service(s) provided, or that are to be provided, to me have been fully explained to me by my treating dentist.
4. I have freely chosen to self-pay for services after having asked clinic about payment options and having carefully considered those options.

I have read this election to self-pay for services form and have had the opportunity to ask any questions I may have had about the form. Any questions I may have had about this form have been answered to my satisfaction.

Patient/Parent/Guardian: _____ Date: _____

OPTIONAL UPGRADED SERVICES

Along with this same concept of the HITECH Act, patients also have the right to choose upgraded options for their dental care. You can find the clause with details about upgraded options if you read your insurance contracts. As an example:

> Delta Dental Contract 2018: "Treat Enrollees with the same quality and provide access to care consistent with the balance of Provider's practice and not differentiate or dis-criminate against any Enrollee on the basis of source of payment."

In other words, you have to provide the same quality, care, and options to insurance patients as you do with your non-insurance patients. The typical ethical rules that come with this have to do with treating all patients the same way when dealing with upgrade options.

First, you must give the "insurance standard" rate option. Upgrades cannot be forced on the patient.

Second, you must charge cash patients the same upgrade fees you do to insurance patients.

The most common example of this is with orthodontists. It is an industry standard that orthodontists will charge more for porcelain brackets than traditional metal brackets as an upgrade to the standard braces package the insurance company offers to pay for. This may come in the form of a $500 upgrade fee above whatever the in-network rate is for braces.

> **Q: But wait, we don't charge our cash patients different amounts.**
> A: If you don't, then you either cannot charge upgrade fees or you need to reorganize how you charge all patients in order to correctly follow the rules. Here is an example of this:

An office's standard fee for braces is $5000 and is inclusive of everything, including porcelain brackets.

The in-network fee averages around $3500.

Instead, the office decides to manage insurance rules more efficiently and sets: braces fee = $4500, porcelain upgrade fee = $50, and in-network fee = $35.

	Office before change		Office after change	
	Cash patient	Ins. patient	Cash patient	Ins. patient
Braces	5000	3500	4500	3500
Upgrade fee	-	-	500	500
Total	5000	3500	5000	4000

The office also understands that itemized treatment plans are not productive, so they give the cash patient a treatment plan that says $5000 (inclusive of treatment and porcelain upgrade). The ledger however correctly states the $4500 base fee and the $500 upgrade fee. Now the office can correctly offer *all* patients, in- and out-of-network, the added upgrade fee for porcelain brackets.

This is the legal, correct way to handle this.

Caution

Upgrade fees are not designed to get you back to your normal full fee. As you can see with the ortho example, the patient is still getting an insurance discount, as they should. Upgrade fees are designed to allow patients to get additional services or options without the office having to take a hit on that added cost of care.

Other Common Upgrade Fees

Rush Fees – On occasion you may get patients who need their lab work back faster than normal. Many labs will accommodate this rush request but will charge an added fee to put you at the head of the line. The patient should be 100% responsible for this added rush fee.

Gold Alloy – Gold crowns from decades ago used to be cheaper than porcelain when porcelain first came out. Since then the process of making a porcelain crown is much more efficient, and the cost of gold has skyrocketed. Therefore, the lab fee today for a gold crown is often a lot more if not double the cost of a porcelain crown. However, insurance rates rarely change, and gold crowns are most often the lowest reimbursement crown option in a fee schedule.

Instead of the dentist not offering gold at all, you can charge an upgrade option for the added cost of the gold alloy, which most labs will itemize separately on your bill.

> **Q: I thought the lab fee was included in the cost of the procedure.**
> A: The lab fee is the base fee for the crown and is part of the insurance crown code. The gold alloy however would be an upgrade fee that is separate and paid 100% out of pocket by the patient.

Cosmetic Upgrades – If you are an in-network office, you probably have noticed that you cannot provide the highest cost care at the lowest cost price. That is not what insurance is about. An office often cannot afford to pay $400 to a lab to make a crown when the total fee for the crown is only $600. Many quality labs in the country can make crowns for near or under $100. However, most of these labs are not staffed by high detail, master lab technicians who can produce the most aesthetic work. The cosmetic labs take a lot longer to make a good cosmetic crown and therefore charge more for that work. The difference in cost between the office's standard lab and the cosmetic lab is an upgrade fee that can and should be charged to the patients if they want that added level of quality.

The same goes for any additional lab costs. Examples include custom shading or staining, all porcelain butt margins on a PFM (porcelain fused to metal crown), full metal occlusion, or any miscellaneous lab fee above and beyond the base lab cost.

Invisalign™ – This is a cosmetic upgrade like porcelain brackets. (See Chapter 18)

Same-Day Crown Convenience Fee – Many CADCAM offices will charge an additional fee for a same-day crown. While technically, the costs to produce this crown are less than a standard lab, the basic concept still applies. As long as this is offered as an optional fee, it is legal.

But Insurance Will Just Disallow These Additional Fees!

If you realize this, then great, you have been paying attention. You are correct in that insurance companies will disallow these additional upgrade fees. One option is to use the HI-TECH waiver to not submit the fees to insurance. The only challenge with this is a full-page additional form the patient needs to sign.

As an alternative, you can have the patient sign a small waiver that can be put inside the treatment plan itself. This will avoid multiple pieces of paper, as well as make the whole process cleaner and smoother.

Below is a copy of the ADA's Sample Consent Form for services not paid by insurance, which is quite acceptable. However, it is a bit bulky to use. The next paragraph has a simplified alternative that can be inserted into a treatment plan easily.

"Treatment plan options have been presented to me. I understand that my insurance benefit will not pay toward the upgraded service(s) that I selected, and I understand that I will be responsible for the fee for this treatment. I wish to waive my insurance plan guidelines for the upgraded service(s) and I release the provider, Dr. _____, from the contractual terms of my plan in this case."

Sample Consent Form: Service(s) Not Paid For by the Benefit Plan

(Practice name) accepts (Plan Name) dental benefit plan, under which you are covered:

By signing below, I (Patient Name), acknowledge that:

- the dental service(s) provided, or that are to be provided, to me have been fully explained to me by my treating dentist.

Patient's name _____ Date_____

Patient, guardian, or guarantor signature _____ Date_____

With respect to charges for services provided, our office will submit claims for the procedures rendered. Dental benefit plans are intended to pay for some but not all dental care costs. You are ultimately responsible for all charges including when the dental plan chooses to reimburse you directly.

By signing below, you acknowledge your understanding that you are responsible for charges for any portion of the treatment rendered on (date of service) that is not paid for by the dental benefit plan,* and that,

- if you choose to have your treating dentist perform a service that is not paid for by your dental benefit plan, you must pay to your treating dentist the dentist's full fees for the service or the fee contractually agreed upon between your benefit administrator and the treating dentist.

Notwithstanding the foregoing, in no instance will you be responsible for paying the costs of any services for which your dental plan is contractually responsible to pay.

Please indicate your understanding and acceptance of these financial policies by signing below.

Patient's name _____ Date_____

Patient, guardian, or guarantor signature _____ Date_____

*Consult your state's applicable laws and regulations for limitations regarding fee limitations and restrictions.

© ADA 2018. Reproduction of this material by ADA member dentists and their staff is permitted. Any other use, duplication, or distribution by any other party requires the prior written approval of the American Dental Association. This material is educational only, does not constitute legal advice and may not satisfy applicable state law. Changes in applicable laws or regulations may require revision. Contact a qualified lawyer or professional for legal or professional advice.

Chapter 19
Understanding Discounts and Fraud - Avoiding Trouble

Let's review the obligations we have as healthcare providers from the aspects of fraud, contracts, and ethics before we discuss how to handle discounts. The term "fraud" is often misused, especially in dentistry. Fraud is a state and federal crime and has specific definitions. In many cases where you may hear the term "fraud," the true term may be "breach of contract" or "incorrect insurance filing."

DEFINING INSURANCE FRAUD

> "An intentional act of deceiving, concealing, or misrepresenting information that results in health care benefits being paid to an individual or group."

What exactly is fraud in reference to insurance billing?

Each state has some modification to what is determined as insurance fraud, but most follow the same basic idea. For simplicity purposes we will focus on Texas as it has one of the easier- to-understand rules. The purpose of posting the entire law (seen on the following page) is not to read it, but just act as a reference point.

Summary of the law
- You can offer sliding scale or charity case fees for the financial or medically indigent (#2)
- You can provide a membership plan (#3 - written policy)
- The fee you routinely charge non-insurance or "cash" patients must be the fee you submit to insurance.

MYTH - AN INSURANCE COMPANY DOWNGRADING, REMAPPING, OR OTHERWISE CHANGING CODING ON CLAIMS IS FRAUD.

This is a common misconception. A dentist or office changing coding or information is considered fraud. What is different about the insurance company?

The reason it is fraud by the provider is the provider and patient are the only ones that know what happened in the treatment room. Lying about what happened is the definition of fraud. However, insurance codes are meant to communicate information TO the insurance company, not FROM. They have the ability to modify that language (coding) for the purposes of processing the claim. This is not fraud.

In most cases, code changes are in lieu of a straight denial, so they often work in favor of the dental office or patient to remove more hoops that you would have to jump through to get reimbursement.

TEXAS INSURANCE CODE

TITLE 5. PROTECTION OF CONSUMER INTERESTS
SUBTITLE C. DECEPTIVE, UNFAIR, AND PROHIBITED PRACTICES
CHAPTER 552. ILLEGAL PRICING PRACTICES

Sec. 552.001. APPLICABILITY OF CHAPTER. (a) This chapter does not apply to the provision of a health care service to a:

1. Medicaid or Medicare patient or a patient who is covered by a federal, state, or local government-sponsored indigent health care program
2. Financially or medically indigent person who qualifies for indigent health care services based on:
   - A sliding fee scale; or
   - A written charity care policy established by a health care provider; or
3. Person who is not covered by a health insurance policy or other health benefit plan that provides benefits for the services and qualifies for services for the uninsured based on a written policy established by a health care provider.
   - This chapter does not permit the establishment of health care provider policies or contracts that violate any other state or federal law.
   - This chapter does not prohibit a health care provider from entering into a contract to provide services covered by a health insurance policy or other health benefit plan with:
1. The issuer of the health insurance policy or other health benefit plan; or
2. A preferred provider organization that contracts with the issuer of the health insurance policy or other health benefit plan.

Added by Acts 2003, 78th Leg., ch. 1274, Sec. 2, eff. April 1, 2005.

Amended by:

Acts 2005, 79th Leg., Ch. 724 (S.B. 500), Sec. 1, eff. June 17, 2005.

Sec. 552.002. FRAUDULENT INSURANCE ACT. An offense under Section 552.003 is a fraudulent insurance act under Chapter 701.

Added by Acts 2003, 78th Leg., ch. 1274, Sec. 2, eff. April 1, 2005.

Sec. 552.003. CHARGING DIFFERENT PRICES; OFFENSE. (a) A person commits an offense if:

1. The person knowingly or intentionally charges two different prices for providing the same product or service; and
2. The higher price charged is based on the fact that an insurer will pay all or part of the price of the product or service.
   - An offense under this section is a Class B misdemeanor.

Added by Acts 2003, 78th Leg., ch. 1274, Sec. 2, eff. April 1, 2005.

MYTH - I CAN CHARGE CASH PATIENTS WHATEVER I WANT BECAUSE INSURANCE HAS NOTHING TO DO WITH IT.

This is a myth that usually just comes from lack of knowledge. Technically it would be true if you never filed an insurance claim. The basic definition of insurance fraud is knowingly charging an insurance patient more than a cash patient. In other words, you are attempting to charge the insurance carrier a premium price. It has less to do with the cash patient and more to do with how you charge an insurance patient.

When you submit a fee to insurance that is higher than your cash patient fee, that is the definition of fraud.

EXAMPLE

"Mrs. Jones, you need a crown on that broken tooth. The fee for that is usually $1500. However, since you do not have insurance, we can lower that fee to $1000."

In this example, what you do for Mrs. Jones is not the problem. However, if you then submit any fee higher than $1000 to an insurance company for the same crown service, then you have committed insurance fraud. This is because $1000 is your crown fee, not $1500. Your standard fee is what you would charge a cash patient, and this is what must be reported when you file an insurance claim.

Just to be complete, charging different fees for different patients also has two other issues.

Breach of Contract

If you are in-network with an insurance company, part of the contract you signed is to provide your normal fee on all claims. Here is an example clause within a common contract from Delta Dental which is a good representation of most insurance network contracts.

EXAMPLE

Online Delta Contract 2018

"Provider agrees to: include the fee regularly charged by the Provider for such services"

Ethics

The American Dental Association also considers charging different fees based on insurance coverage to be unethical. From the ADA Code of Ethics:

5.B. REPRESENTATION OF FEES

Dentists shall not represent the fees being charged for providing care in a false or misleading manner.

5.B.1. WAIVER OF CO-PAYMENT

A dentist who accepts a third-party payment under a co-payment plan as payment in full without disclosing to the third party that the patient's payment portion will not be collected, is engaged in overbilling. The essence of this ethical impropriety is deception and misrepresentation; an overbilling dentist makes it appear to the third party that the charge to the patient for services rendered is higher than it actually is.

5.B.2. OVERBILLING

It is unethical for a dentist to increase a fee to a patient solely because the patient is covered under a dental benefits plan.

5.B.3. FEE DIFFERENTIAL

The fee for a patient without dental benefits shall be considered a dentist's full fee. This is the fee that should be represented to all benefit carriers regardless of any negotiated fee discount. Payments accepted by a dentist under a governmentally funded program, a component or constituent dental society sponsored access program, or a participating agreement entered into under a program with a third party shall not be considered or construed as evidence of overbilling in determining whether a charge to a patient, or to another third party in behalf of a patient not covered under any of the afore cited programs constitutes overbilling under this section of the Code.

What if I Am Not a Member of the ADA?

This question comes up often. "If I am not a member of the ADA, must I use their claim forms and follow their rules?" The first answer to this is that all states consider these practices (waiving co-pays, overbilling, and fee differentials) fraud, and insurance contracts consider them a breach of contract. The ADA is just another reason on top of that to do the right thing.

However, the legal answer is this:

If you use ADA claim forms, you have agreed to abide by the ADA Code of Ethics. This includes either the paper or electronic versions. And since there are no other accepted claim forms in the country, if you file insurance, you are bound by the ADA code of ethics, regardless of whether you are a member of the ADA or not.

Now, this book is designed to offer you an answer to any challenge that has a possible solution. In the next section we will discuss solutions for typical challenges you may face on the topic of discounts to avoid fraud.

UNDERSTANDING DISCOUNTS WITH INSURANCE

Legality

In the previous section, you learned that billing different fees to patients based on insurance coverage is unethical, breach of contract, and a state/federal crime of insurance fraud. Many dentists and offices ask:

"How is this possible, legal, fair? I should be able to charge less for patients who don't require me to go through all the hassle of dealing with insurance and waiting for the payments."

Unfortunately, all I can give you is the truth: Life is not fair.

However, there is a solution for what you likely want to do, which is offer your patients some benefit for not making your life more difficult with insurance. This chapter is going to go through all the possible discounts that you can and cannot offer to a patient and stay legally within the insurance framework (if you file any insurance claims for a patient).

General Rules

Most laws are written in order to hold up an ethical or moral standard that has been decided by society. When it comes to insurance and discounts, there are a few general rules you should always keep in mind.

These rules apply for both in-network and out-of-network offices. If your office ever files a claim, consider these rules as standard practice.

- Always bill your normal, full fee on insurance claims
- Give insurance patients the same access to specials, deals, or discounts as any other patient
- Inform the insurance company of any procedure-specific discounts

The reason for these rules is to ensure you are being truthful and honest in everything you do, keeping you out of trouble with the law and with your contract obligations.

The best way to think about this is in defense of your patients. It is not their fault the insurance company is difficult to work with. It is not their fault that an office signed an insurance network contract with multiple stipulations that are onerous to deal with. It is not ethical or moral to punish the patient for these issues.

Co-Payments and Deductibles

A co-pay is the fee insurance requires the patient to pay alongside insurance, and a deductible is the amount of money that the patient is required to pay first before insurance pays.

It is unethical and illegal to write off a deductible or co-payment without informing the insurance company.

To understand the reasoning behind this, recall how insurance companies function (Chapter 17). Actuaries determine premiums and benefits based on expected use of the insurance policy. They utilize a set of general assumptions, one of which is that patients pay co-pays for more expensive treatments, which may result in the patients choosing less treatment than they would otherwise. If you manipulate the system by not charging the required deductible or co-pay, then you throw off all the calculations that the insurance company ran in order to design the policy the patient has. If this happens too frequently, the insurance company will either increase premiums or decrease benefits for all patients across the board. Again, this all starts with being honest when you file an insurance claim.

Is There Any Circumstance Where Part of the Co-Pay or Deductible Fee Can Be Modified?

For in-network offices the answer is simple, there is no part of the fee that can be modified without informing the insurance company. For out-of-network offices that answer is different.

EXAMPLE CLAIM FOR A FILLING - OUT OF NETWORK OFFICE

Office Standard Fee: $140

Insurance UCR Fee: $100
(UCR: Usual, Customary, and Reasonable)

Policy Coverage on Fillings: 50%

Deductible: $50

The co-pay for this filling is $25, and insurance is going to pay $25.

The copay is part of the UCR fee not part of the full fee. Anything above UCR ($40 in this example) is an optional differential fee to collect from the patient. The reason behind this is because it does not affect what the insurance company would have paid. If the office's fee is $100 or $1000, the insurance company does not care because it is only going to base coverage on the UCR fee of $100.

You cannot modify the copay or deductible in or out of network. The only part of the fee you can modify is the differential above UCR.

You can modify any fee above UCR without needing to inform the insurance company. Any fee below UCR you must inform the insurance company about.
The challenge: What is the UCR if you are out of network? (See Chapter 22: blue book.)

How Do I Provide Discounts to Patients Who Are in Need if I Am Out of Network?

As mentioned in the previous section, you can discount any office fee above UCR for a patient without needing to inform the insurance company.

If you discount the price below UCR, you would then need to inform the insurance company of that change. You can do this by writing a simple narrative attached to the claim.

How Do I Provide Discounts to Patients Who Are in Need if I Am In-Network?

The network contracts that are signed stipulate that you will charge no more or less than the agreed upon fee schedule for covered services. This means any change in fee that you make for an individual must be reported to the insurance company.

The question you might want to ask yourself about making an additional fee reduction is:

> Why would you want to discount more than the already 30–50% discount required by your contract?

If you still choose to further discount the price below your network fee schedule, you would then need to inform the insurance company of that change. You can do this by writing a simple narrative.

Example Remark Notes

Most of the reason offices choose to offer discounts to patients is for marketing purposes. The following are a few examples of remark notes that you can attach to a claim:

> "Patient is not participating in co-pays for this service because of X reason."

> "Patient is being given a $xx.xx discount for use of a marketing coupon."

> "Patient has a 10% discount due to X reason."

These narratives are designed to ensure you are honest with the insurance company and avoid fraud concerns (or breach of contract if in-network). Including these narratives may not affect the reimbursement you receive. However, depending on the service and the insurance company, you may receive a lower reimbursement. This is within the insurance company's right, as they may feel they should participate in the same discount the patient is receiving. If you are going to be discounting fees below UCR, do realize you may be giving twice the discount if the insurance company decides they are entitled to it as well.

What About Dental Care Benefits for My Dental Office Team?

This is the most common question dentists have about the use of insurance and discounts. How do I legally provide my employees with dental benefits if they are already covered by dental insurance through a spouse or family member?

Unfortunately, many offices unknowingly handle this incorrectly, and they open themselves up to audits and fines. The chance of getting caught and paying penalties is low, but when the answer is fairly simple to avoid any issues, why not just play it safe?

Common Office Practice for Providing "Free Care" Dental Benefits to Employees

A number of dental offices have an employee policy that reads something like this:

"Employees get free care from the office, except they have to pay any incurred lab fee."

This is a fine policy to have if the office never files insurance for one of its employees. However, if you do file an insurance claim on behalf of one of your employees, "employee free care" is basically insurance fraud. You essentially lied to the insurance company when you filed the claim. For example, your front admin team has no insurance and gets free care. Your clinical team has insurance through their spouses, and when you file a claim against their spouses' policy, you are now getting paid to treat them. Not disclosing to the insurance company that without insurance, these employees would get free care is what makes this practice illegal and fraudulent.

Now, in reality, an insurance company going after one office legally for this one claim alone is not likely to take place because the cost and effort of the legal process would not make it worth the insurance company's time. However, employee dental benefits can surface during an otherwise larger insurance audit; then this employee claim practice would become a liability for the office as now the insurance company is paying legal costs anyway and adding the small time to investigate what is known to be a common issue in dental offices will come up.

This is not to say you cannot offer dental benefits to employees, just to say benefits should be structured correctly to maintain full legal safety.

Best Office Practice for Providing Dental Benefits to Employees

Here is a better way to state dental benefits offered to your employees:

"Employees get $X per year to use on dental services as a benefit of employment."

By structuring the benefits this way within your employee handbook, you state you are still charging every patient, employee or otherwise, the same exact fees. This removes all potential issues with billing insurance companies. It also means that employees covered by insurance actually have a higher/better benefit, which makes it worth their keeping the insurance and paying for it (and thereby the office getting some reimbursement).

This method also has a few benefits for your practice:

- Employees dental benefits have a knowable max cost for the office each year, which helps maintain a healthy budget and avoid employee abuse;
- These benefits can be shown on a compensation breakdown yearly, which helps illustrate the true value of an employee's compensation; and
- You can still stipulate lab fees need to be covered separately if desired: "Lab fees incurred are not covered by this benefit."

Discount Coupons with Insurance

It has become common practice for dental offices to advertise with postcards, fliers, in magazines, and on websites. And those ads might incorporate one or more discount coupons.

When advertising your practice, you should realize that your state most likely has rules on how to appropriately use coupons within the law. These rules are enforced by the state board of dentistry. Each state is slightly different, but one general theme is that false advertisement and/or fraud are not allowed.

When you publish ads with discount coupons, you want to make sure that you save all documentation with these discounts for both insurance and non-insurance patients. Specifically, a picture or scan of the coupon is enough. This information will be useful if you ever have an insurance audit.

A question that often comes up is:

"I see corporate-run dental offices utilizing this type of coupon, why can't I?"

There are a few concepts that make corporate-run offices different.

- Corporate dental offices are not governed by state dental boards, only individual license holders are (dentists, hygienists, registered dental assistants).
- Corporate headquarters often are located in another state, which may have different laws.
- Corporate offices have larger, more expensive legal teams.

While none of these feels fair, they are a part of the system of laws in America. Often more expensive lawyers win the case before it even starts.

Our recommendation to you is to run your practice and develop your advertisements based on what is right and legal, not what someone else might be getting away with.

Let's show a few examples of coupons that you should be careful with or not use. Afterward, we will discuss solutions you can use without causing potential concerns.

Cash Patient or "Insurance Excluded" Coupons

You are not allowed to offer different fees or specials for patients based on whether they have insurance. It is illegal to have stipulations within an advertising coupon such as:

- Cash patients only
- Only patients without insurance
- Insurance Excluded

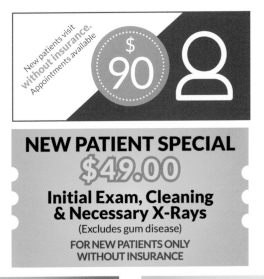

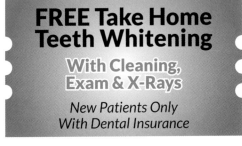

"X off Treatment" Coupons

It is common to see coupons that offer the patient either a flat or percentage discount off a service. The office should use caution with these types of coupons because how they are worded will make a difference in how you legally manage an insurance claim.

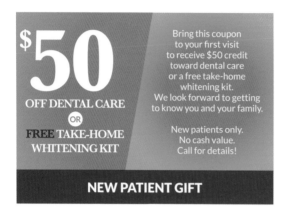

"$50 off major treatment" for instance means you are giving the patient a discount tied to a direct service. In this case you are required to inform the insurance company about this discount when you submit the claim.

"$50 credit toward future treatment" is the improved version of this coupon. Credits prior to treatment are not necessary to report to the insurance company as the credit has nothing to do with the service that is being rendered.

Social Coupons (Groupon)

The basic concept of social coupons, such as Groupon, is that the provider offers at least a 50% discount to the patient, and Groupon collects 50% of the remaining fee. This means that at minimum you are providing a service at a 75% discount.

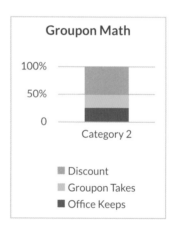

The other concern with systems like Groupon is they are often considered to be "fee splitting," which is illegal in many states. If you look into this type of advertising, be cautious. It might be a good idea to have an attorney review your state laws to see if this practice is legal for your office to consider.

Cash or Check Payment Discounts

It is a common policy for offices to provide a small discount (2–5%) for a patient paying in cash or with a check. The reasoning behind this is that credit cards cost the office somewhere between 2–5%, and they want to pass the savings on to the patient.

The problem with offering a "cash discount" is that insurance companies may also pay in cash (direct deposit) or with checks.

It is therefore fraudulent to provide this type of discount to any patient if you ever file insurance claims on behalf of your patients unless you are also giving your insurance patients and their insurance carrier this same discount.

If you choose to continue offering a cash/check pay discount at your office, then you would need to inform the insurance company through an attached note.

EXAMPLE **NARRATIVE**

"Patient was given a 5% courtesy for paying in cash."

Best Practice for Use of Coupons:
Cash and Insurance Patients

We've talked about how "not to" offer coupons and discounts. In this next section, we'll discuss how you can legally and properly use discounts for your cash and insurance patients.

Either-Or or Pick-One Coupons

You cannot offer coupons that stipulate, "Cash patients only," "Only patients without insurance," or "Insurance Excluded." However, if you want to provide coupons for cash patients, you can do this by offering an either-or coupon.

Cash patients tend to want flat savings.

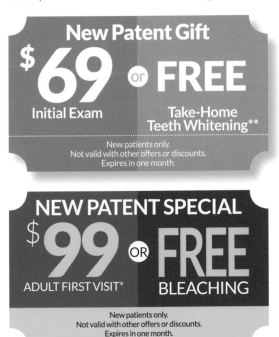

Insurance patients tend to want added value, since insurance is typically covering the costs of routine care.

If you create a coupon that satisfies both but only allows a patient to use one of the two benefits, you will legally create what the office is trying to provide.

The stipulation here, though, is that you must honor whichever part of the coupon the patient wants. For example: infrequently you may have a patient with insurance ask to use a coupon for discounted or free service that insurance would typically cover. If they choose to take this route, you need to honor the coupon and not file their insurance for that service. (It would be prudent to have the patient sign a HITECH/HIPAA release form.)

Pre-Pay or Payment-in-Full Discounts

While many offices incorrectly use discounts for cash patients and open themselves up to fraud or improper billing claims, there is a solution to provide basically the same result the office is looking for without the legal concerns.

If you want to attract more cash patients, patients without insurance, or incent patients not to draw on their insurance plan, then a pre-pay or payment-in-full discount may provide the avenue you are looking for. Just like any special, to avoid committing fraud, the discount must be available to all patients.

These types of discounts are your legal way to provide a "cash patient" discount.

The best part about this form of discount is that you aren't just giving away money. You are trading the patient's discounted payment for security that you are getting paid today, security that you do not need to wait for insurance to pay, and security that they are going to show up for their appointment since people follow their money. If you send AOB to the patient, you also have security against the insurance company ever demanding a refund from the office.

How they work: patient pays you before or at the day of service, and in exchange you provide them a discount on that payment (not the service). The fee for your service is not changing; therefore, the ledger should correctly show the full cost of the service provided.

Insurance companies will never prepay you for treatment; therefore, this discount naturally is unavailable for them to take advantage of. This means there are no legal requirements to inform the insurance company.

As a suggestion, you may want to define the discount to require prepayment of the entire treatment amount to qualify (instead of the co-pay amount). This is what makes it in essence a "cash" patient discount, as in-network patients will usually not want to participate.

In the following example we will use a 10% prepayment discount. The amount you actually decide to use in your office is purely up to you.

Standard office fee for service: $1000.

Cash patient – Patient gets a 10% prepayment discount and therefore gives you $900. The ledger shows the $1000 service and an adjustment for the prepayment discount of $100.

Out-of-network patient – Patient pays you $900 after their prepayment discount. You file $900 with the insurance company. Since the patient has prepaid you, they really are no different than a cash patient to the office.

In-network patients – Most will not want to pay up front. The rare patient who accepts this option will pay the full amount of treatment minus the prepayment discount. This does become slightly complex with your network contracts. Here is a breakdown of options:

If your $1000 service has a $700 network fee, and your patient choses to prepay $630 ($700 – 10% discount), you can either send a claim for $630 or for $700 with a narrative describing why the patient did not pay $700.

EXAMPLE NARRATIVE

"Patient received a 10% courtesy for prepaying."

Your options for the claim are:

1. Preferred: File the claim with assignment of benefits set to the patient (not the office)
2. Acceptable: File a claim accepting assignment of benefits and:

- sign the paper check over to the patient when it gets processed; or
- refund the amount to the patient's account if you get electronic payments.

> **NOTE**
> If you just write the patient a refund check, you will be taking even more of a discount from the patient if they used a credit card or check due to the merchant services cost. Refunds should be processed in the manner the original money was received.

OTHER EFFECTIVE DISCOUNTS

Something to note about the following options is that none of them are tied to a specific procedure; therefore, there is no way or reason to communicate them to the insurance company.

Credits

Many patients may end up with a credit in the office for a variety of reasons: Overpayment for a prior service, a loyalty/referral credit, warranty work, and so forth. There is no reason you cannot apply a prior credit (or balance) to a patient's out-of-pocket cost for their new services being rendered. No mention of the credit is necessary when you file the claim. The claim should reflect the full office fee and be processed as normal.

Multiple Service Discount, Case Fees, or Bulk Discounts

These are basically all variations of the prepay or payment in full discounts. Often, they are used with larger cases that go well beyond the insurance maximum.

Bartering Discounts

Bartering, or trading one service for another, is a common practice among dentists and their families, friends, or vendors. These bartering agreements may have state or federal laws you need to abide by in how you manage the barter, such as the IRS. From an insurance point of view these are basically just like any other credit the patient has.

> **EXAMPLE**
> You agree to take care of your physician's family preventive dental care, and they agree to take care of your family's preventive medical care in exchange.
> A painter needs dental work and is unable to otherwise afford it. As an alternative you agree to exchange his skills as payment or partial payment for his dental care.
> The owner of your lawncare company is a patient, and you both agree to provide a flat credit each year to each other.

Caution: Math with Discounts

When you are looking at what discounts you want to potentially provide to your patients, you want to make sure you understand what you are actually giving them and what the return will be to your practice. A business runs to provide service to a client but also to earn a profit. Profits help provide resources to improve/maintain equipment, give bonuses or raises to team members, and generate a return for the owner for the risk of owning the business.

According to the American Dental Association, the average dental office across the country runs around 70% overhead/30% profit margin. For the following example though we will use what top offices typically generate, which is a 60% overhead and 40% profit mix.

When you have a 60% overhead, that means you are profiting 40 cents on every dollar from your normal fees.

Discount	Profit	Required work
20%	1/2	2×
30%	1/4	4×
35%	1/8	8×

Let's say you then offer a 20% discount on a service for a patient. That means you are now collecting 80 cents on the dollar, with the same overhead, which gives you a profit of only 20 cents: half your normal rate. And the office has to work twice as hard to earn the same 40 cents.

What Happens if You Provide a 30% Discount?

If you collect 70 cents on the dollar, with the same 60 cents overhead, you have a profit of 10 cents. This is one-fourth the profit from your normal fees, meaning you have to work four times as hard for the same money.

It is important that before you consider offering discounts, you should predict the ramifications those discounts may have on your office effort and revenue.

How Can You Make Prepayment or Other Discounts Work Out Well Without Losing Money?

Many offices will say they are uncomfortable adding a 10% prepayment discount because of the above formula for effort versus profit. A possible solution to this dilemma is to raise all your fees 10%. As mentioned before, the prepayment discount is basically a cash patient discount where you are getting your normal office fees without getting into the fraud concerns.

If you raise your fees 10% and then apply a 10% prepayment benefit, it may incent more patients to prepay. With a prepayment discount, your patients who prepay will experience no change in costs. The patients who do not want to take advantage of the discount are possibly telling you that there may be an issue when it comes to collecting money or maintaining their appointment. Therefore, these patients will be the only ones paying 10% more.

Chapter 20
Advanced Insurance Coding

This section is going to review internal coding, multi-coded services, commonly misused codes, and handling insurance audits. It is meant to serve as a good overview to an otherwise extremely complex and lengthy concept.

For ease of reference, here is the list of ADA code groupings. The American Dental Association (ADA) creates and maintains a list of codes that define most of the common services in dentistry. These codes always start with a D and are followed by four digits. The first of the four digits corresponds to the category of service. For example, endodontic codes are also referred to as the D3000 codes.

CDT codes	Category of service
D0100–D0999	Diagnostic
D1000–D1999	Preventative
D2000–D2999	Restorative
D3000–D3999	Endodontics
D4000–D4999	Periodontics
D5000–D5899	Removable prosthetics
D5900–D5999	Maxillofacial (surgical) prosthetics
D6000–D6199	Implants
D6200–D6999	Fixed prosthetics
D7000–D7999	Oral surgery
D8000–D8999	Orthodontics
D9000–D9999	Adjunctive

These codes are designed to be used for communication with insurance companies for the purpose of claims reimbursement.

INTERNAL "SLUSH" CODING

ADA codes are not meant to describe every service that can be done in a dental office, only the ones where insurance may provide reimbursement. Therefore, this leaves a list of services in a dental office that aren't defined by a common code. These additional services can be best described using an internal, or "slush," code. Internal codes are ones that do not necessarily need to be submitted to insurance. Insurance companies will not understand them anyway since they are not ADA recognized codes. Internal codes are developed by the office team to supplement the ADA codes and are best used to provide clarity around a service provided to a patient that is atypical or a modification to another service.

How Do I Code for Upgrade Fees?

The most common example of this is teeth bleaching. While there are ADA codes for bleaching of teeth, insurance never pays for them, and the ADA code is written to be per arch. Since it is rare for a dentist/office to provide bleaching on a single arch, many offices will use an internal code instead of the ADA code.

Common services where you might use internal coding:

- Bleaching
- Rush fees
- Upgrade fees
- Cosmetic lab fees
- In-office products
- Services without a good ADA code
- Bulk services
- Membership plans

MISCELLANEOUS CODES VERSUS INTERNAL CODES

It is a misconception that you have to use an ADA code for everything you do. This myth often leads to the suggestion to use the ADA miscellaneous codes when a better code does not exist. The challenge with using ADA miscellaneous codes is they can create an office nightmare with tracking.

One problem with using the miscellaneous code is the code is not descriptive of the service provided when you look back at a ledger or treatment plan. Another problem is when you classify multiple services within the same code (Dxx99), the fee must constantly change, depending on the specific mix of services attached to that code. Changing fees within a code can lead to errors as well as more potential for embezzlement or fraud by team members.

1. ADA miscellaneous codes are not descriptive of the service. If you itemize a treatment plan or ledger, it will often cause patient concerns and headaches; and
2. Multiple fees under a single code can create billing challenges, tracking problems, and potential for embezzlement or fraud.

Internal codes can often be used instead of a "miscellaneous" ADA code (Dxx99). Here is an example of ADA miscellaneous codes used for restorations with D2999:

DATE	VISIT	TH	SURF	CODE	DESCRIPTION	FEE
11/11/2020	0			D2999	Unspecif restorative proced B/R	75.00
11/11/2020	0			D2999	Unspecif restorative proced B/R	100.00
11/11/2020	0			D2999	Unspecif restorative proced B/R	125.00
11/11/2020	0			D2999	Unspecif restorative proced B/R	300.00
					Visit 0 Totals:	600.00

What are the above fees for? Can you tell?

Sure, you can add a note to them, but that requires extra steps in both their creation and backtracking. The point of being an in-network office and accepting lower fees is to be more efficient, not less. Insurance will never pay for any of these services anyway and will create a nightmare to try to process them, both for you and the insurance company.

Another challenge is that some codes require a tooth number, and others do not. A computer code cannot be set to both at the same time, and typically most systems are not designed to give access to team members for admin capability to make those changes.

Alternative example of the same fees using internal coding:

DATE	VISIT	TH	SURF	CODE	DESCRIPTION	FEE
11/11/2020	0	8		LF300	Cosmetic Lab Upgrade	300.00
11/11/2020	0	8		LF301	Custom Staining	100.00
11/11/2020	0	20		LF135	Survey Crown	75.00
11/11/2020	0	20		LF200	Lab Rush Fee	125.00
					Visit 0 Totals:	600.00

Can you tell what each fee is for now? Is there any question?

Each service is now set to a specific code, with a unique identifier and descriptor, and has a unique fee attached. This prevents the team from ever needing to change fees in the system, which will avoid potential mistakes or abuse.

Best practice with miscellaneous codes is to create your own internal coding system that is more descriptive and better suited for the needs of the office. The ADA does not create these codes because many of them would be too custom to each office, and the ADA code set is designed for national use. The ADA codes are also designed to communicate to insurance for reimbursement; they were never intended for general practice billing.

Internal codes provide the office a more efficient way to explain costs in a ledger as well as providing a set flat fee for the service. This prevents the team from needing to ever change fees in a system and leads to more efficiency and clarity within a dental office.

MULTI-CODED SERVICES

One of the best parts about dentistry is most of our work is fairly straightforward and simple to understand. Unfortunately, working with insurance is not nearly as straightforward and simple. There are several examples of treatments where dentists look for a single ADA code to describe; but in reality, that service can only be described through a combination of several codes.

An easy example of this is a dental implant. When you talk about an implant with a patient, most often what the patient is thinking is the entire process of getting a new tooth. From a coding perspective, however, there are minimally three codes required to describe that process (there could be others).

- The implant itself (artificial root)
- The crown that simulates function and aesthetics
- The abutment that connects the two parts together

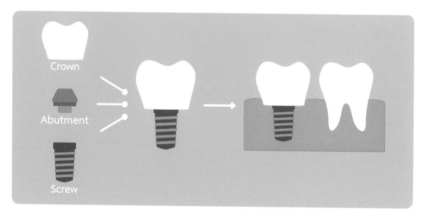

When you describe an implant to a patient, you are likely thinking of three procedures where the patient is probably thinking just one. This can be a concern when the dentist tells the patient they need an implant, and the treatment plan shows three itemized services (implant, abutment, crown). This can also be a concern if the office provides a treatment plan for an implant only, and the patient is expecting a replacement tooth to be included in the cost estimate.

When you prepare a treatment plan for multi-coded services, it is important to plan the entire case as a whole so the patients are aware of everything they are starting. This may take a little more time and effort at the beginning but will save you and the patient potential headaches and wasted time in the future.

The following page has an example treatment plan for an implant that removes the itemization of procedures. Instead of dealing with coding and itemized fees, this example option can devote space to answering some common questions:

- How long will this take?
- How can I make this affordable?
- What are my optional services?

IMPLANT TREATMENT PLAN

Patient: _____   Date: _____

Implants are a three-step process:

1. Implant placement – 60-minute appointment
2. Impressions – 30-minute appointment
3. Delivery – 30-minute appointment

The total treatment time will be _____ months.

The fee for this service will be: $_____

Insurance estimate: $_____

Please check if you would like either of these optional services:

_____Temporary tooth - $

_____Sedation - $

Total treatment fee: _____

We have a variety of ways to help make this treatment affordable; please choose which option is right for you:

___Pre-payment in full discount option: $_____

___In-office payment option (6 months): $_____down and $_____ /month

___In-office payment option (12 months): $_____down and $_____ /month

___Care credit payment option (60 months): $_____down and $_____ /month

_____**I understand if insurance does not pay for any reason that I am responsible for the full amount**.

I acknowledge I have read and understand this form and have received a copy today. I understand the fees in this treatment plan are valid for 90 days but may change after that time. I understand these fees do NOT include general dentistry treatment on other areas or teeth.

_____   _____
Patient signature   Date

_____   _____
Treatment coordinator signature   Date

HOW TO HANDLE "ALL-ON-4"/HYBRID CASES

The most misunderstood and asked about treatment is what is commonly referred to as "All-on-four." Also known as a hybrid denture or hybrid prosthetic, this is a denture that is permanently screwed into place on top of four or more implants. The confusion in these cases is that each case has several codes that are required to correctly describe and bill for the service. It is very similar to an implant with three codes (implant, abutment, crown), just more complex.

Many dentists and offices will misinterpret the coding mix required for a hybrid case.

The ADA codes D6114/D6115 refer to a hybrid prosthetic for the upper or lower arch. However, these two codes alone do not accurately describe the entire hybrid process. And this is where a lot of offices struggle with how to handle these with both patient billing and insurance claim submission.

The patient cost for a hybrid denture can be anywhere from $20,000 to $40,000 per arch, including the surgery, sedation, and prosthetics. Often the lab fees for these are rather high as well, in the $2000–$5000 range per arch. In addition, all the implant and prosthetic parts add up to a lot of initial cost to work these cases.

Insurance companies often have a fee for the D6114/D6115 that is lower than the cost for the lab/materials the office must cover. This is because these codes only describe the acrylic teeth that are attached to the hybrid denture, they do not describe all the other parts of the appliance process.

When you think about a hybrid denture, you must consider all the multiple parts involved in that process. Each part typically is reported by a separate code. Here is a basic list of the most common codes surrounding a hybrid denture, there may be more, depending on the case.

Extractions	D7140–D7251
Alveoloplasty	D7310–D7321
Tori removal	D7471–D7485
Sinus lifts	D7951–D7952
Bone grafts	D7953 or D614
Sedation	D9222–D9248
Implants	D6010
Temporary abutments	D6051
Temporary denture	D6118/D6119
Titanium bar	D6055
Final abutments/attachments	D6056, D6191, D6192
Final denture	D6114/D6115
On-site lab technician	Internal code

*If you are installing a Zirconia hybrid (instead of the normal acrylic), then this should require either an upgrade fee or can be coded as a fixed implant/abutment retained bridge instead of the denture codes.

As you can see, hybrid dentures are *far more* than just the single code that many dentists and offices mistakenly believe. It is important to use all the coding available. Most of these codes will not be covered, and therefore will be at office full fee. There is no reason that an office should be constrained much, if at all, with PPO contracted fees that would prevent you from being able to do these cases at reasonable prices.

Patient Discussions

These hybrid cases are often all-or-nothing approaches. Unlike traditional dentistry, there is not really an option to remove parts of the plan. The above coding list has a level of complexity that can confuse even an experienced dental team member; what do you think the average patient will understand?

Similar to single implant services, it would simplify the process for everyone involved to avoid the itemized lists. Itemizing out an insurance code list tends to only add confusion and a potential for patients to want to "pull things off the menu," which is not really an option in these types of cases. Coding should purely be used to help communicate with the insurance company for any potential reimbursement, not for patient illustration or education.

The other thing to think about with these complex cases is they often include multiple providers, many of whom may not be contracted with the insurance company (specialist, anesthesiologist, on-site lab technician, etc.).

The offices who manage these cases often illustrate treatment with flat case fees to remove the complexity for all involved.

One thought is to make sure that if you do need to itemize out a plan, ensure that the sum total of the individual items far exceeds the full case fee. It helps to remove any ideas the patient might have that it is a menu to pick and choose from.

TIP

Treatment plans for cases like this are much better presented to the patient as full case fees. Itemizing out an insurance code list tends to only add confusion and a potential for patients to want to "pull things off the menu," which is not really an option. Coding should purely be used to help for insurance reimbursement, not for patient illustration or education.

The following page has an example treatment plan that removes the itemization of coding, simplifies the explanation to the patient, and provides patient waivers for any in-network concerns with pricing.

HYBRID TREATMENT PLAN

Patient: _____   Date: _____

Treatment goals: _____

Care covered by this plan:

    Surgery and sedation for the (upper/lower) jaw

    Temporary smile for day 1

    Final customized smile

The total treatment time will be _____ months.

Total investment: _____

Insurance estimate: $_____

We have a variety of ways to help make this treatment affordable; please choose which option is right for you:

10% pre-payment in full courtesy	Save $_____	$_____
Pay at time of treatment		$_____
No-interest payment plan	12 months	$_____
Extended payment plan	60 months	$_____

_____I understand if insurance does not pay for any reason that I am responsible for the full amount.

I acknowledge I have read and understand this form and have received a copy today and that treatment plan options have been presented to me. I understand the fees in this treatment plan are valid for 90 days but may change after that time. I understand that insurance is an estimate, and I will be responsible for the total fee for this treatment. I understand much of the treatment course I have decided to take is beyond insurance coverage; therefore, I wish to waive my insurance plan guidelines for these upgraded services, and I release the provider, Dr. _____, from the contractual terms of my plan in this case.

_____   _____
Patient signature   Date

_____   _____
Treatment coordinator signature   Date

HOW TO HANDLE COMMONLY MISUSED CODES

As dentists, we get a great education in how to provide dentistry but a poor education in how to handle coding and insurance. Team members tend to get even less education, often being trained by the previous person who had that job (whether or not the previous person fully understood what they were doing).

There is not enough space in this book to be able to review every dental code, and other books already go over those in detail. Therefore, this section is going to review only the most commonly misused codes and how to correctly make them work for you and your office for your patient's benefit.

Simple (D7140) vs Surgical (D7210) Extractions

D7210 Description in 2021: "extraction, erupted tooth requiring removal of bone and/or sectioning of tooth, and including elevation of mucoperiosteal flap if indicated. Includes related cutting of gingival and bone, removal of tooth structure, minor smoothing of socket and closure."

Several years ago, the ADA changed the definition of surgical extractions. The D7210 code no longer requires a flap, mostly because of the industry shift toward atraumatic extractions and flapless surgery. As you can see from the above description, to correctly report a D7210 a provider would need to report either:

1. Bone removal required to remove the tooth

or

2. Sectioning a tooth was required to remove it

For simplicity purposes for the dental assistants, if the dentist picked up a handpiece to get a tooth out, it is most likely a surgical extraction, D7210. No handpiece usually means simple extraction, D7140. This is because the main way to either remove bone or section a tooth would be a handpiece and burr.

You want to make sure within your clinical notes you specify at least one (or both) of these two key phrases to justify charging for the higher-cost surgical extraction.

> **EXAMPLE**
>
> "Tooth #3 surgically sectioned and bone intentionally removed in order to successfully remove the tooth and roots completely."

This same line from your clinical notes is best to copy within the narrative you send to the insurance company to justify the service and prevent them from trying to down-code and reimburse you less.

CONTROVERSY NOTE

It is a common debate among dentists that bone can be removed with other instruments (such as an elevator) and teeth can be sectioned other ways (such as a cowhorn forceps). The real answer to this debate is to go back to the original code description. The ADA code for a surgical extraction says if the bone removal or tooth sectioning was required to remove the tooth. Unintentional bone removal with an elevator or unintentional sectioning with a pair of forceps would not fit with the code description.

This controversy often arises with in-network providers because of the fee difference. Because insurance companies often require incredibly deep price cuts, the dentists are trying to find a way to get fairly compensated.

However, what code you use should have nothing to do with reimbursement. Always use the code that fits the description of the service and bill only what you do. This push beyond coding descriptions by dentists is what insurance companies use as justification for down-coding and why many companies may automatically down-code a surgical extraction to a simple extraction. If this happens, it is important to know the exact definition of the code and have the insurance company reprocess the claim.

Periodontal Maintenance (PM D4910) vs Prophylaxis (PX D1110)

The most controversial debate that occurs in dentistry in the US surrounds the question, "What is the difference between a PM and a PX?" On a simple level:

   PM: Cleaning teeth on a patient with periodontal disease and bone loss

   PX: Cleaning teeth on a patient with no periodontal disease or bone loss

But it is far more complex when you look at specifics. The controversy occurs where one code starts and the other ends, since patients often present somewhere in between instead of at the extremes. In order to sort through the complexity, this section is going to focus on some basic details so that you can help determine for your own office how you want to handle these cases. There is no common agreement, best practice, or "standard of care" when it comes to this topic as dentists are often split down the middle.

Can We Alternate Billing Between PX and PM?

The short answer is no, this would typically be considered incorrect billing. While there is debate on whether a patient who develops periodontal disease can later go into remission, no one tends to debate that this actually cannot happen on a recurring three-month frequency from disease to health to disease and back again. When you bill for a service, you need to bill for exactly what you did. You should never bill for what insurance may or may not pay for. The reason this question tends to arise is because some rare insurance policies will cover two PMs and two PXs in a given year.

The correct way to handle this is to always file what you did, the PM. Then every alternate claim you should write a narrative asking for the alternative benefit of a PX (instead of the PM). This will allow the patient to get their four covered cleanings per year (two PMs and two PXs) but still allow the office to maintain the most correct billing.

EXAMPLE **NARRATIVE**

"Please provide alternative benefit of a D1110"

The next concern over coding is due to the way insurance handles the difference between PM and PX. PM is typically a basic service that comes with co-pays and deductibles, whereas PX is unfortunately described as "two free cleanings per year" by employers and insurance companies.

This means that if you code a PM instead of a PX on an in-network patient, it takes their out-of-pocket costs from $0 to $30 or more. It is common for patients to complain about this difference and the dreaded phrase "I just want my free cleaning" gives nightmares to most admin dental teams.

Since there is no universally accepted answer, let's review the three most common options so your team can figure out what works best within your office.

Option 1 - "Once a perio patient, always a perio patient"

This approach revolves around the generally accepted idea that periodontal disease is all about bone loss, and since bone loss typically cannot be reversed, a patient with perio will always need PM. This is more of a clinical mind-set.

Option 2 - "People and circumstances can change, nothing is absolute"

This approach revolves around the analogy that we often see patients who may not have cured their periodontal disease, but with treatment and better home care, the disease will become dormant for years. If a patient has no bleeding and minimal calculus buildup, why would you charge more than a routine cleaning (PX)?

With this philosophy, patients who show minimal signs of perio other than previous bone loss can and should be billed based on the amount of time/effort it takes to treat them, which often is no longer than a non-perio patient. Under this logic, over time PM patients may start to be billed as PX patients if their condition improves and treatment starts to take less time and effort. This is more of a business mind-set.

Option 3 - "We just want to avoid complaints"

This approach is taken by a dentist/team who really want option 1 but do not want to deal with the worst complaints that come from the rather poor way insurance describes hygiene in dentistry. These offices will try to keep patients on PM but end up changing to PX for patients who complain about billing (getting their free cleanings) in order to keep the patients in the office.

No matter which philosophy/approach your team chooses, please realize there is no solid agreement within dentistry, and therefore any of these options will work. The best thing to do is discuss this dilemma with your whole team and determine the philosophy and approach that works best for your office. This is not a topic to use as a reason to accuse or label someone on your team as unethical or uninformed. There truly is no best answer.

Full Mouth Debridement (FMD D4355)

This procedure results in one of the most incorrectly used codes in dentistry. The reason is that there is no clear code to accurately define a patient who hovers between healthy (PX) and full periodontal disease (SRP), given the way the ADA codes are set. To give you a broader, international viewpoint on this, many countries actually charge based on time with the hygienist instead of based on static codes that have very fuzzy lines in between. Until someone in the US decides that several codes to describe cleaning junk off teeth isn't rational, we have to manage with the current flawed coding system.

FMD is not a code for patients who have gingivitis or otherwise are diagnosed somewhere between healthy and perio. The FMD code was originally created to be a code that is rarely used.

FMD is specifically a code that is used when you "cannot adequately diagnose the tissues (teeth and gums)." In other words, if the gross calculus is built up so much you cannot determine the level of periodontal health, then an FMD is a good code to use. Due to being unable to diagnose the tissues, conceptually you cannot file a D0150 comprehensive exam along with an FMD. And many insurance companies will deny claims when you put these two codes together.

The correct way to use an FMD is:

> Visit 1: FMD and D0140 – Limited exam

> Visit 2: (SRP or PX) and D0150 – Comprehensive exam

Gingivitis Cleaning (D4346)

Since FMD was incorrectly used so often, the ADA created this code to be used for patients who hover between healthy and perio, PX and SRP. The problem with this code is that insurance companies do not like it, do not want it, and have tried to kill it. They actually succeeded in 1995 when another code with almost the same description came out and was eventually phased out.

(1995) D4345 — "Periodontal scaling performed in the presence of gingival inflammation."

(2017) D4346 — "Scaling in presence of generalized moderate or severe gingival inflammation."

Why is this code a problem?

The original design of the code was to create something that correctly communicated to the insurance company that added time/effort and therefore cost is involved with treating a patient who is not healthy but is not yet at the bone loss stage. These patients often need a lot of counseling in order to avoid becoming SRP/perio patients. Because of this, the fee for the gingivitis code should be 50–100% higher than a prophy code. However, insurance companies do not want to find reasons to pay more for services, especially routine recurring services such as hygiene.

Many insurance companies currently treat D4346 in one of four ways:

1. Preventive service with the same fee as a PX
2. Basic service with the same fee
3. Basic service with a higher fee
4. Major service under the periodontics category with a higher fee and lower percentage

With option 1, there is zero reason to use this new code. Clinical notes describe the health of the tissue and what was done to treat it, not insurance codes. If the price and results are the same, why even have a different code? (Remember, ADA codes are purely for insurance reimbursement, not for describing clinical cases.)

With option 2, the patient now goes from a free cleaning to something with both a co-pay and deductible. This approach requires a lot of admin team time to get the patient to understand why, and since there is no increased fee, an office is actually worse off for trying to correctly use this code.

With option 3, you still get the added time hassle to explain to the patient why they don't get their free cleaning, but at least you get paid more for it. The problem is often the amount of increased reimbursement does not justify the added headaches and complaints, not to mention the added time of the hygienist. To truly be a valuable code, the reimbursed fee for it needs to be significantly higher (e.g., 50–100% higher).

Option 4 has the same challenges at option 3 but is now even worse because insurance is helping at a lower percentage rate.

Unless the way this code is treated by insurance companies changes dramatically, we are likely to see it disappear, just like its sister code years ago.

If you are going to try to use this code, it would be a great idea for your team to role-play all the complaints that patients will have with its use so that you can be prepared to answer the questions patients will inevitably have.

Scaling and Root Planing (D4341/D4342)

This is a reference point to follow the discussion points about periodontal disease coding. Often offices will have challenges with reimbursement on these periodontal services, so it is incredibly important to document these cases well with complete perio charting (pocket depths, gingival margins, furcation involvement, mobility, suppuration, etc.), photos, narratives, and so forth. A majority of denied cases with scaling and root planing services provide inadequate documentation for the claims examiner to be able to approve a case. Pocket depths alone will often lead to denial.

Please see Chapter 23 for a detailed discussion and example cases on how to get paid for this commonly denied service.

Implants, Bridges, and Dentures

Many insurance companies are requesting a pano or FMX before paying for any of these three services. You should plan to always acquire recent x-rays taken before treatment for all insurance patients in anticipation of this common request. Whether you submit them with the claim or not depends on the insurance company and your experience with which ones do and do not prefer that information up front.

The reason behind this requirement is because of a LEAT (least expensive alternate treatment) clause in many insurance policies. The insurance company typically is looking to see if a partial denture would be an alternative option. The x-rays are to show if there are missing teeth on the contralateral side—opposite side, same arch (top vs bottom). If there are missing teeth on both sides, a partial denture technically is an acceptable option, and therefore that is what the policy will cover instead of the actual service provided.

As you learned from the previous chapter, the office will collect in full (network fee if in-network) the amount of the service provided. The insurance company will only pay the amount they would pay on the partial, making the patient's out-of-pocket portion higher. See Chapter 6 for a review of why insurance companies have LEAT policies.

Also make sure to check for missing tooth clauses (MTCs) when creating estimates (details in Chapter 6).

Palliative Care (D9110)

Palliative treatment is often either a misused code or an unused code because many offices do not understand it. However, insurance companies may cover this code, so knowledge and effective usage of it would serve you well. In the simplest terms, this code is for:

> Physical treatment of a painful/uncomfortable problem without solving the underlying condition, treating symptoms more than cause.

Since D9110 is treatment of a condition (pain), this code is generally not acceptable to be billed out with other definitive treatment codes (fillings, crowns, root canals, etc.). With many insurance plans D9110 can be reimbursed as often as needed, but occasionally you may find plans with frequency limitations.

Palliative care does not include the exam/evaluation or the x-rays; therefore, you can bill an exam and x-ray alongside this D9110 code.

Examples of when you should use this code:

- Smoothing a sharp edge of a tooth/restoration
- Adjusting occlusion on a painful tooth
- Removal of impacted foreign object causing gingival irritation
- Cleaning inflamed tissue around partially erupted wisdom teeth

Examples of when there are more descriptive codes:

Problem	Code
Placing temporary fillings in broken teeth/ partially removing soft decay and placing a temporary filling	D2940 – Sedative filling
Opening abscessed tooth to relieve pain	D3221 – Pulpal debridement
Incising an abscess	D7510 – Incisal and drainage
Admin local anesthetic to relieve pain	D9210 – Local anesthetic not operative/ surgical
Apply desensitizing medicament to exposed root	D9910 – Desensitizing meds

Examples of common misuse of this code:

Misuse	Use instead
First step of a root canal	1) Internal code, or 2) D3221 Pulpal debridement (not reimbursed in addition to root canal)
Definitive treatments	Code for the treatment (filling, crown, extraction, root canal, etc.)
Office visit for post-op observation	D0171 – Re-eval post-op visit
Office visit for non-post-op observation	D0170 – Re-eval non-post-op visit

Exam Codes

Most offices understand the common D0120, D0140, D0150 exam codes. The other exam codes that exist require some explanation. These other exam codes are designed to provide a more complete array of codes that are more indicative of the treatment provided. Realize in most cases insurance companies will only ever pay for two exams per year, regardless of the type of exam. Once the patient has used up their frequency of exams, the patient would be responsible for paying 100% of any subsequent exams within the year.

Failure to use these codes due to insufficient insurance reimbursement levels or feeling bad for the patient is not justified and is a disservice to the office and provider. It is not the job of the office or team to make up for inadequate coverage on the part of the insurance company and/or employer. You have no control over what coverage a patient is offered; therefore, you should take no part in ownership of that problem. The group of exam codes that follow are the codes which describe the various types of exams that are conducted by a dentist.

Exam code	Descriptor
D0170	Re-eval, non-post-op visit – assessing the status of a previous condition
D0171	Re-eval, post-op visit (if for perio treatment, better reimbursement comes from D0180)
D0180	Comprehensive eval (with full perio charting) on a patient with perio or risk factors for perio
D0190	Screening of a patient
D0191	Assessment of a patient

TIP

It is not the job of the office or team to make up for inadequate coverage on the part of the insurance company and/or employer. You have no control over what coverage a patient is offered; therefore, you should take no part in ownership of that problem.

Teledentistry (D9995/D9996)

Virtual consults are a more modern concept in dentistry and these codes came out in 2017 to help provide a way for offices to get reimbursed for any additional time/costs incurred from use of virtual technology to confer with a patient. These codes are billed in addition to the exam codes (D0140, D0170, D0171, D0190), though they are often not covered by the insurance carrier.

> D9995 teledentistry – synchronous; real-time encounter
>
> D9996 teledentistry – asynchronous; emails, recordings, and so forth

See Chapter 31 to learn more about teledentistry codes and how to use them.

REMAPPING

Remapping (previously called down-coding) is a process in which an insurance company recognizes the submitted code, reviews the case, and then decides to provide reimbursement based on an alternative benefit code.

This is often a confusing and seemingly unfair concept for offices because it would be fraud for an office to change codes. How can it be legal for an insurance company to remap codes?

One has to understand with this situation that insurance companies have a different set of rules. The reason changing codes is a problem for an office is that a code is the communication you have with the insurance company. They are not in your office when treatment is rendered, so the only information they have to go by is the coding and documentation you submit. By submitting an incorrect code, you have essentially lied to the insurance company, and they have no way of knowing.

However, insurance companies are all driven by the regulations they have in place and the policy that was purchased by the patient or employer. Any remapping of procedures is based on contract language, not whims.

When an insurance company remaps a code, this is their way of communicating to the office information contained within the contract. Often remapping is because the employer decided they wanted to lower the premium paid for dental benefits for their employees when they signed up for the insurance policy. Therefore, the insurance company reduced the benefits available to the subscriber based on the new, lower premium budget. Remapping is one of several ways that the insurance company can reduce costs in order to reach the budgetary needs of the subscriber or employer.

It might also help to understand what would happen if insurance companies did not remap codes. If the insurance company did not have the ability to remap codes, you would see far more denials with notes that the policy does not cover that procedure mix. The process of remapping is the insurance company's way of still being able to process the claim without additional headaches for both the office and insurance company.

In short: yes, it is legal for an insurance company to remap fees for reimbursement.

What follows is a discussion around several common scenarios where remapping or down-coding tends to happen.

Insurance Challenges with Remapping X-Rays

If you are out of network, all this means is the insurance company will reimburse less, and the patient is responsible for more. But overall, the office still collects the same amount of money.

If you are in-network, often the contracts are written such that any remapping of x-rays is what the office agreed to accept as payment in full for the services provided. This is why it can be incredibly important to understand these common remapping scenarios so the office can be aware and give patients a good estimate.

How Does Insurance Define an FMX?

While dentists and the ADA define an FMX as 14–20 x-rays, insurance companies often re-map a much lower number of x-rays to an FMX. The most common number to get remapped is either 7 or 8 x-rays (4 BWs and 3–4 PAs). Each insurance company is a little different, so it can be important to know this distinction with each company.

The more accurate way of knowing whether a series of x-rays will be remapped to an FMX is based on cost. When you add up the cost of 4BWs and the individual PAs, whenever that number goes above the insurance fee for an FMX, typically insurance will remap. Again, this is not a set rule everywhere, just the most common rule of thumb used by insurance companies and the easiest for teams to understand.

EXAMPLE X-RAY SCENARIO

4 BWs – $41
1st PA – $17
Additional PAs – $14
FMX - $90
7 x-rays (4 BWs, 3 PAs) = $86
8 x-rays (4 BWs, 4 PAs) = $100

In this case, seven x-rays are most likely to be paid as submitted, but eight x-rays would be remapped to an FMX since the individual costs would go above $90 (the price of the FMX).

Understanding the FMX pricing distinction makes a difference for the office in terms of what is likely to be collected. However, the larger difference will be for the patient due to frequency issues. FMX and pano almost always share frequency, meaning if one is paid, the other will not be during the time frame. The typical time frame is three to five years.

Here are some common scenarios that come up that cause confusion and challenges with this issue of remapping and reimbursement.

FMX and Pano Scenario

Let's say you submit x-rays, which is not an FMX according to the ADA. Insurance may likely remap the reimbursement to an FMX. If the patient needs a pano next year because of erupting wisdom teeth, the pano will not be covered because it will exceed the frequency limitation. The patient will have to pay out of pocket for the pano.

Two-Providers Scenario

As a different scenario, let's say you have a new patient. This patient just saw another provider seven months ago and had eight x-rays taken but now wants to switch to you. BWs and PAs are likely to be reimbursed because BWs often have a six-month frequency, and PAs often have no frequency. However, if you take eight x-rays or more, the insurance is likely to remap those x-rays as an FMX, so the patient will have no reimbursement for those x-rays and will need pay out of pocket. If you instead only took seven x-rays, the patient would have coverage and no out-of-pocket costs. As you can imagine, this might make a big difference for the patient.

Same-Day FMX/Pano or BWs/Pano

If the dentist decides that the patient needs both an FMX and pano on the same day, one of the two will not be covered. When submitting both, the insurance company is likely to pay on the lower cost service and disallow the higher cost service to an in-network provider.

A more common scenario to the FMX/pano is when dentists will want to see four bitewings and a pano for new patients. The challenge with this x-ray mix is the same as with remapping to an FMX, insurance will remap any number of x-rays that add up to be more expensive than the FMX fee. This means that the bitewings will often not be paid, and the bitewing frequency clock will likely be started.

A common incorrect solution that offices take with this problem is to split the claims. It would be fraudulent to change the date of service, so it is advised not to do this. Another route would be to take the x-rays on the same day but file the claims on separate days (with the same date of service). This second route is not fraudulent, but it is deceptive. The insurance system will likely process the claims separately and pay separately. However, this error is often caught later, and insurance will demand their overpayment back (see Chapter 12 for insurance refunds).

The most correct solution to this problem is to physically take the pano on a separate day. This way both the bitewings and pano would be processed on separate claims, cannot be remapped, and therefore the office gets paid more in line with the services provided. This would also not be in error; therefore, insurance will not ask for refunds later.

How to Enter Payment for a Remapped Service

It is common for an insurance company to remap the individual x-rays that were taken to an FMX instead for reimbursement. This can cause some confusion with the team on how to enter payments into the office ledger (or system).

First, you should understand that what the office submitted was completely correct, and therefore nothing should be changed within your system or ledgers. Remapping is purely for the insurance to reimburse the service, not because the office did anything wrong.

Next, enter the actual reimbursement payment received as you would any other. If you are asked to set specific numbers to each service, just split crediting the payment for the FMX between the pano and bitewings to add up to the amount reimbursed. Make sure that each allocation of payment does not exceed the cost of the service for the pano or bitewings.

An in-network office would then adjust off the fee difference between the pano + BWs and the FMX as an insurance adjustment.

An out-of-network office would have the choice on whether to write off as a courtesy or to bill the patient the remaining balance (see Chapter 19 on discounts).

Within the adjustment, best practice would be to write a note that "insurance paid on D0210 - FMX."

EXPERT TIP

Insurance often has a three to five-year frequency limitation for reimbursement of an FMX or pano. Best practice would be to create an internal code for "FMX/pano payment." This would allow the office to track back the last time either an FMX or pano was covered, allowing you to more quickly advise the patient on their potential benefits for a new x-ray.

This code would need no fee attached to it as it would just be for tracking.

CBCTs and Panoramic X-rays

CBCTs are usually not covered by insurance. Therefore, a common concern for offices is whether they can help the patient by submitting a pano instead for partial reimbursement for the patient's benefit. CBCTs most often come with a rendered pano included within the readout that is generated.

When one looks at the ADA dental coding, the code description does not specify how the x-ray was acquired.

Therefore, yes, an office would be able to capture a CBCT and submit a pano to insurance for partial payment.

EXAMPLE

If your office has a CBCT fee of $300 and a pano fee of $150, you may submit a claim for the pano and charge the patient for the remaining $150 that will not be covered by insurance.

Q: Our patient had a pano four years ago. The patient today needs a CBCT. Will the patient get reimbursement?

A: Depends mostly on the frequency. If there is a five-year frequency limitation, likely the patient will have no expected reimbursement and will need to pay 100% out of pocket. Commonly, coverage for an FMX, Pano, or CBCT have shared frequency.

Panoramic Bitewings – What to File?

This works the same as CBCTs and panoramics. ADA coding does not specify how the x-ray is acquired. Regardless of whether you use a film, intra-oral sensor, or a pano machine if the result is to obtain bitewings, the office should file a bitewing code.

The code should depend on the dentition of the patient, just like traditional bitewings.

If the twelve-year molars have erupted, a pano BW would be submitted as:

D0274 – Bitewings – four films.

If the twelve-year molars are unerupted, then a pano BW would be submitted as:

D0272 – Bitewings – two films.

Since panos will only take the entire mouth at once (both sides), there should be no instance where a pano BW should be filed as a single bitewing code.

Chapter 21
Insurance Audits

If you are in-network with an insurance company, you may occasionally get an audit letter like the one shown here.

Why we're contacting you
You are receiving this letter because we have identified a claim submission pattern from your dental office that does not appear to be consistent with other dental practices. We recognize there are unique characteristics of a dental practice that could result in different claim submission patterns. Our analysis has been adjusted to account for the mix of patients specific to your practice receiving these services.

What you need to know
Our billing pattern analytics are based upon claims submitted and services rendered between 06/2017 - 06/2018.

A total of 97,032 general dentist practices were analyzed, and it was determined that you are submitting a greater percentage of claims for Large Fillings than most general dentists. Your office has one of the highest utilization rates of Large Fillings registering at 69%, while most other offices that provided these services had a rate of 24%.

Additional information
We are including the ADA's Current Dental Terminology Descriptor for the indicated procedure(s). Large Fillings:
Direct restorations that include three or more tooth surfaces. Large fillings include CDT Codes D2160, 02161, 02332, 02335, 02393 and 02394.

MetLife has a responsibility to ensure that claims are appropriately processed, and as such, we will continue ongoing review of claim submissions. This could include a request for clinical documentation on future claims for these specific services if this claim pattern continues. In that instance these claims will be reviewed for necessity by a specific MetLife dentist consultant. Such information will enable us to continue to ensure that claims are appropriately processed. In addition, we can use the results of our claim reviews to inform Dentists of our findings, as well as to help design and manage our benefit plans to help accommodate the needs of our clients and their members.

Sincerely,

Dental Product Management

These letters typically state something like "You are doing significantly more of this procedure than an average provider." This information/data shared is usually presented as a percentage of patients treated. For example, "You are providing more D7210 surgical extractions vs D7140 simple extractions than the average provider."

A common feeling or concern expressed by dental office teams is that these letters are designed to scare the dentists into providing less expensive care.

While this view may have some truth to it, do realize that the people who monitor trends in an insurance company often have the training and belief they are revealing potentially adverse trends, thereby providing helpful "early warning" to offices. If there are billing issues you are unaware of, it can be valuable to know and have an opportunity to correct before it develops into an investigation that could cost the office/dentist a lot of money.

The reality is the process of reviewing and uncovering trends does help to curb overall costs. Insurance companies continue to maintain these types of systems because they are shown to save money in the long run. Dental offices do take notice when trends are pointed out and often reduce billing errors, translating into lower cost claims.

These letters are typically computer-generated, though, just following a formula. If you receive a computer-generated letter such as this example, there is no general response expected or necessary to the insurance company. If you have a billing system error, just correct it, and move on. If you feel these letters are pointless, you are not required to respond.

The important understanding for the team is that receiving a computer-generated audit letter does not necessarily mean the dentist is doing anything improper. Here are some example scenarios which reflect positive office procedures that may generate a trend outside of the average:

- The hygienists have better-than-normal training on spotting and treating periodontal disease early. When you treat the expected amount of perio according to the ADA and AAP, you will have a significantly higher amount of SRP claims than the average office/dentist.
- You work in an area with a lower-than-average dental IQ. As a result, patients go to the dentist for preventive care less often, and you will naturally have a higher incident of treatment needs.
- Your dentist has advanced surgical training and therefore will be doing more surgical extractions compared to an average dentist who refers many of the more difficult cases to specialists.
- Your dentist has advanced training in root canals and therefore treats more of them in office than the average dentist who has received minimal training from dental school.

These letters are helpful to use as a reminder to review your systems and make sure everything is being done correctly. If you cannot find a concern within your procedures, especially if you have a similar situation to any of the above scenarios, then you are likely fine continuing to work as normal.

If you feel like it is important for you to send a response, the best practice is to send something descriptive but brief. Be nice, professional, and provide reasoning to why your office will naturally have a different outcome/trend than normal. It also helps to provide a definition of the dental code that is in question and that you follow this code based on the exact ADA description.

Here is an example of a potential response:

> "We received your letter dated <Month/Day/Year> letting us know you have detected a distinct claim submission pattern from our office, specifically a higher level of surgical extractions. Thank you for your review. We are proud to respond with the explanation that our dentist has more advanced training in surgical extractions, and therefore you will see us treating a higher proportion of D7210s. Unlike the average dentist, we rarely refer out these types of treatments. We only submit them when intentionally sectioning and/or removing bone as the dental code requires."

Chapter 22
Treatment Planning with Insurance

Insurance can be complex and confusing to many dental professionals who deal with it every day. Can you imagine how much more confusing it can be to a patient who has no training or experience?

Many of us understand our patient's confusion but often make it worse with the approach that is commonly taught in dental offices. Have you ever gone to get your car fixed and had the mechanic try to explain what was wrong with the car? He or she starts rattling off words you don't understand or referencing parts in the car you never knew existed. Your brain starts to fog up, and you end up thinking of other things while they are talking, such as how much all of this is going to cost or whether it is all really necessary. For those who understand their car well, you can probably imagine a similar situation with a CPA trying to explain IRS tax law or a lawyer trying to explain legal language. The problem in all these scenarios is our natural tendency to try to help someone understand our profession and instead end up making the situation worse.

Dentistry alone can be hard to explain at times; then adding insurance makes it far worse. In order to appreciate how to help our patients the best way possible, we need to think about what they really want to know. Here is the short list of typical patient questions before a dental treatment:

- What is the problem that needs correction?
- What is the proposed solution?
- How many trips will it take to fix?
- How much time will it take to fix?
- What level of discomfort can I expect?
- How much will it cost?

We can answer all these questions without giving the patient a crash course in dental terminology or a 20-minute diatribe on the details of the insurance breakdown we spent an hour on the phone trying to retrieve. Most patients just want the basics. They want to be talked to like a normal human being, not a dental professional.

We need to realize when people don't ask for certain information, it is often because they do not need or want that information. This is especially true for dental insurance.

What does this mean when it comes to insurance estimates?

Less is more!

The fewer details we give, often the more clarity we provide the patient. This not only helps the patient better understand treatment but also takes less time for the team. Here are some ways you can accomplish this:

- Do not give insurance details without being asked
- Avoid itemization of the treatment plan
- Be more confident in your estimate

Let's discuss each of these for better clarity.

Insurance Details

Many offices spend a long time obtaining and preparing a complete breakdown of an insurance policy's benefit to be able to give an accurate estimate. It is only natural to want to convey all that information we learned. That is the wrong approach for most patients.

Example case: Mrs. Jones is your patient with insurance. She has a few cavities and a broken tooth, and prevention of future problems is a large concern for her. The dentist presented a treatment plan, which included a few fillings, a buildup and crown, and a couple of sealants.

Common Discussion

"Mrs. Jones, your dentist diagnosed you as needing a mesial-occlusal filling on No.3, a distal-occlusal filling on No.4, a crown on No.14, and sealants on tooth 2, 15, 18, and 31. Your crown is going to need a buildup to be able to stay on.

"You have a $50 deductible. Your insurance covers your fillings at 80%, your crown at 50%, and your sealants are not covered. Your insurance downgrades composites to amalgam, and downgrades crowns to base metal, which means you have to pay more for each of the fillings and crown.

"Your first filling is going to be $90 because of your deductible and co-pay; the second one will be $40. Your buildup will be $150. The crown is $600 because of your downgrade. And the sealants will be $40 each.

"Do you have any questions?"

Now, I don't know about you, but I got confused even having to write this. Can you imagine what the patient is thinking at this point? You threw a dozen numbers at them as well as several dental terms they don't understand. They are confused about the entire thing and therefore don't really want treatment anymore because when the brain becomes confused, it has a very hard time processing information and coming to a decision. In these scenarios, you often have two outcomes:

1. The patient gives you some excuse of why they cannot make a decision today, such as needing to talk to their spouse (even though they came specifically today to fix the broken tooth)

2.   They schedule the recommended appointment, the confusion never really goes away, and they end up last-minute cancelling or not showing up at all

Is the patient a problem patient or do you think you could have had something to do with why that patient did not move forward with treatment?

Best Practices Discussion

With the same patient and treatment as the previous example, let's try to make this easier on the patient.

"Mrs. Jones, Dr. X is amazing and is going to take great care of you. Do you have any questions about the plan he gave you before I talk about your insurance and finances?

"No? Great.

"To get your concerns/teeth fixed and back to a healthy condition as Dr. X advised, it will require one visit of two hours with a short follow-up visit three weeks later. After applying your insurance benefits, your portion will be $1040. Do you have any questions before we find a time that works for you to be able to take care of your teeth?"

Notice how in this scenario you answered the main patient questions in less time:

- How many trips will it take to fix?
- How much time will it take to fix?
- How much will it cost?

The other three questions about problem, solution, and discomfort should have been handled by the clinical team. You also reiterated to the patient a sense of confidence by confirming the doctor is amazing and is going to take great care of them. The patient now has clarity about what she needs, in simple, easy to understand language. Now if she has any additional questions, she can ask, and you can be prepared to answer. Every patient is different in what they want to know, and many want to know a lot less than we naturally are inclined to give them.

Mrs. Jones is far more likely to walk away with an appointment that she will show up to. More importantly, she will have better clarity about her treatment plan and therefore will be happier with her experience with you.

Itemization

"But I always have patients ask me about more insurance details and each item on the treatment plan."

Yes, often this is because you invited them to do so by itemizing out their plan and going into all the details before you answered the patient's main questions about time and money. You basically told them insurance details are more important than their treatment needs.

Patients understand their money; they don't often understand dentistry. Therefore, when they are confused, they are going to drop back to what they do know: money. When you confuse a patient and then hand them an itemized estimate, of course they are going to start picking apart the treatment list.

The moment you start having to defend each treatment item, the chance that the patient is going to show up for all the treatment and be happy about it has dropped significantly.

When you remove the itemization as with the examples with Mrs. Jones before, you simplify your process, and you often have happier patients. The few patients who still want more details will ask for them, but when they do, you will spend less time because you will be only answering the questions they want answered.

How to Create Good Insurance Estimates

One of the most common complaints about a dental office revolves around billing practices. When you have to tell patients that they owe more money than the estimate they were given, they are typically upset. It does not matter how clearly you explained it was just an estimate, they are often going to think you did something wrong. In many cases, they would be correct. The main rule to remember when it comes to an insurance estimate is: You cannot be right 100% of the time. So which of these two phrases would you rather tell a patient?

1. I'm sorry to tell you that your insurance did not pay as much as estimated; you owe an extra $100.

or

2. I'm happy to report that your insurance paid *more* than they originally told us they would; therefore, we are issuing you a credit on your account—great!

The chance of you having a patient upset with No.2 is very low, especially when you word it this way. Happier patients stay with offices longer and cause the team less hassle. It should be the goal to have far more of conversations about No.2 instead of No.1.

If in doubt, err on the side of *overestimating* how much the patient will owe.

When an insurance company tells you that it is going to pay 80% on a filling, expect a downgrade and estimate 60% instead. Or when the company tells you that it will pay 50% on a crown, estimate 40%.

This is a great starting point if you aren't 100% certain of what a particular insurance plan will pay for the treatment.

Always remember refunding money is easier and makes for happier patients. Collecting unexpected balances is a hassle and often ends up with unhappy patients. Most of us want happy patients.

When you process a claim and end up with a credit on a patient's account, you need to have a system for what to do with these credits. Credits cannot just stay with the office indefinitely according to state laws. Having multiple credits on accounts can also skew the numbers when running accounts receivable reports, which can ruin the ability of the office to stay functional.

How can you be more confident in your treatment estimates if you are out of network and do not have a fee schedule? Read the next section on Blue Books.

HOW TO ESTIMATE OUT-OF-NETWORK BENEFITS (BLUE BOOK)

The term "blue book" comes from 15th-century England because important records were often kept in blue covered books. A blue book in today's world typically refers to a collection of stats or information to serve as a guide. In this case, we are talking about a guide for what insurance will pay for out of network patients.

As you receive insurance EOBs and claim reimbursement checks in the office, you can start developing your own "blue book" guide for how each insurance company pays. Your in-house guide captures those details you really want to understand, such as how much exactly each insurance company pays for each treatment code. Insurance companies are often very predictable once you see their patterns because they operate by a defined system of rules. Each insurance company has its own internal rules; hence, keeping your blue book, organized by company and treatment code within that company, will become a great resource.

For example: if you see that Cigna should be paying $500 on their crowns based on the breakdowns you get, but you only seem to be getting $450 on the EOBs, this is information you need to keep track of.

This is especially important for out-of-network offices when you cannot get the insurance UCR fee schedule easily. The blue book becomes your basic fee schedule for each insurance company.

Most practice management software packages can keep track of this information for you so you do not have to manage it on paper. It should only take a few months to develop a fairly good start on a blue book that supplements your normal procedure codes.

Once you know exactly how much each insurance company will pay on specific procedures, you can use that number directly instead of needing to calculate an educated guess for estimates.

UNDERSTANDING PRE-DETERMINATIONS/ PRE-AUTHORIZATIONS

How to handle pre-determinations is a fairly controversial topic in dentistry because of the differences in state laws that you will see around the country. State laws directly influence how this topic is handled in individual dental offices and whether pre-determinations are worth the effort. The first thing to understand is the distinction between these terms. Both terms refer to a written estimate given before treatment is performed. The difference however can mean a lot:

Pre-determination: "not a guarantee of payment or estimate"

Pre-authorization: "guarantee of payment with adequate documentation"

Pre-authorizations are common in medical care. This is when the insurance company reviews the case/intended treatment in advance and not only tells you what it will pay, but they are also required to pay that much by law when the treatment is performed.

Dentistry is different. Pre-authorizations are not common, we instead have pre-determinations, which are not guarantees of payment.

Insurance companies aren't very fond of pre-authorizations because they have to basically agree before a treatment is done that they will pay for it as well as exactly how much they will reimburse. Pre-authorizations work to increase the acceptance rate for treatment because the insurance carrier has agreed in advance to pay for that treatment. Pre-authorizations mean the insurance company will likely have more claims to pay out.

A pre-determination is a free, optional service provided by an insurance company before a treatment and is in essence an estimate of what the patient should expect to owe. In contrast to a pre-authorization, a pre-determination is not a guarantee of payment.

Pre-determinations often work against the dental office in favor of the insurance company. Claims data show that 70% of pre-determinations in dentistry never end up with a claim being processed. This data flags the inherent problem with pre-determinations. So why does this problem happen?

A pre-determination submitted to an insurance company may take days or weeks to come back with a response. And like any other business, when clients walk out the door, there is a high chance they will not come back to complete a purchase. In retail, this usually means the client went to another store to buy, but they bought the item somewhere because they *wanted* it. In dentistry, this often means the patient just put off getting the treatment done because most patients do not *want* dental work until they *need* it.

When you tell the patient that they must wait days or weeks for a pre-determination, without realizing it, you have basically told them that the insurance coverage is more important than the treatment itself. This is why a majority of pre-determinations never result in a claim, nor the patient getting the treatment that they really need.

> **TIP**
>
> When patients are asked to wait days or weeks for a pre-determination, without realizing it, you have basically told them that the insurance coverage is more important than the treatment itself.
>
> Claims data show that 70% of pre-determinations in dentistry never end up with a claim being processed.

So Why Would an Office Champion the Use of Pre-Determinations if They Are This Problematic?

State Law

The state has a law that forces insurance companies to honor a pre-determination as a guarantee of payment (just like a pre-authorization). If you are in one of these states, a pre-determination can be an amazing thing because you have a 100% accurate estimate since the insurance company must comply (e.g., Texas enacted this law to take effect in Sept. 2020). It is important to understand that currently ERISA-based plans are not subject to state laws (see Chapter 3). Since ERISA plans often make up about half of the plans you will encounter, this law is only partially effective.

Misunderstanding

Many office teams don't understand how pre-determinations are hurting them, or they don't understand how to prepare good estimates without using them. This is the most common misunderstanding we have observed at Practice Whisperer. If you run the data for offices in non-favorable states, the treatment acceptance rate is significantly lower than average because they overuse pre-determinations, and as a result, many of their patients don't return to get treatment. The team mistakenly believes the pre-Ds are helpful because they don't track the lowered treatment acceptance rate resulting from their use.

What Are the Pros and Cons to Using Pre-Determinations Regularly in a Dental Setting?

There are a few times when pre-determinations work against the office. Most often, it is because of a lack of knowledge about insurance, and therefore, the quick fallback is to do a pre-determination on all treatment instead of learning how to develop insurance estimates more effectively. Instead of becoming skilled at managing insurance claims, the pre-determinations can become a crutch for the office.

The worst times to use pre-determinations is when the process will delay necessary treatment, and you have a patient with infections, pain, large cavities, broken teeth, and so forth, especially when you can get the treatment on the schedule today or this week. The pre-determination process delays getting your patient the care they need and also significantly lowers your acceptance for treatment.

However, there are a couple of situations where it makes good sense to take advantage of pre-determinations no matter which state you are in.

First, is to use pre-determinations on work that has to be delayed anyway. If you are booked out for weeks or if the treatment otherwise has to wait (such as waiting three months after you just removed a tooth, and the patient wants an implant). These are great times to use a pre-determination because you are not artificially delaying the timing for patient care.

Second, is when the patient did not otherwise schedule treatment. When you send out a pre-determination, both the patient and the office will get a written copy of it. You can use these letters as a great reason to contact the patient back at a later date and revisit the conversation about getting them on the schedule for treatment.

> "Your insurance company agrees you need this treatment, and great news is they are going to cover $X of it! Are there any other questions you have before we look for a good time for you to come get that treatment done?"

Pre-determinations can either be a detriment or a boon to the office, depending on how you use them. When used correctly, they can boost treatment acceptance, provide more clarity, and provide you with more ways to contact patients that have not yet scheduled treatment.

Chapter 23

How to Get Paid for Commonly Denied Services

Some of the most commonly denied procedures revolve around crowns and periodontal treatments. Often the reasons for denial can be traced to the difference in perception between a dental provider and an insurance claims examiner. Insurance companies build entire provider packets explaining what they need to see to process claims correctly. Commonly dental offices either have no idea these exist or unfortunately have never read them.

Here is a basic breakdown of how to get reimbursement on 99% of your claims involving fillings, crowns, buildups, and scaling and root planing (SRP).

FILLINGS

It might seem odd to have fillings listed here. Most fillings are auto-adjudicated and paid without human involvement at all. This means that they do not require x-rays, photos, or narratives.

However, some fillings will be flagged in the automatic system to be pulled out or auto-denied. This is where many teams get confused. "None of my other fillings get denied; what happened here?"

Many insurance policies will have an exclusion against paying for treatment resulting from abrasion, abfraction, erosion, or cosmetics. They tend to see these reasons as "elective," and therefore payment responsibility is entirely on the patient. Cosmetics is the obvious reason that many do not argue. However, many dentists and offices forget about the other reasons (abrasion, abfraction, erosion), which can cause concerns with reimbursements as well.

Every insurance company system will flag different issues. However, the generic view is that anterior fillings that include the incisal edge, especially multiple fillings, will often be pulled from the automatic system. This is because the computer system is assuming that these fillings were done as cosmetic or other non-covered reasons.

To combat this view, the team must be prepared for when such denials do happen. If the teeth were truly being treated for decay and/or fractures that were not from bruxism, then documentation with x-rays or photos should be prepared and sent with the first appeal. As long as the office can show necessity due to decay or fracture, the treatment will get reimbursed.

If the case is because of abrasion, abfraction, erosion, or cosmetics, then the best practices solution would be to advise the patient up front when presenting the estimate that insurance may not help with reimbursement. The patient should be prepared to pay 100%.

BUILDUPS

The most common reason for buildups to be rejected is that different insurance companies assess crown codes differently. Most companies treat the crown code as your "prep date," or the day the dentist prepares the crown and does most of the work.

Alternatively, some companies (such as Cigna) treat the crown code as the "seat date," or day of delivery of the crown. Contrary to some myths out there, the code itself does not define whether the treatment is prep or seat date. This determination is up to the insurance company to define. The insurance company is only defining when the company will pay for the treatment. The insurance company is not allowed to define when the office bills the patient for the treatment.

Why Does Prep Date vs Seat Date Matter with the Buildup?

Think about the procedure itself. If you place a buildup and prep a traditional crown, you then send the impressions to the lab for a couple weeks to make the crown. The crown then must be seated on a second visit, weeks after the original prep date. So, by definition, if crown codes are considered seat date, you cannot code out a crown and a buildup on the same day since that would be physically impossible to do. This is the reason you may notice companies that consider the crown codes as "seat date" seem to deny every buildup. The denial is not about the service itself and whether it was needed; it is about the timing of the procedure not matching up with how the insurance company defines the code and process.

But the Denial States "Service is Inclusive of a Crown"

Realize, as discussed in Chapter 11, that the computer systems insurance companies use to run their EOBs aren't designed to know why the service was denied. It is also true that insurance companies see many dentists misuse the buildup code D2950.

D2949 code is defined as a "Placement of restorative material to yield a more ideal form, including elimination of undercuts." This code was developed in 2014 because of the misuse of the D2950 buildup code, which is only about creating "retention" for a crown. D2949 is considered inclusive of a crown as it is either considered required to get a good impression or not necessary at all to support the crown. If the insurance company cannot tell why you needed a buildup specifically for "retention," it will assume you did a D2949 and deny it as "inclusive of a crown." This does not mean a true D2950 buildup is inclusive of a crown, just that they are assuming you used the wrong code.

Whether it is fair or whether the insurance company should assume this about buildups, you can have your opinions about; but ultimately this is what current dentists have to work with.

The way to correctly avoid problems with claims for buildups is to show the insurance company that you did a true D2950 buildup. This is why you will often see companies that request before and after x-rays of the buildup.

Also see Chapter 18 on disallowed services for more information on codes like this that are considered inclusive of other services.

What if The Insurance Company Requires Before and After X-Rays of the Buildup?

As mentioned before, the insurance company is really asking for proof that you did a D2950 buildup instead of a D2949 foundation. Either photos or x-rays will work. The insurance company communication may say x-rays only, but photos are interchangeable with x-rays for this purpose. Photos are typically faster and easier to take and provide much better views of what you are doing. Taking good photos can be a replacement for the requested x-ray in this circumstance.

What Documentation is Required to Receive Reimbursement for a Buildup?

In order to be considered a true buildup, many insurance companies will have some internal qualifiers they are looking for. Each company is slightly different, but most use a combination of the following:

- > 65% missing tooth
- < 2 mm ferrule height
- at least 1 cusp missing

If you provide documentation of all three scenarios, then you should be covered for almost any insurance company. Good photos with clear narrative go a long way to eliminating most of your denials on buildups. The best two pictures to obtain are:

1. Pre-decay removal
2. After the build-up is placed

Pre-decay removal photos will ideally show decay, fractures, missing structure, and anything else justifying both the need for the crown as well as the buildup.

After buildup photos ideally have a noticeable color difference compared to the surrounding tooth structure to make it show clearly. Here are a couple of good examples of great before and after photos for necessary buildups.

Case Example 1.   **Significantly Missing Tooth Structure**

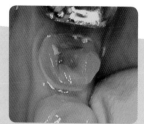 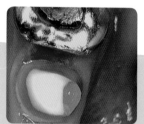

Mid-Op photo –
notice there is no question this tooth needs a BU

Post-BU photo –
notice the easy-to-see BU

Case Example 2.   **Decay Under a Prior Buildup**

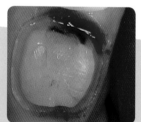 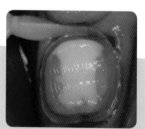

Mid-Op decay photo –
this decay would not show up on an x-ray

Post-BU photo –
notice the easy-to-see BU

The reason for this clear documentation is to show the insurance company what we see clinically that often won't show up in an x-ray. We all know that pictures are worth far more than any amount of words you can write, which makes good photos worth far more than any narratives you could write.

In case one, since the buccal part of the tooth still exists, it often won't show as broken enough on an x-ray to convey the need for a build-up.

In case two, the decay under a buildup often won't show clearly on an x-ray like it would in a photo.

When you send the correct documentation for your buildups, you will notice a significant drop in the denials you have to handle from the insurance company.

CROWNS

Crowns are some of the more expensive day-to-day procedures that dentists will provide. Naturally claims for crowns will draw the attention of the insurance company to make sure it is only paying for necessary treatment instead of elective treatment. Over the years the number of claims for crowns have increased, and insurance companies have noticed. Multiple factors affect why we are doing more crowns now than 50 years ago, but the main point to remember is if you want to get paid on crowns, you should make sure to send as much of the correct information/documentation as possible.

Realize that crown claims are processed by a human agent. The agents usually have zero dental training and are minimally trained to look for a list of specific items. If you provide that list, they generally process and accept your claim. If you do not provide good documentation consistent with their list, you get denied. So what are insurance examiners trained to look for? It depends on the company specifically, but here are the main items that most typically look for:

- Missing/broken cusps (decay or fracture)
- Previous broken/decayed crown
- Cracked tooth syndrome
- Insufficient tooth structure for a direct restoration (filling)
- Prior root canal (posterior tooth)

The more of these items you provide as reasoning, the more likely your claim will get paid.

Now, also realize what we submit to the insurance company in the form of photos and x-rays can hold more weight than anything you write in a narrative. Therefore your narrative and the visuals need to match up. You can find a great narrative checklist form on page 220.

Caution! There are on occasion dental offices that will send the exact same x-ray/photo/narrative combos with their claims (i.e., from a previous patient), and insurance companies will pick up on this as an act of lying or fraud (an example of why insurance companies do not trust every dentist).

When it comes to getting both buildups and crowns reimbursed, the following pages contain some case examples of the common reasons why the information submitted often leads to the denial of the case.

Case Example 1. Internal Fractures

One of the common reasons a tooth needs a crown is because of a fracture and/or cracked tooth syndrome. Cracked tooth syndrome is when a tooth becomes cracked deeply and everytime you put pressure on it, the tooth hurts because the fracture is being pushed apart, harming the nerve. The problem with these cases is that these fractures won't show up on an x-ray.

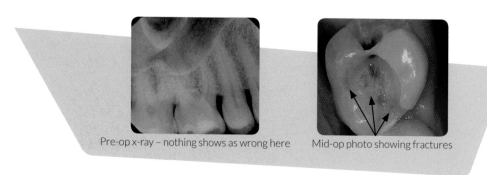

Pre-op x-ray – nothing shows as wrong here   Mid-op photo showing fractures

As you can tell from this x-ray, there is nothing to indicate tooth #3 needs a crown. However, the photo clearly shows the internal fractures as well as the missing DL cusp once the prior restoration is removed.

The x-ray alone, even with a good narrative, may get denied and end up requiring a dentist-to-dentist discussion after the second denial. This is a waste of the team's and doctor's time. Adding the photo above would move this case directly to acceptance.

Important Notes to Include in the Narrative:

- Missing DL cusp
- Internal fracture from mesial to distal along pulpal floor
- Cracked tooth syndrome (patient reports pain to tooth sleuth on ML cusp)
- Insufficient tooth structure for direct restoration
- Crown required to stabilize fracture and prevent loss of tooth

Summary: This case has an almost 100% chance of denial based on the x-ray alone. The photo and resulting narrative would individually increase the chance of reimbursement some, but in combination, these give the claims examiner the information they would need to approve the claim without delay.

Case Example 2.   **Broken Cusps**

The bad part about trying to put a three-dimentional object like a tooth on a two-dimentional x-ray is that often you cannot see everything clearly. This makes x-rays unclear to the claims examiner and will cause claim denials. Here is a great case in which the x-ray could be interpreted a couple of different ways and is likely to be denied by x-ray alone.

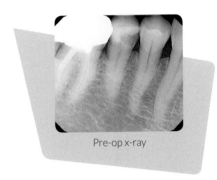

Pre-op x-ray

However, the photo is clear as day because the lingual cusp completely broke off. This is also a great picture to demonstrate why the cracked buildup needed to be replaced.

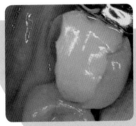 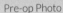 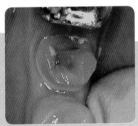 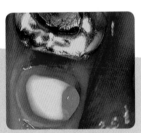

Pre-op Photo   After restoration removal   Post-BU photo

Important Notes to Include in the Narrative:

- Broken L cusp
- Failed prior restoration due to fracture
- Insufficient tooth structure for direct restoration
- Crown required to stabilize fracture and prevent loss of tooth
- 90% of tooth structure missing, buildup required to provide retention and ferrule for crown

Summary: This case has a small chance of getting approved with the x-ray alone but almost zero chance of getting the buildup also approved. By adding photos, this case becomes simple for a claims examiner to approve it immediately without any delays.

Case Example 3.   **Decay on X-Rays**

This patient had a root canal a few years ago and never received the necessary crown. As a result of the food packing between the teeth with the first buildup, the patient developed a cavity under the restoration. Decay is not always visible on x-rays, as you can see from this case. There is no doubt this crown would have been covered because of the root canal, as posterior root canaled teeth are industry standard to need crowns and therefore get almost 100% approval for reimbursement. However, the buildup would likely be denied in this case with the x-ray alone because it doesn't show the decay.

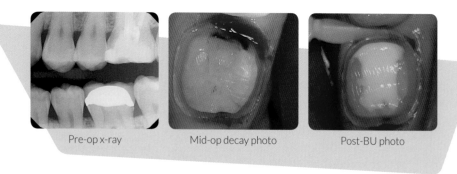

Pre-op x-ray   Mid-op decay photo   Post-BU photo

In order to achieve reimbursement for the buildup, good photography would be required. As you can see from the photos, the decay is obvious when seen clinically, and this infor-mation needs to be adequately presented to the claims examiner. The decay photo and the after-new-buildup photo will provide most of the necessary information.

A good narrative will solidify the case for the claims examiner to approve reimbursement.

Important Notes to Include in the Narrative:

- Failed prior restoration due to food packing and resulting decay on the mesial. See attached photo as decay is not obvious on the x-ray
- Old buildup and decay were removed
- Decay did NOT spread to the root canal orifices
- Crown required for all posterior root canaled teeth
- Buildup completed, see attached photo

Summary: Remember that the claims examiner does not have the luxury of being in the room when the tooth is being treated. They only have the information that you send them with the claim. Providing good documentation in cases where x-rays are not completely clear as to the reasoning for the services is imperative for avoiding claims delays and denials.

Case Examples 4 and 5. Cracked/Broken/Decayed Amalgams

Similar to the first case with the internal fracture, cracked or decayed teeth with large amalgams are often hard to see on an x-ray. Therefore, the x-rays alone don't indicate clearly why a crown would be necessary. See the bitewing x-rays from the cases below that show minimal reason for the necessity of a crown in either case.

However, in the photos you can see the multiple fractures, the missing cusp, and the minimal supporting tooth structure.

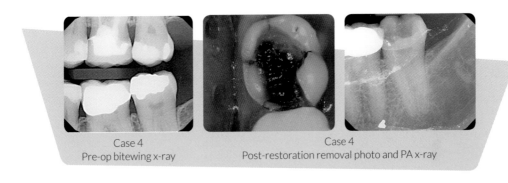

Case 4
Pre-op bitewing x-ray

Case 4
Post-restoration removal photo and PA x-ray

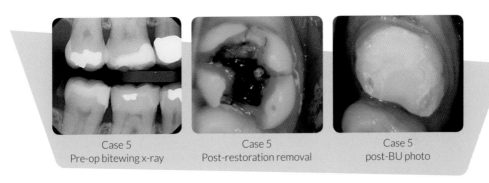

Case 5
Pre-op bitewing x-ray

Case 5
Post-restoration removal

Case 5
post-BU photo

In cases like these, it is best to send the x-ray that is taken at the time of final determination that the crown was necessary, which is the post-restoration removal PA. The insurance company needs to see what the dentist does at the time of that final decision point between direct and indirect restorations.

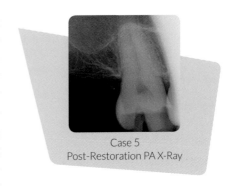

Case 5
Post-Restoration PA X-Ray

Summary: Make sure the photos and x-rays you send help the claims examiner see what the dentist does chairside when working on teeth. Pre-op photos before restoration removal often work against this communication with the insurance company..

BUILDUP AND CROWN NARRATIVE FORM

Patient: _____   Tooth #: _____
Prior Restoration(s): _____   Prior Crown Placement Date: _____

ENDODONTICALLY TREATED TOOTH
__Previous Root Canal: Date: _____

DECAY
__Caries extensive enough to undermine cusps, requiring cuspal coverage: B L MB DB ML DL
__Recurrent caries adjacent to existing restoration(s): at M O D B L surface(s)
__Recurrent marginal caries involving crowns, not repairable: at M O D B L surface(s)
__Caries undermining the incisal angle of an anterior tooth: MI DI

FRACTURE
__Tooth fractured; cannot be reasonably restored with a direct restorative material.
   __Previous fracture, previously restored cusp(s): MB DB ML DL
   __New fracture, with the loss of cusp(s): MB DB ML DL
   __Incisal angle(s) on anterior: MI DI
   __From trauma; __Yes __No   (If yes) Cause: _____
__Prior restoration fractured; cannot be reasonably restored with direct restorative material.
__True cracks and/or fissures with loss or displacement of enamel (not "craze lines"), in these areas:
   a. Horizontal, in dentin at base of these cusps: MB DB ML DL
   b. Mesial to distal, in dentin of pulpal floor
   c. Mesial to distal, across occlusal surface enamel
   d. Across the (__mesial/__distal) marginal ridge(s)
          __ Seen clinically, not visible on x-ray
          __ Stops trans-illuminated light
          __Fractured porcelain on existing crown: Mesial Distal MB DB ML DL MI DI

PAIN – Clinically confirmed diagnosis of Cracked Tooth Syndrome
__Pain on biting and/or release of pressure, on these cusps: MB DB ML DL
__Pain upon thermal stimuli: __hot/__cold/__both
__Clinically reproduced pain goes away in: ___seconds/___minutes

INSUFFICIENT TOOTH STRUCTURE

Inadequate remaining sound tooth structure to support
a direct restoration. Approximate amount *of missing* clinical crown structure:
40%   50%   60%   70%   80%   90%

BUILDUP PLACED
__Build-up material is NOT being used as a filler, to eliminate undercuts, box form, or concave irregularity.
__Insufficient anatomical crown structure for retention of a new crown (see above).
__Tooth has been endodontically treated

ADDITIONAL SUPPORTING DOCUMENTATION ENCLOSED:
__Clinical/Intraoral photographs __X-rays

"I attest to the accuracy of the information based upon my clinical evaluation and chart review."

Dentist Signature: _____ Date: _____

ONLAYS AND INLAYS

Some dentists will do inlays and/or onlays in an effort to be more conservative with a tooth. The thing to remember about these services from an insurance point of view is the LEAT (least expensive alternative treatment) clause (Chapter 6). Inlays and onlays are often seen as more expensive versions of a filling; therefore, insurance companies are typically going to downgrade their payment to the reimbursement they will give for a composite or amalgam of the equivalent number of surfaces.

With inlays, there is no way around this other than to understand what insurance will pay and estimate accordingly. With onlays, the dentist and team need to understand the differences and similarities between crowns and onlays. The best way to illustrate this is with basic geometry.

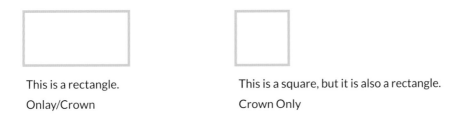

This is a rectangle.

Onlay/Crown

This is a square, but it is also a rectangle.

Crown Only

A rectangle is a four-sided shape with the parallel sides being equal in length and with 90-degree angles.

A square is a four-sided shape with all sides equal in length and 90-degree angles.

When you have a four-sided shape of equal lengths and 90-degree angles, it fits the definition of both a rectangle and a square.

Crowns and onlays are the same.

An onlay is an occlusal coverage restoration that covers one to four cusps. A full crown is an occlusal restoration that covers all the cusps of a tooth.

If you have a tooth that needs all cusps covered, you can call it either a crown or an onlay—it fits the definition of both (like a square is also a rectangle). And since crowns get higher reimbursement, it is in the patient's best interest to code it as a crown, no matter what internal shape you give it.

But there are different types of crowns as well. A three-quarter crown is an occlusal coverage restoration that covers three-quarters of the natural crown surface.

If you have a molar with three cusps covered or a premolar with 75% coverage, you can call it either an onlay with minimal reimbursement or a three-quarter crown with higher reimbursement.

Filing Claims for Inlays and Onlays

If you choose to file inlays and onlays, remember the basics of estimates for the patient.

Example Fee Table	Office fee	Network fee
Amalgam	200	100
Composite	300	150
Inlay	800	500
Onlay	1200	800
Crown	1200	800

If your patient needs an onlay, you should estimate the insurance reimbursement is going to be based on the composite filling ($150). If the insurance has a LEAT clause, it will be based on amalgam ($100).

The $800 onlay will be **$720 out of pocket for the patient** after insurance paid the $80 (80% of $100).

Alternatively, a crown would be **$400 out of pocket for the patient** and $400 insurance reimbursement.

If the onlay is large enough to be considered a full crown or a three-quarter crown, it would be in the best interest of the patient to file coding that will achieve better reimbursement on the patient's behalf.

Can We File an Onlay as a Non-Covered Service and Get Paid More for the Service in Total?

This depends on your state laws. However, in almost every state with non-covered services legislation, a downgrade means the insurance is still paying something toward the treatment, making it a covered service that must be done at network prices.

SCALING AND ROOT PLANING

The service that gets denied as much if not more than crowns is the scaling and root planing (SRP) services. Similar to crowns, most of these denials result from what is documented more than true case denials from a dentist consultant. Realize that most claims that are denied are first seen by a claims agent with no dental experience and minimal training on claims. They are only looking for a list of supporting information to accept or deny a claim. If you send the information, they are going to accept your claim. Understanding these concepts can help you get less than a 1% denial rate on your SRP services.

Periodontal Charting

Periodontal disease is misunderstood by many dentists and office teams. What we've learned about the disease has changed drastically in the last few decades, and the way we classify it has changed a lot as well. The other important point to remember is what was discussed in Chapter 15 about how insurance companies think. The insurance company has a list of criteria they need in order to process a claim that is often different from what the office team has been taught to send.

At Practice Whisperer, we get messages weekly about claims that were denied, especially periodontal claims. The common trend with most of them is a lack of the basic data that a periodontal claim needs to avoid the denial.

According to the American Academy of Periodontology (AAP), periodontal disease is diagnosed and classified primarily by clinical attachment loss (CAL). CAL is a calculation of two data points: pocket depth (PD) and gingival margin (GM, aka recession). If you do not have both data points, you technically cannot have a CAL reading. Without a CAL reading, you cannot diagnose the case, and the insurance company does not get the criteria it needs to process the claim.

Clinical Attachment Loss is a combination of Pocket Depth and Gingival Margin recession.

$$CAL = PD + GM$$

Pseudopocket is a term that is often used in discussing periodontal cases. This term basically means that the tissue is swollen due to the inflammation, which can cause up to 2–3 mm of swelling. When tissues swell, the PD will increase without meaning bone loss has occurred. Remember, bone loss (CAL) is how periodontal disease is tracked and measured, and bone loss is what needs to be documented to get reimbursement for periodontal treatments. If you have not measured GM, then the assumption is that you have 2–3 mm of swelling, which is subtracted from your PD to determine the CAL.

Pseudopockets causing false readings in a perio chart is the first topic that tends to arise if you talk to a dentist consultant at an insurance company when trying to get a claim approved. Without GM marked, the conversation will rarely go the way you want. In order to avoid this problem, it is important to mark every GM site, even if it is zero. No data point should be left empty on a perio chart.

> **TIP**
>
> Mark Gingival Margins (GMs) on every site, even if the GM is 0, to prevent debates on pseudopocketing. No data point should be left empty on a periodontal chart.

"Insurance Is Saying X-Rays Do Not Support SRP"

X-rays provide supportive documentation for diagnosis in a periodontal case, but the only thing that the AAP says tracks and monitors the severity of periodontal disease is CAL in a full periodontal chart. X-rays alone cannot diagnose periodontal disease and therefore cannot be an exclusive reason to deny or approve a claim.

The reason x-rays cannot be legitimately used to approve or deny periodontal concerns is because of the nature of x-rays themselves. In order to see a change in an x-ray, there typically has to be at least a 60% density loss. Dentists know this fairly well when it comes to seeing interproximal cavities, the thing we look for most on bitewing x-rays. This same phenomenon is also true for bone loss. Remember, x-rays take a 3D object and put it on a 2D screen. When bony pockets first start to develop, they will not show up on an x-ray because those bony pockets first start to form right against the tooth, which is going to block the view on a 2D x-ray. By the time you clearly see bone loss on an x-ray, the case has already reached the moderate-to-severe stage and is much harder to maintain after therapy.

You will get these types of narratives on claim denials for SRP because that is the way the system is set up. Insurance dentist consultants will use this line of reasoning because that is part of the script they are trained to go through. This does not mean that the system or the consultant is right in denying the claim from a clinical perspective. Therefore, you should be prepared to push back and take the case back to the only thing that matters, which is CAL.

Discussions with Insurance Dentist Consultants (How to Get Denied Claims Approved)

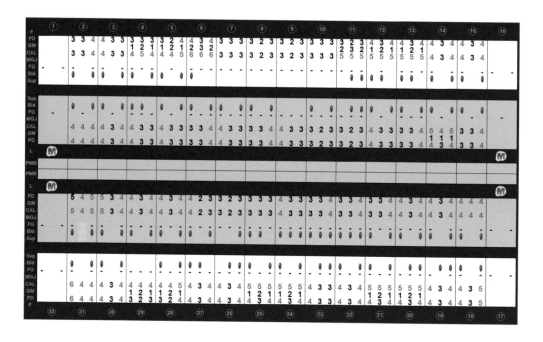

Here is an example case claim that was denied twice with the attached periodontal chart. The case went to a direct discussion with a dentist reviewer after the second denial. The reviewer was pleasant to talk to but was obviously trained on how to fight with every possible comeback. He just picked the wrong person to try to disagree with.

Reviewer: "Let's start with the x-rays; there is not a lot of bone loss here to justify SRP."

Dentist: "While I agree this is not a severe case, there are several points here where you can see vertical attachment loss [list 2–3 spots]. Do you see this?"

Reviewer: "Yes, but it is still not enough."

Dentist: "Okay, let's talk about the AAP definitions of periodontal disease. Last I checked, their guidelines are to diagnose periodontal disease, and resulting treatment recommendations, on CAL. Would you agree with this?"

Reviewer: "Of course. But a lot of these areas could be pseudopocketing, which would not justify SRP."

Dentist: "I agree, swelling with perio is possible, which is why we should look at the areas with marked recession. Tooth 4, 5, 6 have 4–6 mm of CAL; tooth 11–13, 20–21, and 28–29 all have 4–5 mm CAL. It is my understanding according to the AAP that 4–6 mm of CAL requires SRP to get under control; would you agree?"

The conversation went on a couple of more minutes, but in the end, the case was paid.

So here is a basic outline of how to fight these on the phone:

1. X-rays – If x-rays are brought up, you should be ready to discuss areas of obvious vertical attachment loss and loss of lamina dura. It is then also important to steer away from x-rays and fall back on the true definition of perio, which is from CAL.
2. Pseudopocketing – This is why it is so important to mark every gingival margin point, because without those, the claim of 2–3 mm of swelling is normal. Think of this as someone taking your 5–6 mm pockets and subtracting 2–3 mm from each. What you end up with is a patient that has swollen tissue but no bone loss or periodontal disease. Focus on the AAP and periodontists' guidelines for defining perio by CAL, not pockets or x-rays.

TIP

The failure in this case, and why it even ended up at the second denial, was the lack of marked gingival margins on every tooth. This allowed different interpretations of the pocket depths. This case would likely have never made it to this point if all the GMs had been marked in the original claim.

---

3. Photos – We did not talk about this since we had clear photos, but it always helps to have pictures of the *perio probe in place* showing not only the depth but also the blood—one per quadrant. These pictures as well as the bleeding points help show that the PDs are accurate, as well as the bleeding points. Having the pictures in the original claim stopped the reviewer from bringing up the idea of subjectiveness with probing.

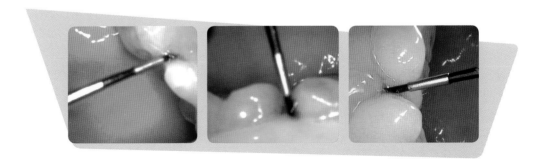

Moral of the Story: Your Perio Chart Is Everything

If you fail to document every point, especially bleeding and gingival margins to have accurate CAL, you will deal with more denials. Have a FULL perio chart, and there is not much to debate.

When talking to reviewers, remember they are dentists. They also happen to be your last chance at achieving reimbursement for the patient. You can have whatever opinion you want about them with what they do, but you will get further being professional rather than being rude. The entire conversation with this reviewer was pleasant, and he nicely at the end agreed to approve the case. These dentists potentially can help you—angering them is not the way to go.

Remember insurance companies are after the low-hanging fruit, offices that are easy to deny because of missing information or lack of pushing back. Push back, and they will go after another piece of lower-hanging fruit.

Part 3

Profitability and Ownership Within an Insurance-Based Practice

Chapter 24
Profitability and Insurance Discounts

While dental offices rarely fail, many offices around the country are barely surviving. This is often because owners don't clearly understand one of the most important business concepts: the critical linkage between overhead and profit. Let's review the basics here.

Overhead is the broad category of expenses for necessary equipment, supplies, and facilities to operate your practice and serve your patients. Overhead is comprised of two components: fixed and variable expenses.

Fixed expenses are those expenses that are the same regardless of how many patients you treat. They are also the largest expenses in an office, often accounting for more than three-quarters of monthly overhead. Fixed expenses include rent, utilities, payroll, marketing, and so forth.

Variable expenses change based on how much work you do or the number of patients you treat. Variable expenses include supplies and lab costs. These expenses will vary each month, depending on how many patients you treat. Variable expenses usually consist of only one quarter of your overhead.

So why are these concepts so important to master?

As you grow your practice and you treat more patients, your variable expenses will naturally continue to grow as well. A healthy dental office will always spend money on supplies and lab work consistent with their patient volume. You can potentially reduce variable expenses somewhat, for instance, finding less expensive labs, using less expensive supplies, and even finding cheaper suppliers. However, this category of expenses will always be linked to your individual patient treatments, a necessary and appropriate expense.

Fixed expenses represent a much higher overall cost to the business and therefore where the greater attention should be focused. Carefully managing these provides the greatest opportunity to improve the office profits.

For example, if it takes you X amount of money in fixed expenses to treat 100 patients, it also takes you that same X amount to treat 200 patients. Yet you are going to bring home more profit in treating patients 101–200 than you will treating the first 100.

See where your office fits in with these examples:

Office A and office B have same-sized teams, one dentist, similar treatment services, and the same fixed expenses.

Office A produces $100k per month and has the normal 60% overhead expense, $45k from fixed expenses and $15k from variable. This leaves office A with $40k profit.

Office B produces $140k per month, pays the same rent, has the same payroll costs, utilities, and so forth. However, office B also has a 40% higher variable expense from doing 40% more work ($21k). Office B, therefore, ends up with $74k profit (140k income – 45k fixed – 21k variable), which is almost double the profit of office A, while doing only 40% more work.

	Office A	Office B
Production	$100,000	$140,000
Fixed Expenses	$45,000	$45,000
Variable Expenses	$15,000	$21,000
Profit	$40,000	$74,000

This is the efficiency that is unique in dentistry, which is why profitability can be so much higher in our industry compared to most others. In most other industries, the variable expenses comprise a much larger chunk of the overhead and therefore doing more work per month does not lead to the same exponential growth.

Think of a restaurant, one of the least profitable businesses in existence. While dental offices can average 30–40% profit, restaurants average around 5%. Why? Their variable expenses (e.g., food and beverages, which have a set shelf life and need constant replenishing) far outweigh their fixed expenses. This means inefficient restaurants fail (90% in the first year), efficient ones only barely succeed, and highly efficient ones do only slightly better than the average successful ones.

Variable vs. fixed expenses are critical concepts to master and remember. It is the foundation of how you need to think about overhead and profit in your own office in order to evaluate what fees do and do not make sense when negotiating with insurance companies.

Why Should Team Members Care About Profitability?

Have you ever met a colleague who works for another office talk about the amazing CE cruise they just took last month? Or how about the fun team shopping spree their doctor took them on? Or how about the $1000 bonus check they just earned? Would you love to have a massage therapist come in monthly to work on your neck and shoulders and relieve the stress?

Offices that are minimally productive don't have the money to be able to pay everyone well, much less have enough for the extra benefits that you might have heard about from friends. Highly efficient and productive offices have the financial resources to provide some great perks for being a team member.

We all have a job to be able to make a paycheck; there is nothing wrong with that. But let's face it, money alone is not what drives most of us. According to Gallup polls, most people would leave a job with good pay in order to find a more positive or less stressful working atmosphere.

What it takes to get an office to produce more often leads to team member satisfaction.

Customer Service: Increasing customer service skills will make patients happier during their visit, which results in less stress for everyone! Think of all the patients that cause you stress during the day, it is the unhappy ones. Happier patients accept more treatment.

Simplicity: More treatment accepted means more efficiency and less wasted effort for the team.

Atmosphere: A more efficient and effective office makes for a more positive and happier employer. A happy boss leads to a more pleasant work environment for the entire team."

And the ultimate answer is the entire reason you work in a dental office. We are there to treat and serve patients. The more treatment we can provide, the better off and healthier our patients will be.

Overall, expenses matter to the team because doing our jobs better will lead to a happier, more productive, less stressful, and more rewarding job.

Achieving Profitability as an In-Network Provider

Now that you understand the basic concepts of overhead and profitability in the office, let's apply that to how we handle procedures and insurance network discounts.

A common concern that comes up for teams and dentists is that they cannot afford to do a treatment for the network discounted fee. First, if it has been a while, it might be a good idea to review Chapters 4 and 16 on the entire reason for being in-network and accepting lower fees.

Once you are clear on why you are in-network, let's talk about how to achieve profitability with lower fees.

The overarching premise one needs to understand when your office is in-network is that **providing discounted care does not mean providing the most expensive care at a lower price**. Providing discounted care means finding ways to provide clinically acceptable care at a lower price. This means not buying the most expensive materials, not using the most expensive lab, and not taking the most amount of time to complete the treatment.

One of the greatest parts about working in dentistry is that there are so many ways to treat a problem. When a patient loses a tooth, they can either replace it with an implant, a bridge, a partial denture, or even do nothing. Take that a step further, and you can assess the costs of individual procedures as well as the related costs surrounding them. A crown can be made by a lab for anywhere from $50 to $500. Composite materials and supplies can range widely in costs. Dentists can do the same treatments in 30 minutes or 2 hours. All these aspects affect the cost of treatment.

Let's review each aspect individually to see what this might mean for an office.

LABS

Dental labs can be as unique and varied as the different breeds of dogs in the world. They come in all shapes and sizes, prices, and services. A highly cosmetic lab will typically charge at the higher end ($300–$500) per crown, but the beauty will often be seen in the result. However, their crown is not going to be functionally any stronger or longer-lasting than most other labs. Having amazing aesthetics has value, but not every patient needs or wants to pay more for the additional cost if you gave them the option. There are amazing labs all along the price spectrum in dentistry. A high-priced lab does not necessarily mean better functional quality.

Just like dental offices, lower-priced labs often can provide the services at that level because of internal efficiencies. Less remakes, higher volume, and better systems make for a less expensive crown.

As a dental office, you cannot and probably should not be providing the same crown from the same lab for $1500 for one patient and $600 for another. It would be rather unfair to the patient paying $1500.

What instead should happen is that the office provides a high-quality, low-cost crown from an economy lab when providing the service for $600, the in-network rate. You can often see this is even the expectation of the insurance company because many of them will recommend labs to their network providers. These recommended labs all have one thing in common: low cost (typically below the $100/unit mark).

If the in-network patient wants a higher cosmetic quality crown, then they can be given that option to use the higher-end, more expensive lab. This option though comes with the added costs associated with providing that treatment, which the insurance company will not help cover. See Chapter 18, "Upgraded Services," to see how to offer this option to your patients in the correct way for insurance patients.

In the end, the insurance patient is getting a discounted price on their treatment because the office can provide a lower-cost product that will still be functional and clinically acceptable.

SUPPLIES

Dental supply costs are like lab costs in the wide variety of options and price ranges. You can find composite ranging from $20 per average filling to $50. Impression materials, bonding agents, infection control supplies, and almost any other supply item you buy in a dental office can range widely in cost for products that in many ways aren't any different.

Think of the last time you went to the grocery store. If you look at the cereal aisle you will find 50 different brands and types of cereal, some of which are almost exactly alike. The store brand can be extremely similar to the name brands. There is a reason for this; many times the store has the same factory make that product as the name-brand item using the same ingredients. The difference is you are paying for the brand name and marketing cost that goes with it.

Dentistry is no different. There are very few manufacturers in the world that make dental equipment and supplies. Name-brand companies pour a ton of money into research, development, marketing, and a larger overhead. Generic companies take over once the patent is gone and make the same or similar product for less.

You can see this in pharmaceuticals as well. Advil and Ibuprofen are the same exact drug down to the molecular structure. The only difference besides price is the packaging and the brand name; the product is the same.

Being in-network often means finding the same quality materials from a generic brand instead of buying the latest, "greatest" composite or material. Just like labs, some of the higher-end composites may have a little better color and natural appearance, but typically, the only people who can tell the difference are dental professionals.

EVALUATING PROCEDURE PROFITABILITY

If you are in-network and concerned that the fee of a service is not gaining a profit, then that is something you need to evaluate. This chapter will help you in the process. Remember, throughout this section, we will be talking about the variable costs associated with providing treatment. Whether you do 1 crown or 100 crowns in a month, your fixed costs are going to be the same.

> **NOTE**
> If you are not a fan of numbers, you might want to skip to the chapter summary. This next section is highly detail oriented.

Fillings

Class 2 fillings are often the least enjoyed and least profitable treatment that general dentists provide. For the normal fees associated with these, the amount of time spent doing them is not proportional to any other treatment. Let's evaluate the profitability of doing a single class 2 filling.

Filling Profitability Example: Assume on the high side that you will be using 1 carpule of composite, 50 uses per bottle of bond agent, and 2 carbide burs. This may overestimate the costs some, but the example will better demonstrate the point.

Class 2 Filling – Material Costs				
	Composite	**Bond**	**Burs**	**Total**
High	$7	$4	$12	$23
Avg	$5.50	$3	$8	$16.50
Low	$4.67	$2.20	$6	$12.87

Variable Cost – Let's use an average insurance price of $120 to determine the difference between what the office collected and what the variable costs were.

Class 2 Filling - Profitability			
	Price	Supply overhead	Difference
High	120	$23	$97
Avg	120	$16.5	$103.5
Low	120	$12.87	$107.23

Time Cost – Now let's apply that difference in cost to the amount of time it took to provide that treatment. Assumptions are paying 1.5 people per hour at $15/hour to account for the RDA and a receptionist.

Class 2 filling time cost	Collections after variable costs		Dollars per hour	Payroll cost	Profitability per filling
	High	Low			
60 minutes	107	97	$97–107	$23	$74–84
45 minutes	107	97	$129–142	$17	$80–90
30 minutes	107	97	$194–207	$11	$86–96

Class 2 Fillings Summary

As you can see from the chart, supply cost does have a small variance, but the biggest impact on profitability for fillings is time. Time is actually the main driver of whether a dentist can be successful with insurance discounts or not. When the dentist and team can provide more dental care per hour, the success and profitability of the office goes up significantly.

> **NOTE**
> In no way is this to suggest sloppy or incomplete work. The speed of a procedure has little to do with the quality of the procedure. There are plenty of examples in the country of slow dentists providing poor quality and fast dentists providing excellent quality. Speed is more a function of efficiency. A thorough consideration of all details of a common procedure can result in a much more efficient and cost-effective result—good for the patient and good for the practice.

Crowns

Crowns are considered the "bread and butter" of dentistry. Unlike fillings, fees associated with crowns are typically much higher and more proportional to the time spent. However, the main cost concern with crowns revolves around what you spend on the lab bill.

HMOs often take this factor out of the equation by allowing the office to charge the lab bill directly to the patient, separate from the crown procedure fee. PPO insurance does not allow this unbundling of the base lab cost.

Crown Profitability Example (with some high-cost assumptions): one diamond bur (assuming multiple that are reused), four crowns per impression cartridge set, ten temps per cartridge, and 0.5 grams of cement used. Average insurance fee of $700.

Crown Overhead and Profitability							
	Burs	Impression	Temp	Lab	Cement	Total	Difference
High	$12	$39	$22	$500	$20	$593	$107
Avg	$8	$25	$16	$150	$15	$214	$486
Low	$5.4	$14	$12.4	$80	$9.5	$121	$579

Now let's apply the cost per hour with different amounts of time taken to complete.

Crown time cost	Collections after variable costs		Dollars per hour	Payroll cost	Profitability per crown
	High	Low			
120 minutes	579	107	$54–290	$46	$61–533
90 minutes	579	107	$80–386	$35	$72–544
60 minutes	579	107	$107–579	$23	$84–556

Crown Summary

Unlike fillings where most of the difference in costs is time, with crowns a lot of the costs includes labs as well. What lab you use can make the largest difference between making no money and a decent margin. With high-end labs and insurance discounts, crowns are less profitable than fillings because they take more time to do. This is why it can be incredibly important to make sure an insurance crown fee covers an insurance crown lab; any reason to increase the lab cost needs to be passed on to the patient (see Chapter 18, "Upgraded Services").

In general, insurance companies not only expect but even go so far as to recommend using a low-end lab. Many will provide you with a specific lab and even potentially a discount for using them.

> **NOTE**
> We are not suggesting use of a cheap lab with poor quality but rather doing your homework to locate a lab with a good reputation, fewer bells and whistles, and more reasonable pricing. They exist in every area. The functional quality of lab work has little to do with the price. The main difference in higher-end lab costs come from the aesthetics side. Higher-end labs can be used, but that additional expense should be paid by the patient (see Chapter 18).

Extractions

Extractions are in an interesting category in that many dentists refer them out routinely; however, the time and supply costs associated with extractions and other surgeries is often the lowest of any dental procedure. The vernacular phrase "as difficult as pulling a tooth" is interesting, since in most cases with trained dentists, it can be one of the fastest, least technique-sensitive treatments provided in dentistry.

Extraction Profitability Example: Assumptions are one suture, one bur (if surgical), two carpules of anesthetic, and miscellaneous disposables. Assumed average insurance fees of simple vs surgical extractions of $100 and $150.

Extraction Overhead						
	Disposables	Suture	Bur (surgical)	Total	Simple difference	Surgical difference
High	4	20	6	24-30	76	120
Avg	3.5	6	4.5	9.5-14	90	136
Low	3	2	3	5-8	95	142

Now let's apply the same concept of time differential to the mix.

Extraction time cost	Collections after variable costs		Dollars per hour
	High	Low	
60 minutes	142	76	$76–142
45 minutes	142	76	$101–189
30 minutes	142	76	$152–284
20 minutes	142	76	$228–426

Extractions are profitable almost no matter how long you take; however, they can often be the fastest procedure for a well-trained dentist.

Root Canals

Root canals are the most likely procedures to be referred out by general dentists. While they do tend to take a long time to complete compared to other procedures, they are similar to extractions in that they have low overhead costs compared to their fee.

Root Canal Profitability Example: Assumptions for a molar root canal are two carpules of anesthetic, rubber dam, and misc. disposables, three files, and three to four canals. Assumed insurance price of $700.

Molar Root Canal Overhead					
	Files	Obturation	Disposables	Total	Difference
High	30	36–49	8	74–87	$613–626
Low	15	18–24	6	39–45	$655–661

Now let's apply the same concept of time differential to the mix.

Extraction time cost	Collections after variable costs		Dollars per hour
	High	Low	
120 minutes	661	613	$306–330
90 minutes	661	613	$409–441
60 minutes	661	613	$613–661

Root canals may be one of the most time-consuming treatments, but it can be profitable, nonetheless.

The huge improvement to root canal profitability, however, comes when you can prep the crown on the same day. If a patient is already in the chair and numb from finishing the root canal, adding the crown prep might take the dentist 5–10 extra minutes and the assistant an extra 20 minutes for impression and temporary.

Root canal + crown time cost	Collections after variable costs		Dollars per hour
	High	Low	
150 minutes	1240	720	$288–496
120 minutes	1240	720	$360–620
90 minutes	1240	720	$480–827

Chapter Summary

It is a common myth among dental providers that "we cannot be profitable with fees so low." However, as this chapter seeks to show, that belief is unfounded.

At the end of the day, every procedure in dentistry can be profitable if you base the materials and labs you choose proportionally to your fees. Low-end fees and high-end expenses do not make sense, which can greatly hurt insurance-based offices. When the office carefully determines what materials and labs used will be proportional to the value of the treatment, it can become a win. The overall goal with dental treatment is to be able to attract enough treatments per month to offset the high fixed costs of running a dental office. Obviously, it is easier to have an office reach the break-even point with a higher profitability on procedures. This does come down to the Walmart concept of higher volume can make up for lower fees.

This same concept works in the other direction too. If a dentist or team wanted to work with fewer patients per hour, they would need to increase the profitability of each procedure by raising fees. Providing quality work with lower expenses, however, can help any dentist in any type of office setting.

The profitability of a dental office has far more to do with understanding and overcoming the fixed costs of the office (rent, payroll, utilities, loans, etc.) and much less to do with the variable costs (dental supplies and labs). Time and efficiency during procedures is often more effective to improve than the cost of materials. It is possible to provide fast, quality care.

If you would like more insight into running an efficient office, look for my first book, *The Practice Whisperer: Practical Steps to Decreasing Stress and Increasing Profit in Your Dental Practice.*

Chapter 25
Does Third-Party Financing Work with Insurance Discounts?

When an office accepts a lower price for a treatment or service, it is natural to be concerned about any expenses that might add to the mix. Financing is a common concern, especially with companies that charge a percentage fee.

For example: if an office takes a 40% price cut to be designated in-network, it can be difficult to also accept a 10% cut from financing that care.

So can an in-network office still offer third-party financing to patients even with the percentage fee required?

When determining whether something is a good idea or not, one often will look to those who are more successful and see what they are doing. Corporate offices and DSOs have spread throughout the landscape of dentistry consistently every year. Almost every one of them offers one or multiple forms of financing. When you look at the most efficient offices in the country (as well as the ones that have the best perks for their team), they almost all have patient financing options as well.

Dentistry is expensive—we hear this myth all the time. In reality, dentistry is cheap for what we do in comparison to general medicine, where a similar surgery would cost five to ten times more. The difference is that in dentistry, insurance has minimal effect on helping patients afford more than the most basic care. When it comes to the more significant procedures, most of our patients do not think ahead enough about their dental needs to save for dental care up front. This is why having one or more financing options can make a big difference in the lives of our patients, by helping them to afford the treatment within their monthly budget.

In the previous chapter we discussed how best to achieve profitability as in-network office. We learned that one needs to focus on both the fixed and variable expenses. And the most significant profitability boost in a dental office's budget is going to come once your collections surpass your fixed expenses for the month. To surpass your fixed expense level will most likely require your office to increase the number of patients you see and/or procedures you complete within that time period.

How Can Financing Aid Profitability?

Think about the last time you presented a $5000 treatment plan to a patient. Let's say it was for several fillings and crowns. Did the patient want to do it all at once or in stages? Often in stages, right? But why? Is it because they want to come back to the office multiple times? Take off from work multiple times? Be numb multiple times?

Not likely.

The patient wants to break up treatment because of cost. If you find a way for the patient to afford the treatment on their budget, most likely they will want to get all their treatment completed in one visit. Dentistry is much easier when you can have just one appointment, one session of numbing, and even more ideally, one visit with nitrous or sedation.

So we can understand why patients would prefer fewer visits in an ideal world; what about dentists and the office?

One treatment visit means less supply costs, less PPE costs.

One treatment visit means less dentist chair time. If completing one crown takes your dentist 90 minutes, adding a second crown won't take an additional 90 minutes. Often the second crown might only take an additional 30 minutes. The same goes for fillings; the first filling may take 30 minutes, while any additional fillings may only take 15 minutes. When you have the patient in the chair, there are many efficiencies that come with additional treatment in the same visit. You only need to wait for anesthetic once. You already have all the materials out and only have one setup and cleanup time. If working in the same quadrant, the dentist gains even more efficiency by doing each step of the process on multiple teeth, saving time, energy, and movements.

The hallmark of a higher-producing dentist is not always about how quickly they can complete a single procedure. Just as often, it is about dentists who do more work in a single visit, thereby gaining a ton of extra time during the day. Dentists are less stressed as well. Doing four crowns and ten fillings in a day on two patients is much easier and less stressful than doing the same work on ten different patients.

Overall, doing more work in a single treatment visit is commonly easier for both the patient and the dentist alike. This is a true win-win arrangement. And often the only barrier to conducting treatment in the way that both prefer is money. If financing helps solve the money issue, then everyone wins.

Offering Financing as an In-Network Insurance Provider

Coming back to the original question of how an office can provide financing even when it cuts a percentage off collections, let's look at some real office scenarios.

SCENARIO A

Dr. Smith has been working in the same office for several years with the same team. The office has collected an average of $50,000 per month during that time period with an average 80% overhead. Dr. Smith's patients are similar to many in the country; they are rarely prepared to afford multiple thousands of dollars in treatment. Yet, Dr. Smith's office is in a working-class community, and his patients often need lots of work done. Dr. Smith not only desires a more fulfilling career, but he is also concerned because many of these patients end up on an endless cycle of treatment since they never devote enough resources to achieve a cavity-free mouth. He always seems to be trying to control the next infection or emergency, instead of getting ahead of the problem.

Dr. Smith takes the advice of a mentor and decides to bring in a third-party financing company. He is apprehensive about how his patients will accept a financing plan, and he is also concerned with how he will afford to provide the financing when it will cost the office money. However, his mentor is a trusted friend, so he tries it despite his concerns.

The first month Dr. Smith offers financing, several patients take advantage of the plan, and he has a $10,000 increase in collections. He is thrilled that he was able to help so many more patients; however, he is concerned that it cost him 10% of that $10,000 just in financing fees. He goes to talk to his CPA to see if he can afford to keep offering this service to his patients.

	June (before financing)	July (after financing)
Collections	50,000	60,000
Rent	5000	5000
Payroll	15,000	15,000
Labs/supplies	7500	9000
Misc. overhead	12,500	12,500
Financing fees	0	1000
Total costs	40,000	43,500
Profit	**10,000**	**16,500**
Profit percentage	**20%**	**27.5%**

In the month before Dr. Smith added financing, he made 20% profit, or $10,000. The month he started financing treatment he made $16,500, which was a $27.5% profit. He was shocked that he made a higher profit margin even with the added costs associated with the third-party financing company. This is when his CPA started explaining how fixed and variable expenses work—the whole reason his mentor suggested adding financing in the first place.

How Was an Increase in Profit Possible?

With Dr. Smith's office, his fixed costs were $32,500. This is money he had to pay regardless of whether he treated one patient or one hundred patients. His variable costs, labs and supplies, did go up by completing more dentistry, but the additional variable costs were a small percentage of his overall expenses.

Every office has a break-even point—that point where the office finally collects enough money so that collections equal expenses. Now the office's fixed expenses are paid. The beauty after this point is that the only expenses left for any subsequent dollar collected are the variable expenses. Variable expenses in dentistry are typically labs and supplies, which range from 10 to 15% of total expenses depending on the office. This means every dollar you collect under the break-even point is still a loss, and every dollar you collect after the break-even point is 85–90% profit.

Financing allows an office to increase production over what they would be able to do without financing. Therefore, the percentage cost of financing is what is driving the office to be above that break-even point. When you add financing, you aren't losing 10% on your total overhead. You are giving away 10% in order to rise above your break-even point, to where you are making 85% profit or more.

Businesses should strive to be as far above their break-even point as possible, and financing is one of many tools that can help you reach that goal.

This is why providing financing in an insurance-based practice works well, often even better than OON or FFS offices, which don't generally have as hard a time surpassing their fixed expenses and break-even point. The math will almost always show that an in-network office needs patient financing even more than a non-insurance-based practice because the in-network discount requires the office to do more work per month to succeed.

"What if All My Patients Want to Finance Care?"

This is a great question, but one that never actually happens for a variety of reasons.

First, many people do not like the idea of owing money or going into more debt. A majority of your patients who have been perfectly happy without financing aren't going to suddenly want it because you offer it.

Second, many patients have treatments that are small and below their insurance maximum. These patients often have a few hundred dollars they could come up with to pay for treatment. The topic of financing may not come up or be enticing to them.

The main patients who want or need financing are those who either need a lot of work done or who would not get any work done otherwise. If a patient would not have gotten treatment otherwise, and financing allowed them to move forward, everyone wins. If the patient used financing in order to get all of their treatment done at once instead of stringing it out over multiple visits and years, everyone wins, just like Dr. Smith's story.

Most of your financed care dollars are going to be for those procedures that fall above your break-even point, and therefore the 10% "cost" to financing is allowing the office to pay for all their fixed costs and keep increasing their profit margins. This is the point at which the office can start being able to afford team perks and bonuses.

Let's run Dr. Smith's scenario again just so you can see what can happen in this potential worst-case scenario where a large portion of patients accept financing. Instead we will show that Dr. Smith collected an extra $10,000 for the month, with twice the amount of collections that was financed by patients who otherwise were not doing financing before. That is $30,000 financed, resulting in a $3,000 finance cost.

	June (before financing)	July (after financing)
Collections	50,000	60,000
Rent	5000	5000
Payroll	15,000	15,000
Labs/supplies	7500	9000
Misc. overhead	12,500	12,500
Financing fees	0	3000
Total costs	40,000	45,500
Profit	**10,000**	**14,500**
Profit percentage	**20%**	**24.2%**

Even after 50% of the income came from financed care, the office still had better profitability and extra resources. This is an extreme example that rarely happens but still comes out as a win for the office. Data from Dental Intel, one of the largest data-gathering programs in the country, shows that the most financing a dental office has ever done is 38% of collections. The offices that produce the most amount of income per dentist hover around 20% financed care.

"What if My Patients Default on Their Financing?"
This can be a real concern. With any kind of financing comes the risk that the person will not pay it back. The easiest way to mitigate this risk as a dental office is to offer only those financing options where the office is paid immediately. These are the options that come with the highest percentage cost but have the most safety.

Companies, such as CareCredit, will finance patient care and pay the office immediately. Any default on the patient's part now become CareCredit's problem instead of the office's. This means that there is no risk of default for the office.

Percentage Cost
One thing to think about, too, with financing costs is that the office often takes a hit on this anyway. If you accept credit cards, the office pays between 2% and 5% on credit card and merchant service fees. The lowest-end cost on programs like Care Credit is 5%, which is not that much higher than your credit card fees. Yes, you can get up above 10%, but the office has the option on which financing options they want to provide, allowing you to mostly control the percentage cost that the office must pay to accept financing.

"My Financing Company Rejects Many of My Patients"

This is a common concern as well with financing companies. They don't like taking risks on patients they are not certain will be able to afford to pay off the balances. Therefore, they have checks in place that drop the highest-risk patients out of the equation, allowing them to safely take the risk on the more secure patients.

There are two main options at this point.

1. **Find alternative financing**. Many financing companies exist from CareCredit to local banks. All of them have different levels of fees to the office and risk tolerance they will allow. Other companies, such as Compassionate Finance, will leave the decision completely up to the office with guidance on who gets accepted. In exchange, the office now takes the risk of defaults. Since this risk exists, these companies have the office charge a fee on top of the treatment fee to offset the default risk. This additional fee is acceptable to include for insurance patients at in-network offices.

2. **Change the treatment plan**. Just like you would without any financing option available, if a patient cannot afford treatment, the dentist and patient should come up with an alternative solution. This solution could be either opting for a less-expensive treatment or stretching out the length of time to complete (and pay for) treatment.

Chapter 26
National Provider Identifier (NPI)

To check eligibility on insurance or submit claims, you will need a National Provider Identifier (NPI). NPI is a nationwide standard 10-digit numeric identifier for either a health care provider or entity, for example, a dentist or a dental office. The numbers are completely random with no identifying coding. These numbers are free and quick to obtain.

You can apply for an NPI number here:
Website: https://nppes.cms.hhs.gov/#/
Email: customerservice@npienumerator.com
Phone: 800-465-3203/800-692-2326
Mail: NPI Enumerator
P.O. Box 6059
Fargo, ND 58108-6059

When you change locations or specialties, your NPI will stay the same.

When you apply for your NPI, you will be asked to provide your 10-digit taxonomy code. For quick reference, here are the dental taxonomy codes:

General Practice – 1223G0001X

Dental Public Health – 1223D0001X

Endodontics – 1223E0200X

Oral and Maxillofacial Pathology – 1223P0106X

Oral and Maxillofacial Radiology – 1223X0008X

Oral and Maxillofacial Surgery – 1223S0112X

Orthodontics and Dentofacial Orthopedics – 1223X0400X

Pediatric Dentistry – 1223P0221X

Periodontics – 1223P0300X

Prosthodontics – 1223P0700X

Denturist – 122400000X

NPI numbers come in two groupings: type 1 and type 2.

Type 1 is an individual provider, and type 2 is an incorporated business, such as group practices and organizations.

Which type do you need?

	NPI
Solo practitioner	Type 1 only
One location, one dentist	Type 1 for dentist Type 2 for practice if claims are in the practice's name
One location, multiple dentists	Type 1 for each dentist Type 2 for practice
Multiple locations	Type 1 for each dentist Type 2 for each practice with unique TIN

If I Am a One Location, One Dentist Office, Why Would I Need or Want an NPI Type 2?

In most cases, insurance companies will negotiate with an entity or dentist. If that negotiation is through an entity with a type 2 NPI number, then you can add additional dentists or change dentists far more quickly and easily. It may take weeks or months to credential a new dentist NPI 1 but only days to add another provider to an existing NPI 2 entity.

Chapter 27
When and How to Drop Insurance Contracts

Many dental offices sign up to be in-network with insurance companies in order to attract a higher volume of patients for their practice. However, sometimes there comes a point at which the office wants or needs to drop a particular network affiliation.

When to Investigate Dropping Insurance:

There are two common reasons that offices decide to no longer participate with an insurance company:

1. The insurance company becomes too difficult to continue working with; or
2. The dental office becomes too busy.

The first point, difficulty to work with, often results from multiple challenges: claims process, payment process, and communication process.

The **communication process** can be different depending on the company. Some insurance companies have invested good resources into becoming more accessible online. This allows an office to locate patient eligibility and sometimes breakdown information online, which can save the office a ton of time instead of waiting on hold forever. Companies that do not have this online availability therefore become harder to work with and might be a reason an office decides to drop networks.

The **claims process** is often the most stated reason for frustration from dentists about working with an insurance company, so much so that some insurance companies have developed a reputation within the profession for being difficult to work with. In general, most of these concerns typically are office-based problems. This textbook will give you the tools so that the claims process becomes simple with most, if not all, insurance companies.

The **payment process** is the last main concern. In recent years there have been several larger organizations and states that have had self-funded plans go bankrupt. Self-funded plans are those where the insurance company administers the policy but is not the source of the money. Refer to Chapter 3 for more background information on self-funded plans. When something happens to the money source, such as a state going bankrupt, the plan no longer pays out claims that have been approved. The challenge is that the insurance company takes the blame, even though it had nothing to do with the problem. Do be wary of using this as a sole reason to drop an insurance company, as the insurance company may not be the problem at all; the insurance company is often as frustrated as the office in these situations since they have to field all the complaints.

The second reason is the office is too busy.

This is the most common reason to terminate an insurance network affiliation. If the office has too many patients, there is little reason to take a network discount for the patients they do see. The best way to increase office profitability when you have a completely full schedule is to get paid more for the same work, which can be accomplished by either raising prices or dropping insurance networks. There are multiple factors to consider before taking this step, however. It is easy to terminate a network contract, but it is far more difficult to restart one because you will need to go through the entire credentialing and negotiating process again. An office would want to make sure it is the right decision for the long term before dropping contracts.

What Steps to Take to Drop an Insurance Contract:

Step (1) Evaluate the Need

The average dentist and office typically want to have an almost full doctor schedule around two weeks out and a full hygiene schedule around three months out. In addition, if an office is to maintain a good life span, it will want to make sure you can get new and emergency patients in within a short time period. This is because new patients will often find another office if it takes too long to get a first appointment with you. The general timing that most patients will be happy with (so they will stay with an office) is up to two weeks for hygiene or treatment and up to two days for an emergency. If an office schedule does not allow this scheduling opportunity, the office is likely to start losing patients due to timing.

The most common way to free up appointment times is to lower the number of patients you see, which can be accomplished by dropping an insurance network and basically choosing which subset of patients you are willing to lose. Having better scheduling opportunities will allow an office to get in more patients who would be paying closer to your normal fees.

CAUTION

If an office does not have a full hygiene schedule three months out and a treatment schedule two weeks out on a regular basis, dropping insurance could cause a lot of challenges that will ripple through the business.

Step (2) Choosing Which Plans to Drop

If you have made the decision to drop an insurance plan, the next big decision is to determine which insurance plan to start with. Dropping all your insurance plans at once often does not work out well for an office. Just think about what might happen if suddenly half your patients decided never to come back.

There are a few different methods to evaluate what insurance network makes the most sense to leave first.

Number of Patients

One of the simplest reports to run is to evaluate the number of patients that see you under each insurance contract. You can expect a percentage of patients to leave the office when you drop an insurance network. By knowing how many patients you have with each company, you can quickly gauge the expected loss of patients after you drop a network plan and therefore what the potential effect would be on the business.

Starting with the insurance companies where you have fewer patients can be a good place to begin. There is value in knowing how insurance companies respond in or out of network, and therefore the networks where you see a minimal number of patients typically will take more team time and effort to manage. Starting with the lowest number can also help the office and team try out dropping insurance with minimal losses and be better prepared when you drop future insurance plans with more patients involved.

Network Discount Price

The most common cited reason for dropping an insurance network is due to the discount that you must provide patients. If you can collect $1200 for a crown instead of $800, it can mean a big difference in the ability of the office to manage expenses. Writing down a list of the average network discount percentage each insurance company requires of your office and dentist can give you a great tool to evaluate which plans need to go first.

As this book mentioned earlier with the math of discounts (page 178), additional discounts to a service mean an exponentially higher number of patients you need to see to make up for the fee difference.

If your smallest insurance patient participation is the one with the highest fees, it may not make as much sense to drop it first.

Insurance Write-Offs

A more complex but more accurate view than either of these two options will be a combination of the concepts. Instead of only looking at the number of patients or the fee schedules, look at the actual financial data of the different networks. If you have two insurance companies with the same fee schedule and the same number of patients, which one should you drop first? How about the one that is causing the most loss of income? If you run a report that also factors in what collections the business is bringing in with each network of patients, you will find out which company you lost more money with. This can allow you to increase the profitability of the office more quickly by dropping the insurance company that is costing you the most.

As an example, let's see the following hypothetical chart:

Insurance	Number of patients	Average network discount	Total collections	Total write-offs
Aetna	300	28	100,000	38,000
BCBS	150	22	200,000	56,000
Cigna	200	20	200,000	50,000
Delta	400	30	400,000	171,000
Guardian	100	41	80,000	56,000
Humana	50	34	30,000	9,000
United	200	35	200,000	107,000

Based on the previously discussed methods, an office might compare plans based on the following criteria:

Patient numbers: Drop Humana first, which has the least number of patients; therefore, having the least impact on the business.

Discount percentage: Drop Guardian first as the largest discount at 41%.

Largest Write-Off: Drop Delta as being the discount that is losing the business the most amount of money. Instead, devote a good amount of that money to marketing, to drive new replacement patients into the office.

The goal of having this level of information is to be able to make the most informed decision possible to be able to plan for what consequences might result from network changes. The team might see Aetna as the most difficult insurance company to work with, but in no numerical situation would it be the most beneficial company to drop.

However, if you find that you need to write off more than the network discount with a company because of company policies, denials, disallows, and so forth, that may be another aspect to look at. If for example, you find that you should only be writing off $107,000 with United, but you are actually writing off $170,000 because of policy problems, this might move it up in a priority list to consider dropping.

Taking Action

Once you have prioritized the list of which insurance company contracts you want to evaluate, then it is time to take action. Dropping all insurance companies at once might be a hard challenge to cope with, but planning to drop one at a time would allow the office to mitigate any losses.

The general message you might hear from offices that have transitioned from in-network to out-of-network is to drop one or two insurance companies at a time. Give the office time to stabilize, especially with hygiene schedules, and then move on to the next one. This timing may be 6 or 12 months in between each phase.

One final step you might want to consider before picking up the phone to cancel is to determine whether it would make sense to stay with a company if they were able to raise the fee schedule. Some insurance companies will respond to a termination notice with a fee increase offer. You want to be prepared to know at what point a fee increase might change the equation about which insurance company to drop next.

For example, with the previous chart:

Insurance	Number of patients	Average network discount	Total collections	Total write-offs
Aetna	300	28	100,000	38,000
BCBS	150	22	200,000	56,000
Cigna	200	20	200,000	50,000
Delta	400	30	400,000	171,000
Guardian	100	41	80,000	56,000
Humana	50	34	30,000	9,000
United	200	35	200,000	107,000

If you were looking at deciding between BCBS and Cigna, which have similar collections and write-offs, and BCBS came back saying they would give you an increase in fees that would drop your discount rate from 22 to 18%, then staying with BCBS over Cigna might make more sense.

Team Preparation Before Dropping Insurance

Patients go to an office for a variety of reasons. These reasons can range all along a continuum from relationship with the office to following their insurance plan. When you drop insurance, an office will lose the patients on the far end of the right side of the spectrum. The more preparation and additional value you can provide to the patients, the smaller that loss will be. A few of the most common forms of preparation are strengthening the relationship, communication training, increasing customer service, having a niche, and offering an alternative option to insurance (such as an in-house savings plan).

Strengthening the Relationship

The doctor-patient relationship is one of the strongest business-to-customer bonds that exist within most industries. Patients often will stick with their doctor through thick and thin a lot more than they will with other companies. Keeping this relationship strong can be the best way to mitigate any patient loss from office changes, such as dropping insurance. The bond is not just with the dentist, though; it can often be the entire team. In general, a patient will emotionally attach to one team member more than the rest. Half of the patients tend to see their dentist as this strongest bond, and for the other half it would be another person on the team. A strong team effort means more than anything toward keeping this bond from breaking.

Train Your Team How to Communicate with Patients

Life and relationships often come down to communication. The Number 1 reason marriage counselors cite as cause of problems is a lack of good communication. This is why it can be so important to plan, rehearse, and role-play the conversations you will have with patients about why you are no longer participating in their insurance network. One wrong word or phrase can be enough to end the relationship. The better you can be at communicating with your patients exactly what you want, the happier and more appreciated they will feel. This will create a strong sense of loyalty to keep them coming to you.

Insurance companies will send your patients letters when you decide to cut network ties with them. These letters will be strongly worded messages trying to persuade the patient to find another in-network provider. Insurance companies do this because in most cases an out-of-network dentist gets more reimbursement, therefore costing the insurance company more. It is in the insurance company's best interest to have fewer patients going out of network.

This is why it is important to get ahead of this problem. Before you drop an insurance company, it would be best to personally talk to all your patients. Let them know why you are dropping months before it happens; this way you can control the conversation instead of the insurance company. Having this conversation in person gives you the best possible chance of keeping the patients.

Here is an example of some language a successful dentist used to keep his patients while dropping insurance networks:

> "A contract with an insurance company is like a relationship. If you were in an abusive relationship, I would tell you to get out. If you stayed, knowing you could leave, that would be your fault. My relationship with your insurance company was abusive, and I put up with it for too long, and it was just getting worse. It's not that I don't care for you, I just don't care for your insurance company. They are abusive to dentists, and I can't support that kind of relationship".

—Dr. Ryan Dunlop

The "Why," or Niche

When you drop an insurance network, typically your patients will have to pay more per visit. An office will want to think about what you are doing to increase the service and care for your patients that will justify the increased cost. Many offices and dentists tend to think that excellent patient care is enough; however, in most cases patients cannot judge the quality of dental care. Quality of care is often not enough because patients have no basis for comparison. You typically need more to balance the equation of cost vs value.

Having a well-defined niche can be one option. In 1986 the movie *Highlander* popularized the saying, "There can be only one." Most dentists think and say they provide great quality, but there can really be only one "best." If you can be the best implant dentist, Invisalign dentist, smile designer, sedation dentist, and so on, then you can attract patients regardless of insurance. Patients will pay for perceived value if it is something they want. The smaller the town you are in, the easier it is to gain this type of reputation. The entire team should be on board with knowing your target niche and being able to articulate it well to patients.

Alternative Options to Insurance (Membership Plans)

Many patients aren't in love with their insurance plan, but there is a general mentality that one needs a plan of some kind or they are overpaying. A membership plan can also attract new non-insurance patients. As a general concept, a membership plan is similar to insurance in that a patient pays a monthly or annual amount to get access to a lower price. These can benefit both the patient and the office in a variety of ways.

Benefits to the patient:

- No maximums
- No restrictions, denials, waiting periods
- Easy to understand
- Saves money

Benefits to the office:

- Higher patient retention
- Hygiene visits are essentially pre-paid
- Fewer missed appointments
- Less third-party involvement in treatment decision-making
- No claims process
- Get paid immediately

Common Plan Language

For a monthly or annual fee, the patient gets access to two free hygiene visits, any exams or x-rays needed, and 10–15% off most other treatments done in the office.

Patient Preparation: Frequently Asked Questions

Once you have pinpointed your niche and can articulate everything you can do to increase value to the patient, you should be prepared for the common questions a patient might ask. It is a great idea to write down every question you hear, so you and/or the team can build a reference sheet with prepared answers. Here are a few common questions with example answers to get you started.

"Why are you not on my insurance company's list of in-network providers anymore?"

The limitations and restrictions of that insurance company kept becoming more stringent, thereby decreasing our ability to provide the quality care that our patients needed. You deserve better than that! Most of our patients decided to stay because of [list top reasons].

"Will I have to pay more than I have in the past?"

In some cases, there is a difference—but most of the changes have to do with what your employer is choosing to pay for (or not to pay for) and not the insurance company itself. Most patients report the difference has been minor, and we still do everything possible to help maximize your insurance benefit.

"Do you have a membership plan?"

Many of our patients aren't as happy with their insurance as they have been in the past and are looking for alternatives. We have a membership plan available that many of our patients have preferred instead of insurance because there are no claims, maximums, restrictions, and the like. A lot of our patients find this is a great supplement to their dental plan and in many cases even a better value! The plan includes two hygiene visits per year, X% off any pre-paid treatment, and any emergency exams or x-rays in the event something unexpected comes up.

"Do you take my insurance?" (patient calling on the phone)

It is important to realize that in many cases, insurance/money is the only measuring tool that prospective patients have when calling a dental office. The immediate goal is to connect with the patient—bypass the insurance for a moment while you gather their name and find out how you can help them. Use common sense and focus on the relationship.

If the office wants to increase new patient flow, just getting patients "in the door" by removing all obstacles often works. If you have created a better customer service experience or niche, the patient is far more likely to stay once you get them in. If money/insurance is an issue, it can help to offer a "new patient special" that might offset any balance that might be left after insurance reimbursement. (See Chapter 19 on discounts.)

"You aren't on the list for my insurance company—do you accept this plan?"

Offices will get this question often. Here are a few answers that offices might give:

Answer 1

Yes, you are able to draw on your insurance plan and receive reimbursement for services at this office. In fact, we serve many other patients with this same insurance plan. We are not on your list simply because this year we are not in-network. All that means is there may be a slightly different rate for any service. And I can absolutely do a benefit check for you to let you know what that difference might be. What our patients who carry that insurance tell us is that they love our team, our dentist, our convenient location, and ease of getting an appointment, so they prefer staying with this dental family over going to another dentist. We also happen to have [offer additional reasons]. In any case, we would love to have you come see us.

It may also be helpful to know that insurance contracts, benefits, and rates change each year. We have worked with your insurance carrier for many years and anticipate we will do so in the future.

Answer 2

You may not find us on that restricted list, but we still have patients in our practice who have the same dental plan, and they do receive reimbursement. It may be a few dollars difference depending on the plan, but we happen to have a "new patient offer" right now that will likely offset any additional cost.

We have had several patients who were curious about what it would look like to go to a dentist of their choice instead of being told by their insurance where to go—they actually found that the fee difference is surprisingly small, while the difference in quality and attention is great. Our dentist made a decision that we would never compromise a patient's treatment decisions and options because of limits on their plan. I would be happy to do a benefit check and see what it would mean for you to come to us.

Answer 3

We have searched and searched and cannot find any dental plan that's willing to provide our patients with the kind of care they deserve. As a result, we're committed to helping our patients maximize whatever benefits they have, but we're not willing to compromise the care we give to our patients for any insurance company. We think patients deserve better, and that's why you came to us in the first place. We're glad you chose us.

> **TIP**
>
> Just because the patient asks about insurance does NOT always mean it is the only determining factor in what dentist they choose. When the level of service/experience supersedes their expectations, oftentimes the insurance becomes secondary.

What to Be Aware of after Dropping Network

The first challenge that offices come across after they drop insurance networks is how to handle estimates. In-network, you have a set fee schedule and know exactly what the insurance fee should be. Out-of-network insurance payments are based on UCR (usual, reasonable, customary) instead, which are not fee schedules that insurance companies will provide.

The way to obtain these fees is slowly, over time, based on EOBs that come in. As you receive and begin to track these fees, your office can build what is referred to as a blue book, as previously explained in chapter 24. A blue book is a list of estimates on the value of something. In this case, it is the value that insurance companies place on each procedure.

Each insurance company will be different with a different UCR; therefore, you will need a blue book listing for each. However, the UCR for each company will be the same company-wide for your area.

The second challenge is even more problematic, but thankfully does not show up as often. This challenge comes from insurance companies that have a different set of benefits for in-network vs out-of-network.

Example: Your patient's employer policy might pay a breakdown of 100/80/50 for in-network and 80/60/40 for out-of-network.

In some cases, this can be a huge problem, where the insurance company pays less to an out-of-network provider, especially on hygiene and preventive services.

It is important to understand why you need to look closely at the insurance company benefits and fee schedule and breakdown. When it determines benefits for an employer client, the insurance company must estimate the cost it will pay out to patients so it can determine what to charge the employer for that policy. They project how many of those employees are going to go to an in-network dentist versus an out-of-network dentist. The insurance company needs to determine that if out of network, they are going to have to pay more per procedure.

Or instead, the insurance company can simplify the process and pay about the same in-network versus out-of-network. They do this by changing the percentage breakdowns.

Example: Delta pays $700 for an in-network crown. The office full fee is $1200. The UCR for a Delta out-of-network crown is $900.

Delta would have to pay $350 in-network but $450 out of network if the breakdown was 50% for both. Instead, if Delta sets the out-of-network major benefit to 40%, they would pay $360. Now the payment Delta has to send out is almost the same regardless of in-network versus out-of-network status.

So why is all this important to determine before dropping an in-network contract?

At Practice Whisperer, we have seen many offices collapse because they have tried to go out of network without preparation. When an office is unprepared to drop a contract, it can cause long-term ripples within the business. Preparation can make the difference between losing a small number of patients versus most of the patients. Not every office can handle being out of network.

Chapter Summary

There are many aspects (or variables) to consider when deciding to go out of network. The goal is to be able to understand what all these aspects are so that you can make the correct decisions for the office when needed, as well as for you and your team to be prepared to handle the consequences of those decisions. It is important to think through every aspect of changing an insurance relationship: from what to tell patients to how to handle estimates. When you plan ahead, you can avoid losing many patients in the process.

Chapter 28
Treating Family and Employees Who Carry Dental Insurance

Many offices offer team member perks for working in a dental office, one of which is dental care. This can be a great thing for a dentist to be able to provide for their team. However, if any employees have dental insurance available through another source, it can lead to a lot of confusion about how to handle the process.

The main questions to think about are:

- Can the office file insurance for team or family members?
- How do you manage a benefits perk without potential insurance fraud?
- Is it possible to bill insurance but not the employee?

The challenge with discussing this subject is that the standard way of handling employee benefits falls into the gray area.

This chapter will discuss the common options, the challenges they present, and best ways to reach your goals *and* avoid getting into legal trouble.

In many dental office employee handbooks, you'll final this common wording for team member dental benefits:

Team Benefits for Dental Care

Team members are eligible for free dental care after their initial three-month period of employment. Full-time team members, spouses, and their immediate children receive free preventive and basic restorative care at no charge.

These appointments for dental care must only be delivered during normal business hours when there is availability on the schedule.

Major treatment and complex cases must be approved ahead of time. Costs will vary based on the case. If approved, lab and specialist fees are to be paid by the team member or family member. The definition of complex is at the sole discretion of the dentist.

Team members receiving dental care must ensure they are not "on the clock" when receiving any kind of dental or hygiene care.

This policy works well until you start bringing insurance into the picture.

Here is a question that came up recently in one of the dental groups. It was from a doctor who genuinely wanted to take care of his team but was unsure how to manage the process.

> **EXAMPLE**
>
> I saw an employee's daughter for an exam, and she needs several crowns. She was ecstatic that I was going to provide it at no charge, as I provide no-cost dental care for children of my employees. A few days later, she found out that she has dental insurance. Insurance requires a co-pay of $500 for each crown.
>
> So I have the choices of:
>
> 1. Charge the co-pay, which she cannot afford, so she won't end up getting the crowns done
> 2. Not charge her the co-pay, and consequently not receive the other $500 from insurance
> 3. Write off the co-pay and collect insurance's portion of $500.

This is a question that comes up often in dentistry. As employers and dentists, we naturally want to take care of our team members. However, when insurance enters the picture, the situation can become more complicated. There are a few aspects to this scenario that you should be aware of. There is an issue of potential fraud, team perception, and obviously money sitting on the table. Let's look at each of these aspects, and then we can talk about some of the best practice solutions to this common dilemma.

Potential Fraud

According to all in-network contracts, an office should not be writing off anyone's co-pays: family, employees, and so forth. However, an extremely large number of offices in dentistry do. This leads to the general perception that writing off co-pays for a small number is okay. This happens too often and is why many insurance companies will not pay dentists to work on their own family at all. The insurance company expects this to happen and therefore decides not to get involved with reimbursement for family.

First, fraud is fraud. Lying to an insurance company is never a good thing to do and may potentially come back to bite you, sometimes years later. Even if you are not in-network with a contract, there are state and federal laws against fraud. See Chapter 19 for more details.

Insurance Perspective: Co-pays are designed to create a barrier (skin in the game) for patients. The insurance company does this to mitigate their potential losses. If the patient cannot afford the co-pay, then the patient declines the treatment, which saves the insurance company from having to reimburse anything. If the dentist waives the co-pay, he is effectively helping the patient to steal from the insurance company a benefit they would not otherwise have been able to legitimately claim.

Dentist Perspective: The dentist feels it is okay to lose the co-pay to get the often-larger portion that insurance pays. The dentist may see it as losing some money, but that is the kind and compassionate thing to do for patients to ensure they receive the care they need.

"But I Know Other Offices that Do This and Have Not Been Penalized."

To understand the reason so many aren't penalized for this, you have to look back at the inner workings of an insurance company. Investigating a dentist for potential fraud requires a lot of manpower to get the details and evidence. Insurance companies are not enforcement agencies; their primary goal is to make money. In this instance, that primary goal works to the benefit of the dental office because an insurance company is not going to spend the massive effort and cost of starting an investigation if the potential payoff is small. A handful of employees and family members who get co-pays waived does not add up to enough dollars to justify the expense to the insurance company.

This is why most dentists can get away with the practice without many repercussions. However, just because you can get away with a crime, no matter how small, does that mean you should still do it?

Where dentists will find themselves in trouble with small issues like waiving co-pays for employees/family is when the dentist becomes under investigation for other concerns. If the insurance company is already looking and spending the effort, then it just adds to the chargebacks and penalties that would come with the process.

When these fraud issues become large enough to involve the court system, you typically work with a judge. Judges aren't usually very sympathetic to insurance companies wanting to charge employees more for treatment. However, if there are additional fraud issues along with those claims, it becomes less about the employees and more about recurring patterns of illegal actions. This can make what seems like a small issue of employee co-pays to escalate to a larger fraud issue.

"What if I Just 'Cannot Collect' from the Employees/Patients?"

Technically, we are not collections agencies, and we cannot gather all the money that is owed to us from patients. So sometimes offices may take the approach that they tried to collect the co-pays, but the patient did not comply. The co-pay eventually gets written off as "uncollectible."

While this may seem like a good idea, it is all about patterns. If you have a pattern of never being able to collect co-pays from certain procedures or from certain people, then it becomes a history of fraudulent actions instead of a simple inability to collect.

Best Practices to Handle Insurance and Employees

The good news is there are a couple of ways to handle this scenario without any hint of fraudulent activity, thereby avoiding potential problems.

1) Just Inform the Insurance Company on the Claim.

"Patient is an employee and is not participating in the cost for this treatment."

This simple statement will absolve you of any fraud issues completely. The insurance company can decide for itself if it is going to pay for treatment or not with the information.

Remember, fraud with an insurance company is about being untruthful to them. If you freely give all the information, what the company does with it is up to the company now, and you have no illegal actions.

Doing this means there is no need to change your benefits policy; however, you do run the risk of an insurance company deciding it doesn't want to pay anything either.

2) Modify Your Benefits Policy.

If instead of committing to completely free care, you instead offer a yearly dental credit benefit, then the insurance issue no longer becomes a concern. Here is how this works:

With this method, you are technically charging the employees to satisfy the insurance company, but it also protects you against some employees taking far more benefits than others. There are occasional sad stories of dentists doing thousands of dollars of work on a new employee, and then the employee quits soon after.

With a benefit/credit system, there is less opportunity for the office to be taken advantage of by an employee. This system also allows employees who are covered by insurance to actually receive a larger benefit, and their insurance has some use to them. And since you would essentially be charging your employees full normal prices, there are no issues with insurance or fraud at all. In many aspects this is the gold standard for offering team dental care benefits. Here is how this can be worded in your employee handbook/benefit plan.

Team Benefits for Dental Care

Team members are eligible for dental care benefit credits after their initial three-month period of employment.

Full-time team members, spouses, and their immediate children receive $X/month (or $Y/year) credit to use toward their dental care.

These appointments for dental care must only be delivered during normal business hours when there is availability on the schedule.

The credit cannot be used for lab or specialist fees, which are to be paid by the team member or family member.

Team members receiving dental care must ensure they are not on the clock when receiving any kind of dental or hygiene care.

Dental insurance now becomes an extra benefit to the employee. If all employees receive, say, $2000 office credit, those with insurance also have another $1500 of coverage. Insurance pays what it would normally, and the co-pay comes out of the employee's credit. This also helps avoid any possible fraudulent issues with billing insurance on a patient that would otherwise not have to pay for treatment.

Chapter Summary

Providing dental benefits for employees and their families helps to attract and retain team members. It is a good thing. However, it pays to understand how that benefit should best be implemented in order to avoid any legal problems. The first place an investigation tends to start in a dental office is with team members. Investigators know that offices are typically the laxest on the charts and ledgers of employees. If your employee files are perfect, often it may stop an investigation before it moves further. If you keep the files of your team members as clean as possible, you can avoid many claims of fraud, misrepresentation, and other legal concerns.

Chapter 29
The Role of Insurance Coordinator

It is clearly important that one or more individuals on your team be well-versed in all aspects of dealing with dental insurance claims. If your practice is large enough, a full-time insurance coordinator would be ideal. So, let's start by discussing what the role of an insurance coordinator would look like in a perfect world.

What Is the *Purpose* of the Role?

The insurance coordinator plays a key role for the dental office. The ADA claims that 65% of patients carry some form of dental insurance. Their research also shows that patients who carry dental insurance will visit the dentist far more often and will accept more treatment than patients who don't carry insurance. For the typical dental office, 65% of their patients represents a large portion of their revenue stream. Therefore, the twofold purpose of the insurance role is to ensure:

1. **Your patients receive the maximum benefit from the insurance policies they are paying for**. First and foremost, we are in the business of serving the oral health care needs of our community. We offer our patients the best health care we can provide. If the greater majority of our patients carry some form of dental insurance benefit, we want to ensure that they receive the care they need, while at the same time maximizing the benefits that they are already paying for. Patients don't always fully understand their benefit plans, and since we work with insurance every day, we can provide a more experienced eye to educate them, help them make informed choices, and navigate a complex system.

2. **Your business is promptly paid for the services you provide**. Insurance benefits and claim procedures play a key role in treatment decisions even before a claim is filed. Treatment plans developed, materials or supplies determined, labs chosen, and timing selected can all be influenced by a patient's insurance benefit plan. Having expertise in the nuances of insurance becomes an important planning assist. Then later, when the claim is filed for benefits from their insurance carrier, the claim payment is usually assigned to the dental office. That means we must wait until a dental claim is processed and approved before we are paid for the services we provide. The completeness, clarity, and accuracy of a dental claim submitted makes the difference as to if, when, and how much the office is ultimately paid.

What Are the *Responsibilities* of the Insurance Coordinator?

An insurance coordinator is an insurance specialist, a patient educator and advocate, and a claims expeditor.

Insurance Specialist - Serves as onsite practice specialist in all aspects of dental insurance.

- Develops strong knowledge base of typical insurance plans utilized by the office's patient population
- Understands all aspects of the claim process: patient information required, how to complete all details of claim forms, where/how to submit claims, how/where to contact insurance companies for questions and follow-up, how to respond to requests for more information, claim denials, insurance audits
- Consults with team members during the treatment planning effort to educate them on the insurance ramifications of specific treatments, supplies, materials, timing, and so forth.

Patient Educator and Advocate – Works directly with patients regarding their insurance benefits.

- Collects information needed for verification of a patient's dental benefits
- Contacts insurance carriers to verify patient benefits before office visits and treatment
- Educates patients about their dental insurance plan and how to maximize their dental benefits
- Answers patient questions. Conducts research if needed for complete clarity
- Serves as patient advocate with insurance carriers to ensure they receive all benefits due from their insurance plan

Claims Expeditor – Submits insurance claims as a service to patients; proactively follows up to ensure timely resolution and payment.

- Prepares claims on behalf of the patient. Thoroughly completes all information according to insurance company requirements, attaching appropriate clarifying documentation such as x-rays, photos, etc.
- Submits claims promptly according to insurance company requirements
- Develops a systematic follow-up process to ensure claims are promptly handled, identifying problems early
- Responds readily to questions and additional requests from the insurance carrier
- When claim denials are received, researches potential issues and resubmits as appropriate with additional clarifying information
- Notes trends with specific insurance companies and/or benefit plans. Changes or modifies approach to best resolve any difficulties
- Educates the team about new or outstanding insurance related issues. Raises larger issues to the dentist/practice owner

What Job *Skills* Are Important for Success in this Role?

- **Detail Orientation**. Ability to organize and work with data and information with a strong attention to complete itemization and accuracy
- **Follows Instructions/Plans**. While not difficult, insurance plans are extremely specific and concrete. Working with many insurance companies and their processes and

requirements necessitates a comfort level of compliance with multiple policies, contracts, and procedures

- **Multi-tasking**. This is a critical skill. It requires the ability to keep many "balls" in motion and move back and forth between tasks (e.g., handle waiting on hold with insurance and completing other tasks at same time)
- **Comfortable Navigating Ambiguity**. Although insurance plans, patient benefits, and network contracts are generally straightforward, there are many moving parts involved to ensure benefits are achieved and claims paid. Ambiguity (uncertainty) in the insurance field surfaces when different departments or different insurance representatives convey differing instructions. Frustrations can arise. Therefore, insurance coordinators are most productive and successful if they are comfortable with ambiguity, able to persevere through moments of conflicting information, and reach positive outcomes
- **Follow-Through**. This is a job where follow-through matters. The ability to stay on top of status for multiple open claim cases, follow up on a timely basis, and achieve prompt resolution is a hallmark of a great coordinator
- **Able to Broker Solutions**. The insurance coordinator must be a good listener, ask good questions, be assertive in seeking answers (often from multiple sources), able to speak clearly, educate others, and ultimately achieve positive outcomes for all parties involved. The individual must be tenacious in reaching resolution, as well as know when to raise more complex issues to the attention of practice management

What Are the Measures of Success in This Role?

- **Patient Feedback**. Patients who carry a dental insurance plan expect to receive the level of benefit for which they are paying. Although their contract for dental insurance is really between them and their insurance carrier, they do rely on their dental office to best understand their benefit plan, ensure planned treatments are covered by their plan, know in advance what their financial obligation will be, file claims on their behalf, follow through, and resolve any difficulties which arise. When the process goes smoothly, the patient may have little feedback. However, when the process does not go well, it can result in frustration, anger, poor feedback, low referrals, and/or loss of a patient.
- **Claim Approval Rate**. This is another critical measure of success. A fully trained insurance coordinator (and/or well-trained office team) should achieve a high percentage of approved claims and flow of realized revenue for the practice. Conversely, the number of claim denials or requests for additional information should be low. Metrics should be available for all claim data within your dental system. We recommend you regularly track this data.
- **Claim Write-Offs**. A strong insurance coordinator will minimize the number of claim payment write-offs that are incurred in any year of operation.
- **Regulatory Compliance**. A strong coordinator will help to ensure that the practice avoids any problems, complaints, or audits from the insurance company or insurance commission.

How Insurance Coordination Works in Smaller Offices

The challenge within many dental offices is that they aren't large enough to justify a full-time insurance coordinator. Quite often we see offices where one individual assumes several roles/responsibilities.

It is common occurrence for the front office team member to serve as greeter, scheduler, insurance coordinator, treatment coordinator, and collection coordinator. In some practices, the insurance coordinator is less generalized combining only treatment and financial coordination. In yet other practices, a dental assistant or hygienist might serve as insurance coordinator and/or treatment coordinator in addition to their chairside roles. Any of these options can work. The key to success juggling multiple roles is dependent upon the strengths of the individual involved.

Any of these role combinations do share one commonality: They require someone who is great at multitasking. For the small office, assembling a group comprised of strong multitaskers makes for a nimble team. How best to combine roles does call for a bit deeper look at the strengths of individual team members.

Let's look at a real example to illustrate.

> Years ago, we had an insurance coordinator in the office who did a great job, Jessica. She was a happy person, followed our systems and procedures to the letter, and was detail-oriented enough to make very few mistakes. However, a few months into her employment, she had a bad day. While on the phone with an insurance agent to obtain a breakdown, she was told completely contradictory information. She just blew up. She threw the phone down on the receiver, screaming at the phone about being tired of being lied to and stormed off to the break room to cool off. She resigned as insurance coordinator that week.

The fact is Jessica would have been great at several other positions as she was always friendly and a hard worker. However, the insurance role was not right for her because it burned too much mental energy handling tasks that were not her strength.

Selecting the *Right* Insurance Coordinator

In order to achieve the best efficiency in an office, you want to build a team who is well suited for the tasks that need to be handled every day. Most people can be taught to do just about anything. The questions to ask are, how long will it take them to learn it and how efficient they will be when they work on the task?

Anyone can learn to handle insurance, estimates, and claims. However, some team members could work with insurance all week and be efficient and happy. Others may be slower and/or go home drained even after only a day. With the right training, either person can achieve the same results, but the outcomes over time will be much different. One team member may come in happy and get more done every day, while another may come in unmotivated and will accomplish less each day.

Many candidates you come across could be great team members who want to work for your office and contribute to the benefit of your team and patients. However, if you place someone in a position that is not well suited for her, she could burn out like Jessica. She may be more stressed, less efficient, and eventually either resign or cause office team issues, whereas if you assign someone else to that position who is better suited for the task, she will be efficient and happy for years.

So how do you recruit and/or recognize who might be best for the insurance coordinator role?

As previously discussed, there are multiple roles necessary to handle by the front team of a dental office. Let's differentiate some of the key strengths that make each type of role most successful in an office.

Insurance Coordinator. As we have just discussed, this role is best suited for someone who is very detail oriented, can follow instructions/plans well, and is a good multitasker (can handle waiting on hold with insurance and completing other tasks at same time); however, the role does not require a strong ability to adapt to change as insurance rules don't often change. Relationship-building skills would also be less important.

When recruiting for this role, if a candidate does not have related dental background, a background in any form of employee benefits processing or experience in an insurance organization can make for a strong candidate.

> **POTENTIAL INTERVIEW QUESTIONS**
> **FOR AN INSURANCE COORDINATOR CANDIDATE**
>   What do you consider to be your strongest skills?
>   What tasks do you most enjoy?
>   What tasks do you like to avoid or prefer someone else complete?
>   Which do you tend to prefer: To follow a good plan? Or to create a good plan for yourself?
>   What do you find most frustrating in the workplace?
>   Do you prefer to work with a lot of detailed information? Or are you more of a big-picture individual?
>   What would your colleagues likely cite as your strengths, your best skills?
>   Give me an example of a time you were required to work with a lot of detailed information and numbers. What was the situation? The outcome?
>   How would you handle a situation where a patient called the customer service department of their insurance company and were given one answer, though when you called provider relations from the same company you received a quite different answer? How would it make you feel?
>   Do you feel more energized from learning new tasks? Meeting new people? Or completing tasks already started, checking off your list?

Treatment Coordinator. In contrast, someone serving as treatment coordinator is often better suited if they are not as detail oriented because most patients get confused with too much detail. A candidate for this role, too, must be a multitasker. Yet they should be strong at adapting to change—every patient is different. Relationship-building skills are essential for this role. The treatment coordinator should be your best salesperson. Those adept at sales can adapt to each patient/client individually and recognize what is needed to close the sale. An ability to follow through is not as important, as someone else can usually handle the follow-up.

Many general practice, in-network offices have a low acceptance rate with large treatment plans (> $5000). Someone on your team needs to be a great relationship builder as well as adaptable to different types of people and be able to persuade someone to spend a large amount of money with the office. In some cases, that person may well be the dentist.

POTENTIAL INTERVIEW QUESTIONS
FOR A TREATMENT COORDINATOR CANDIDATE

What do you consider to be your strongest skills?

What tasks do you most enjoy?

What tasks do you like to avoid or prefer someone else complete?

Which do you tend to prefer: To follow a good plan? Or to create a good plan for yourself?

What do you find most frustrating in the workplace?

Do you prefer to work with a lot of detailed information? Or are you more of a big-picture individual?

What would your colleagues likely cite as your strengths, your best skills?

Do you see yourself as a natural salesperson? Able to help others see things more clearly in order to make a decision?

Can you give me an example of a situation where you convinced another person to take a specific action? What was the situation, what did you do to convince them, and what was the outcome?

Do you feel more energized from learning new tasks? Meeting new people? Or completing tasks already started, that is, checking off your list?

Collections/Financial Coordinator. For this role, you would look for someone who is very detail oriented, enjoys working with spreadsheets and numbers, and of course a multitasker who is tenacious with a strong ability to follow through. Adapting to change and relationship-building skills are less important.

POTENTIAL INTERVIEW QUESTIONS
FOR A COLLECTIONS/FINANCIAL COORDINATOR CANDIDATE

What do you consider to be your strongest skills?

What tasks do you most enjoy?

What tasks do you like to avoid or prefer someone else complete?

Which do you tend to prefer: To follow a good plan? Or to create a good plan for yourself?

What do you find most frustrating in the workplace?

Do you prefer to work with a lot of detailed information? Or are you more of a big-picture individual?

What would your colleagues likely cite as your strengths, your best skills?

How do you feel about spreadsheets and numbers?

Tell me about a time when you assumed responsibility for tracking a large volume of numbers, perhaps within a system or spreadsheet. How did that assignment turn out? How did you feel about it? Did you make any changes or improvements?

Do you feel more energized entering data? Analyzing spreadsheets? Creating spreadsheets? Or reading reference manuals? Other?

Front Office Greeter/Scheduler. This role serves as your "brand ambassador." The greeter usually establishes the first impression and "tone" of your office/team as well as your tone, as the dentist. Relationship-building skills is of top importance. High energy, a "smiling voice," positivity combined with professionalism are an important blend of traits and skills. While also a multitasker, of lesser importance would be the ability to adapt to change and need for a high level of critical detail.

POTENTIAL INTERVIEW QUESTIONS
FOR A FRONT OFFICE GREETER/SCHEDULER CANDIDATE

What do you consider to be your strongest skills?

What tasks do you most enjoy?

What tasks do you like to avoid or prefer someone else complete?

Which do you tend to prefer: To follow a good plan? Or to create a good plan for yourself?

What do you find most frustrating in the workplace?

Do you prefer to work with a lot of detailed information? Or are you more of a big-picture individual?

What would your colleagues likely cite as your strengths, your best skills?

Tell me about a time when you encountered a difficult situation over the phone. What was the situation? How did you handle it? How did it make you feel?

Do you consider phone calls and questions an interruption in your day? Or your favorite time of day?

There are few people who have strengths in every arena. Most individuals experience some tasks that will drain their energy far faster. Think of yourself during the day, think of the tasks that empower you and you could literally do all day long and not get tired. Contrast that to tasks that you naturally avoid because they are more draining—the thought of doing only those tasks all day is not pleasant, and if you did do it all day, it would make you go home mentally exhausted.

Realize that we dentists tend to possess similar traits. We are often known as very detail oriented, seeking a wealth of information before making a decision, following instructions and planning very well, but we are not necessarily good at multitasking and are reticent to change or adapt to new situations. And as business owners, we can lean toward hiring a team with people who are just like us.

The challenge is that each position in our dental office really requires a different mix of skills. The trick for the dentist/owner is to recruit, select, and then assign the roles that best fit a team member's strengths.

Everyone in my front team can create a treatment plan, come up with the numbers and details surrounding it, and understand the insurance portion that is involved. However, one of my team members (let's call her Molly) handles the large treatment cases far better than anyone else. This is because Molly has a great ability to adapt to each patient's situation differently. Each team member has a different set of needs/wants, a different financial situation, a different scheduling situation, a different view on the value of dentistry. When I ask Molly to do something new, she jumps on it. Her ability to adapt is high. However, I have learned not to go over highly detailed information with Molly—I can see her mind wander, she gets frustrated easily when I do.

One last point: Every role needs a backup, someone crossed-trained who can help with overflow or handle tasks during illness and vacations.

Assessments Can Help

So how do you find out whether someone will be well-suited for the task of insurance coordinator? (or any other key role on the team?) Trial and error can certainly work; the challenge is it takes a lot of time and energy to run through people until you find the right fit. Targeted interviews to learn an individual's strengths, experience, and preferences is another viable approach. An alternative option is to find a way to learn how to assess a person's strengths and match them to the position you need.

If you are struggling to find the right individual(s) on your team who can assume primary responsibility for coordinating insurance for your office and patients and at the same time be successful, productive, and effective handling the majority of claims, then there are some additional steps you might consider.

There are assessment tools that can help to identify strengths and skill sets most suited to the type of tasks required of an insurance coordinator or any other role on your team. One of the more effective assessment tools is the Kolbe Assessment method.

Kolbe works from the premise that there are three parts of the mind that control our thinking, feeling, and doing. The **thinking** part defines our basic intelligence. It grows as you learn and is therefore ever changing. An IQ test is one way in which intelligence can be measured.

The **feeling** part of your mind affects emotions. Assessment tools such as Myers-Briggs measure a person's reactions to circumstances and assigns a personality type. Myers-Briggs can sometimes be useful in understanding the personality mix and appreciating the different personality styles of your team.

The **doing** part of your brain contains the instincts and innate attributes that define your natural method of operation (MO). When you work in your natural style, you are more productive, more comfortable, and more successful. The Kolbe Assessment tool identifies an individual's natural work style. Understanding what type of work comes most naturally to a team member can be very helpful in determining which duties and responsibilities they will be most successful performing.

Let's look at an example that demonstrates how this assessment might work from Dr. Christopher Phelps, who is a dentist and a long-time Kolbe certified trainer.

Dr. Phelps had two strong RDAs who were constantly in conflict. Both were complaining that the other always changes their room setups. The typical dentist response is often to either fire one of them or to assign them specific rooms so they never have to work together. However, in assessing the strengths of these two individuals, we learn there is another option.

Dr. Phelps found with his two RDAs that both have a high follow-through strength. While normally having the same innate strength might be perceived as a good thing, in this case it actually put them in competition. Both had the desire to create a structure or plan for where the supplies were positioned in the operatory. The conflict came into play because their plans vastly differed. Once their respective profiles were revealed, the solution became readily apparent. They were simply asked to work together to come up with a unified plan, one they could both agree on. Once they did this, they worked well together for years. Knowing the Kolbe scores of each person allowed him to find a solution that worked for everyone.

For more information about the Kolbe assessment, simply refer to https://Kolbe.com.

Chapter Summary

Employers tend to want productive team members, and employees tend to want to feel appreciated and have a sense of fulfillment in their careers. When you can fit the right person to the right position, both the employer and the employee will be more satisfied with the arrangement. This allows a stronger and longer-lasting relationship that ultimately serves both the office and the patients more effectively.

Part 4

How Covid-19 Changed the Dental Landscape

Dentistry has always had its challenges, but nothing has affected the industry like the Covid-19 pandemic in 2020. The volume of regulations and changes that happened was unprecedented. There are so many new topics to consider after Covid-19, such as aerosols, infection control, and teams. The changes from the pandemic hit the industry hard enough to deserve special discussion. This section is going to stay on topic with how the insurance landscape has changed and what you as an office can do about it.

Chapter 30
PPE Fees and Insurance Companies

After the pandemic panic hit in 2020, the price of most of the infection-control products used in health care and dentistry skyrocketed. Some of these products became 10 times more expensive. While the idea of low-cost items, such as masks and gloves, going up in price may not sound like a big problem, they can be some of the most expensive supplies in a dental office because of the frequency we go through them. Gloves for our office were one of the top five most expensive supply items before Covid-19. Yet they were only pennies apiece. Masks were under 50 cents apiece. It is unexpected that we will ever see those low prices again. During the Covid-19 pandemic shutdown of dental offices, a host of new changes came about quickly. One of the first immediate reactions was the ADA redefining an existing code to help offices find a way to manage these additional PPE costs.

> "The American Dental Association recognizes the extraordinary circumstances dentists and their patients face as we navigate the COVID pandemic. The cost of infection control procedures has skyrocketed, and dental offices are facing a significant financial challenge navigating this environment. Further, costs of personal protective equipment (PPE) including N95 masks, surgical masks, face shields, gowns, and shoe covers, has increased due to supply shortages with prices variable across the nation. Operatory protective barriers, protective equipment for front office staff, additional disinfection protocols and other administrative or engineering controls (e.g., isolation systems, air purifiers, filters, etc.) are adding overhead for dental offices."

—ADA COVID-19 Coding and Billing Interim Guidance: PPE

The ADA urged insurance companies to either increase procedure fees or allow for a per visit PPE standard fee to account for the massive increase in PPE overhead costs. We will see with time what effect this will have on insurance reimbursement for dental offices.

Currently code D1999 – unspecified preventive procedure by report has been redefined by the ADA to be D1999 – Covid-19 PPE code. You would use this code if you want to bill for the increased costs of PPE for patient care.

The common questions surrounding use of this code are:

What Should I Charge for D1999?

Every office is different with respect to their supply costs, and therefore in offices around the country, fees have been set anywhere from $0 to $150 for D1999. The average fee reported has been between $10 and $20. What you decide to do for your office should consider the added costs you have picked up from PPE supplies, forced decrease in volume due to patient flow restrictions, or increased time needs for procedures.

How Do I Document Additional PPE Costs?

You can notate the additional costs and supplies in both your clinical notes as well as the claim narrative or notes section of a claim. It would be important to document every new or increased cost since March 2020 for both justification of the fees and possible education to the insurance companies.

Example documentation:

"Additional costs represent the collective expenses of the increased supply cost of gloves, gowns, masks, disinfectants, shields, air purifier maintenance, extraoral vacuum, UV lights, etc."

What Will Be Reimbursed?

Every insurance company has treated this code differently. Here is a list of what has happened so far with insurance company response to the D1999 PPE code. Realize that private insurance companies only reimburse any PPE fees to in-network providers:

Company	Code	Allowed?	Reimbursed?	Fee	End date
Washington State Medicaid	D1999	Yes	Per visit	$15	
MCNA Nebraska Medicaid	D1999 or Auto	Yes	Per visit	$10	June 30, 2020
Humana	Auto	Yes	Monthly	$7	Sept 30, 2020
Anthem BCBS	Auto	Yes	Per visit	$10	Aug 31, 2020
CareFirst BCBS	D1999	Yes	Per visit	$7	Aug 31, 2020
Cigna	D1999	Yes	Per visit	$8	July 31, 2020
GEHA	D1999		Per visit	$7	Dec 31
United Concordia	D1999	Yes	Per visit	$10	Sept 30, 2020
UPMC	Auto	No	Per visit	$7	Sept 30, 2020
Lincoln Financial	D1999	In & Out, exclude ortho	Per visit	$10	
Principle	D1999	Yes	Per visit	$7	Dec 31, 2020
HealthPartners Dental Plan	D1999	No	Per visit	$10	Sept 30, 2020

Company	Code	Allowed?	Reimbursed?	Fee	End date
United Healthcare	Must enroll in program http://www.uhcdental.com/	No	Monthly	$5-10, see program details	Dec 31, 2020
Dominion National	Auto		Per visit	$5	Dec 31, 2020
Dental Care Plus Group	Auto	No	Monthly	$10	June 30, 2020
Florida Blue/ Arkansas BCBS/ HMSA	D1999	No	Per visit	Per policy	Dec 31, 2020
Empire BCBS	Auto	No	Per visit	$10	Aug 31
BCBS Kansas	Auto	No	Per $	1-3%	Dec 31, 2020
Delta Dental	Auto	No	Per exam	$10	Oct 20, 2020
Delta Arizona	Auto	No	Monthly	$10	July 31, 2020
Delta Missouri	Auto	No	Lump	Based on past claims	
Delta Idaho	Auto	No	Lump	Based on 2019	
Delta Mass.	Auto	No	Per visit	$10	Aug 31, 2020
Delta Virginia	Auto	No	Lump	Patient #s	
NorthEast Delta	Auto	No	Monthly	$10	June 2020
Delta Kansas	Auto	No	Monthly	$10	July 31
Delta Colorado	Auto	No	Monthly	$10	July 31
Hawaii Dental Service	Auto	No	Monthly	$10	July 31
Delta Arkansas	Application grant	No			
Delta Rhode Island	Auto	No	Lump	Volume	
Delta Wyoming	Application, call	No	Lump		
Delta Wisconsin	Auto	No	Lump	2019 volume	
Delta Iowa	Auto	No	Monthly	$10	Aug 31
Delta Minnesota & Nebraska	Increase base Exam code reimbursement	No			
Delta South Dakota	Increase base exam code reimbursement	No			

Company	Code	Allowed?	Reimbursed?	Fee	End date
Delta Tennessee	Henry Schein Credit	No			
Delta NJ/CT	Auto w/ EFT	No	Per visit	$10	2 months
Delta MI, IN, OH	Henry Schein Credit	No			
Principle	Auto		Per visit	$7	
Premera	D1999		Per visit	Variable	Nov 1
Florida Combined Life	D1999		Per visit	Variable	Dec 31

What if This Code Is Disallowed?

ADA's stance is stated in the Statement on Third Party Payer Reimbursement for Costs Associated with Increased Standards for Personal Protective Equipment (PPE) April 21, 2020.

"When adjudicating such claims, the ADA believes that it is inappropriate for any third-party benefit program to unfairly place the cost burden on dentists by disallowing or bundling charges for PPE on the pretext that the payment for additional required PPE is included in the payment for any other procedure billed for the visit. Denied claims are typically billable to the patient."

This has not stopped insurance companies from ignoring the ADA's public statement. See Chapter 18 on disallow and what to do.

Chapter 31
Teledentistry and Insurance Claims

WHAT IS TELEDENTISTRY?

"Virtual Healthcare," that is, the ability to have a doctor diagnose or help a patient from a remote location, is a concept that has been around since the phone was invented. The actual term "teledentistry" was first used in 1997, when J. Cook defined it as "the practice of using video-conferencing technologies to diagnose and provide advice about treatment over a distance" (https://www.ncbi.nlm.nih.gov/pmc/articles/PMC3894070/).

Even then, the limitations of the technology and the low level of interest/necessity kept teledentistry more as a side option than a true mainstream choice. The Covid-19 pandemic and closure of dental offices brought the need for virtual dental consults and care to the forefront. Many state boards that had left the topic of teledentistry on the sideline now faced an immediate and massive need to decide how best to scale and capitalize on the new trend. Thankfully, the ADA dental insurance codes had already been in place since 2018 for teledentistry. There are two codes:

D9995 Teledentistry – synchronous; real-time encounter. This code is used for direct, virtual consults.

D9996 Teledentistry – asynchronous; information stored and forwarded to dentist for subsequent review. This code is used for email or text correspondence.

You might be thinking that D9996 happens often in dentistry already, and you would be correct. Dental offices conduct electronic correspondence daily with labs, other providers, patients, and so forth. The expectation is this code will rarely be used for normal day-to-day activities and mostly used only in conjunction with other billable services. D9995 is the dental code that most offices will likely use for a live electronic consult over the phone, Zoom, Skype, Facetime, and so forth.

Now, one important point to understand here is that these codes are not intended to reflect procedures, as teledentistry is not a standalone dental service. These are codes intended to define how something is done, such as a consult or exam. When you go to a restaurant and dine in, order to go, or get delivery, those are methods for how you got the food. Teledentistry is the same. This means the codes should never be used alone. Teledentistry is just the method through which you are delivering some other form of dental care.

Please keep in mind that since teledentistry is just the method of delivery, all the normal rules and regulations apply. HIPAA is still fully in force, so as an office you need to make sure that whatever technology service you use is compliant and secure.

Coding

The teledentistry codes can be used with a variety of other codes, most often in the diagnostic arena, such as exams: D0140 – Limited Exam, D0170 – Re-eval non-Post-op Exam, D0171 – Re-eval Post-Op Exam.

*Notice the periodic and comprehensive exam codes are not listed. Typically, without being in-person, these codes would not be reasonable to use with a service that could be provided virtually.

Claims

You may want to refer to Chapter 8 and review the ADA claim form. Item 38, the entry "Place of Treatment" on a claim form is often ignored because it never changes. It is traditionally the dental office. However, with teledentistry it is possible this line might be different. The POS (place of service) code is typically 11 for claims where treatment is rendered in the office. However, in 2017, the POS code 2 was added for "Telehealth Services." If you are providing virtual teledentistry from somewhere outside of your dental office (your office at home as an example), you would want to code a 2 instead of an 11 in this line item on the claim form.

ANCILLARY CLAIM/TREATMENT INFORMATION		
38. Place of Treatment ☐ (e.g. 11=office; 22=O/P Hospital) (Use *Place of Service Codes for Professional Claims)		39. Enclosures (Y or N) ☐
40. Is Treatment for Orthodontics? ☐ No (Skip 41-42) ☐ Yes (Complete 41-42)		41. Date Appliance Placed (MM/DD/CCYY)
42. Months of Treatment	43. Replacement of Prosthesis ☐ No ☐ Yes (Complete 44)	44. Date of Prior Placement (MM/DD/CCYY)
45. Treatment Resulting from ☐ Occupational illness/injury ☐ Auto accident ☐ Other accident		
46. Date of Accident (MM/DD/CCYY)		47. Auto Accident State
TREATING DENTIST AND TREATMENT LOCATION INFORMATION		

Reimbursement

Every insurance company is going to be different with how it handles the teledentistry codes. However, a general rule that most companies use is that the "method in which the service or procedure is provided is not a reimbursable item." Whether you complete a filling with a drill or a laser, the insurance company is just paying for the filling itself. The same applies for teledentistry in most cases, insurance will pay for the exam, but not the method by which the exam was provided (virtual).

The D9995 code is therefore more of a reporting code than a reimbursement code from most insurance companies. This means if you incur a cost to provide your virtual consults and you want the patient to help offset this cost, your D9995 fee is something you would need to bill to the patient directly.

You can expect that most insurance companies that you are in-network with will disallow a fee for D9995/D9996 if you add it to a claim. Please see Chapter 18 on how to handle disallows and the ADA's stance on this topic. As an in-network dentist, the easiest way to handle patients paying for virtual consults is to have the platform you use (e.g., Simplifeye) to charge the patient directly, which some of them can do.

Many offices have also used teledentistry as more of a marketing cost than a reimbursable fee. Several extraordinarily successful dentists have created an entire model around first impressions being gained through a virtual platform, which has appealed to a much larger audience since the Covid-19 pandemic.

EXAMPLE

Example Teledentistry Scenario
Your long-term patient Julie develops severe pain over the weekend. Naturally, the dentist is out of town at a CE course at the time. Therefore, the RDA, Suzie, comes to the office to help Julie with her problem. Suzie sets up a computer so that the dentist can virtually consult with Julie about the concern. The dentist then prescribes for Suzie to take a PA x-ray of the problem area as well as a digital photo. Based on the findings, the dentist determines that Julie has an infection around a decayed tooth and needs antibiotics and an appointment for treatment the following week.

What codes would be used for this scenario?

D0140 – Limited exam
D0220 – 1st periapical x-ray
D0350 - 2D oral/facial photographic image obtained intra-orally or extra-orally
D9995 - teledentistry – synchronous; real-time encounter

*Note – some states require exam codes to have a "dentist's hands in mouth." If you are in one of these states, it would be more appropriate to instead code a consult instead of an exam.

Orthodontics and Teledentistry

Another large industry shift in dentistry that came about through Covid-19 was orthodontics. Do-it-yourself (DIY) orthodontics had been around for a few years prior to 2020, like Smile Direct Club (SDC). As a response to both SDC and other DIY orthodontic programs that tried to remove the dentist from the equation, many aligner companies started providing platforms for dentists to be involved with orthodontics virtually. The general idea is that the software or app would prompt the patient to take photos with and without the aligners in at set intervals (weekly, monthly, etc.). This would allow the dentist or orthodontist to keep track of the progress of the orthodontic treatment without needing to directly see the patient. By conducting the visual viewing virtually, it greatly increases the convenience to the patient and reduces the time and cost to the provider.

Virtual-based orthodontics is a segment of the dental industry that is likely to continue growing rapidly.

Chapter 32
How to Thrive in the New Landscape

Suffice it to say that the changes that have come about due to the Covid-19 pandemic drastically changed the dental world in 2020. Many of these changes are going to be long-lasting or permanent to the industry. It is unlikely we will see a reduction in PPE costs to pre-pandemic levels. Patient perception of dentistry due to unfortunate early and false fear about the safety of dentistry is likely to be felt for years. While it is rare to see a dental office completely fail, there are many offices struggling under the impact of all these unforeseen changes and their associated financial implications. So how can your office not only cope, but thrive in this new landscape of dental care? This chapter will discuss some of the tactics and changes that dental offices have made to survive and thrive.

One of the most proactive actions you can take for your business is learn as much as you can about dental insurance practices, techniques for navigating, and how to get legitimately paid for everything you do. Private offices often have a better capacity to run efficiently with the right training and systems in place. The more the team involves themselves with forming strong relationships with the patients, the less of a challenge you will have with almost every aspect in a dental office.

Virtual Marketing

Today's top marketing techniques are designed to showcase your business, helping it stand out from the rest by highlighting the goods and services no one else provides. Virtual platforms available today can provide dental offices the opportunity to stand out and offer something different over their competitors, not only offering virtual dental consults but also online scheduling, more convenient hours, online education, and so forth. These virtual consults can be done either simultaneously through live programs or asynchronously through recorded videos and email. Many platforms have arisen to provide the compliance and technology to make this option legal and easy to use.

Use of virtual consults could help your office stand apart from others, especially if the concern about viral spread continues in the world. But even after a pandemic is no longer an issue, it could become a differentiator in sheer convenience of being able to meet virtually.

Possible Benefits of Teledentistry and Virtual Consults

Safety – While historically, dental offices have been proven not be a source of viral spread, a virtual setting provides a **completely** safe environment for communication with and minor evaluation of patients..

Cost Savings – Virtual consults do not require gloves, masks, or chair space. There are no costs of PPE or room setup or breakdown.

Accessibility and Convenience – Many patients have challenges with scheduling appointments within their busy work/home schedules, especially during normal office hours. Virtual consults provide a patient with more options to access the dental office and can provide the office a new stream of patients they may not get otherwise.

For example: surgical post-op visits can now be accomplished by the dentist/assistant virtually to assess the patient and provide irrigation instructions. The improvement in patient care and satisfaction can lead to more patient referrals and reviews.

Another option would be non-simultaneous information exchange. Some platforms now exist to conduct video-based messages back and forth. This allows the patient and doctor to not only see each other but be able to communicate on different time schedules, such as the doctor during the day and the patient at night after work. The main feature of using a platform is to have ease of access to past information as well as a HIPAA compliant system.

Virtual gives an office the option to not only reduce costs, but also to stand out from others and be able to gain more patients to counteract the dips in the industry.

PPE FEES – TO CHARGE OR NOT TO CHARGE

Many practices around the country added PPE fees to their patient visits during and even after the Covid-19 pandemic. While these were understandable and justified, the concept has received a rather negative response from many patient and dental groups. Some states, such as Maryland and New York, have tried to legally stop dental offices completely from passing on PPE fees to patients.

Offices need to weigh the value of the PPE charges with the potential negative response from patients and other groups. One alternative many FFS and OON offices implemented was just to raise their prices across the board, to hide the new costs within the normal pricing structure. This is a great option if you are not contracted with an insurance company but does not work for the in-network office.

Alternative Method to Fees

An alternative method is to take the opposite approach and explicitly state that you will not be charging added fees. Use this message instead to market your practice and drive patients to want to see you instead of the dentist down the street. An example message might read:

> Patient Safety Measures
> Our patients' safety is our Number 1 priority. You will notice on upcoming visits that our procedures and equipment have changed during this pandemic.

> This is for your safety and ours. What you won't notice is a charge for additional PPE supplies to keep our patients and team safe. To cover the rising costs of this, some offices will be charging more to cover this added expense. This is absolutely their right, and we respect their autonomy on how to operate their practice. We have decided not to pass along this additional expense to our patients.
>
> We have taken more steps for your safety, but these costs will not be passed on to you! During the close, we have worked on several projects to allow patients better care and accessibility, which we will be announcing soon. We love our patients, and we are choosing to focus on the positive during this time.

Every office is unique; however, many of those differences patients might not notice. A message highlighting the fact that costs won't be passed on to patients can be a difference that is readily recognizable.

Change Insurance Participation

Rethinking your level of insurance participation is another potential response to increased fees. Dropping insurance providers is often a tactic discussed in dental groups; however, there are some hurdles an office might want to think about before taking this step. Refer back to Chapter 30 on PPE fees and insurance coverage and evaluate what costs were not covered with how insurance companies responded to their in-network providers. Also make sure you understand what impact dropping an insurance company might have on your patient population. Many patients may stay, but others will only go to an office that is in-network, and if you drop that coverage, they will leave. It is important to evaluate what the impact might be for dropping an insurance network. You might be able to renegotiate your insurance contract and get higher fees without dropping your network patients. See Chapter 16 for how to evaluate and renegotiate with your insurance providers.

No matter what decision is best for your office, it is important to consider what you will be comfortable with today and in the future.

Membership Plans

A common dynamic during a recession is that many people lose or change their jobs, which means they usually lose their insurance coverage. The consequence for dental offices is that many patients will often choose to avoid going to the dentist completely if they don't have a "plan" in place.

If you provide a viable alternative for patients instead of insurance, they will likely keep coming to your office. Membership plans are very easy to design and implement and can be managed internally by the team or with the help of third-party software. It is important to keep in mind that many patients pay for insurance monthly, through an automatic withdrawal from their account. The closer you can simulate this process with your membership plan, the more successful it will be.

The basic idea of a membership plan is straightforward and simple, making available discounted services—with no waiting periods, deductibles, claims, and so forth. While it may seem counterintuitive to reduce your fees for diagnostic and hygiene services through a membership plan, if you keep your restorative and treatment fees higher than insurance-negotiated fees, the plans will often provide a better option for the office with the added opportunity of gaining more uninsured patients than you might otherwise get.

Patient Financing

Many workers in America live paycheck to paycheck, or close to it. It is often difficult for many to come up with thousands of dollars to get dental work done. Providing ways for patients to pay for their care over time can greatly increase the office's service to the patient as well as the collections the office would not otherwise obtain.

If you were not providing patient financing before, adding financing options can help provide a new source of patients as well as treatment income. See Chapter 25 for more information on patient financing, third-party companies, and whether they might be right for your office.

Dental Work Warranties

There are no guarantees when working with a complex system such as the human body. Many times, procedures done by the book can turn out with results that are completely unexpected. Nerves and teeth don't always respond "normally."

Often dentists will shy away from providing a warranty on their dental work because of this unknown aspect about dental care. However, the concept of a warranty is not about guarantees but about faith and trust in a product or service (dental care).

Implied vs Explicit

One key point to think about is the difference between an implied warranty vs explicit warranty. Explicit warranties are what we normally think of that are written down in detail. Implied warranties are ones that are unspoken and expected based on the situation. In dentistry, most of what we do comes with an implied warranty, meaning that by providing restorative care, the patient assumes that the work will last for years or for life.

We all know in dentistry that everything we do eventually fails due to the environment we are working within. Patients do not understand this unless we inform them. We also have no control over what the patient might do (trauma, chew on objects, bruxism, etc.). The most important point about offering a warranty is not about what you do cover, it is about what you do not cover. Patients will assume the implied warranty, so your explicit warranty helps guide them toward what you want them to know.

What Patients Want to Hear

Customer service is all about giving your patients what they want as much as possible, often services, information, or conveniences that have nothing to do with dentistry. There are a variety of things that clients want to hear from any business, and dentistry is no different.

Confidence – People want to hear confidence in their providers as well as the team. They want to know that you have experience taking care of the things that concern them.

Reduction of Risk – Everything in life has risk associated with it. Often this risk is more worry than reality, that is, a perceived risk. When you can reduce your patient's perceived risk, they will be happier and more confident with your work.

Reliability - People want to know that you stand behind your work and you can take care of any concerns they might have after the fact. Verbal confirmation of this confidence is great, and an explicit written confirmation is even more powerful.

All these desires of your patients can be improved with having a formal, explicit warranty statement for major dental work. A written statement can help solidify their loyalty to the office as well as help them be more comfortable accepting new, high-dollar treatment.

How to Discuss with Patients

"Dr. X does amazing work, and patients love him. However, occasionally life happens, and unexpected events occur, such as injuries or trauma that your teeth were not designed to handle. This is why we are proud to offer our warranty program."

"We cannot guarantee how well anyone will take care of their oral health at home, or how much life will throw at them. What we can guarantee is that we will do everything possible to provide the highest quality care to give you the best chance of your dental work lasting for a long time."

Benefits to the Office

The first and main benefit to both the office and patient is clearly defining expectations for the patient. When a patient is aware that a crown is only supposed to last X years, then they will not unrealistically expect a lifetime out of it.

The second is that patients will get a greater sense of trust with the office if there is a defined policy on how you handle replacement work. This can contribute to higher treatment acceptance when utilized correctly.

The last benefit is more long term. When a patient does have work that eventually has to be replaced, the doctor and office are not stuck with possibly having to do free work.

Sample Plans

There are a variety of ways that offices have managed a warranty program for their patients. Here are some of the more common examples:

Service Policy with your New Crown

Your new crown was built and installed with one of the strongest restoration techniques in dentistry. Under normal circumstances, it should last for years. However, despite the best materials, crowns can fail due to factors outside our control: cavities, excessive grinding, or biting on hard objects such as forks, pencils, ice, or bone. Most insurance policies will not cover a replacement crown in the first 5 years. In the unlikely event that your crown should require replacement in the first few years, this schedule outlines how we will help you with replacement costs.

First year of service – 100% coverage
Second year of service – 80% coverage
Third year of service – 60% coverage

Fourth year of service – 40% coverage
Fifth year of service – 20% coverage
Sixth year of service – 0% coverage

As an example, if your crown requires replacement 14 months after delivery, that would fall in the second year of service. If the new crown at that time costs $1500, you will only pay $300, and we will cover the remaining $1200.

Thank you,
Dental Office Team

LIMITED WARRANTY*

IMPLANT CROWNS: For a period of **5 years** from the date of restoration, we will replace an implant crown or abutment that is damaged due to breakage at no cost to the patient.

GOLD CROWNS OR ONLAYS: For a period of **5 years** from the date of cementation, we will replace a gold restoration that is damaged due to breakage, misfit, or decay at no cost to the patient.

PORCELAIN VENEERS, CROWNS, AND BRIDGES: For a period of **5 years** from the time of cementation, we will replace or repair a porcelain restoration that becomes damaged due to porcelain fracture, misfit, or decay at no cost to the patient. Some teeth are not recommended to have porcelain due to normal requirement for material strength or heavy grinding. If the porcelain breaks due to metal refusal or failure to wear recommended occlusal guard, the crown will be replaced at 50% original fee to patient.

ROOT CANAL THERAPY: Root canal therapy has a 95% success rate, but occasionally does not succeed. If your root canal treatment is not successful, we may send you to a specialist in difficult root canals. If this occurs during the first year, we will refund you 100% of the fee paid for the root canal. After the first year, and for a period of five years from the time of treatment, we will credit the patient portion paid for the root canal treatment toward future care.

COMPOSITE (WHITE) FILLINGS AND SEALANTS: When a tooth has a cavity, we remove the infected area and seal the hole with a composite filling that should not be more than 50% of the tooth. It is the remaining tooth that supports the filling. When a cavity destroys more than 50% of a tooth, a crown is needed to hold the tooth together. Sometimes we place a filling, thinking the tooth is still strong enough when it is not. In this case the tooth begins to break under chewing forces. If this breakdown should occur within a period of two years, we will credit the cost of the filling toward the cost of a crown. We will replace a composite filling or sealant due to breakage, misfit, or decay at no cost to the patient if there is enough tooth structure remaining.

*LIMITATIONS:

1. This warranty will be null and void if the patient does not maintain his/her recommended professional dental cleanings (either every three, four, or six months).
2. If a tooth becomes sensitive after dental treatment and requires root canal therapy, this is a possible complication. There are many reasons a tooth requires root canal therapy that are beyond our control (deep cavities, fractures, and individual patient sensitivities).
3. This warranty does not cover breakage due to accident, trauma, or inappropriate use (chewing ice, opening bottles, etc.)

Third-Party Warranty Companies

An alternative to providing internal coverage for your work is to get an outside company to handle this for you. Generally, these third-party warranties help the office far more than you would think. The basic concept is similar to any extended warranty program you see in other industries. The patient pays an extra percentage of the treatment fee, and the insurance/warranty company covers any damage to the restoration/service for X number of years.

The benefit to the patient is this warranty coverage is provided by an outside company, which means it can be redeemed anywhere in the country. If the patient moves or otherwise is no longer seeing the dentist who provided the treatment, they still have full coverage.

The benefit to the office is any replacement work is now paid for at 100% full fee. The office no longer must conduct free work. An additional benefit is these programs often require the patient to pay a higher fee than the office is charged for the warranty. The difference becomes additional funds for the office. (Example: the patient is charged 14% of the service cost to get the warranty by the office, and the office is charged 10% by the warranty company. The 4% becomes extra income.)

Chapter Summary

Different systems work for different offices. The main idea to get out of this is to consider the options and choose a system in advance of the need. When you plan ahead for all eventualities, you become prepared. When you fail to plan, the outcomes are not what we want and often lead to upset patients or offices losing money.

Part 5

Case Studies

Case Studies
Explained

Many aspects of dealing with insurance companies can be complex, and dentistry is a very visual field. The case studies in this section are designed to help illustrate some common questions and challenges that arise daily for offices and providers. The best way to use this section is as a test for yourself to see if you understood the concepts taught throughout the textbook. It can also serve as a good reference for when you have similar cases arise within your practice.

The case studies are all real-life situations that have been treated by the submitting doctors. Many of these dentists are top of their field and do some amazing work and have beautiful documentation. Many of these dentists are Fee-for-Service and therefore did not deal with insurance in their specific case. Added within each case are insurance-based questions that happen every day in other offices to help better illustrate how to manage insurance. This section should help you better understand these intricacies.

Each case will present the situation and pose questions on the first page. This section is best used as a quiz to see if you understand the concepts discussed in the textbook. We recommend you try to answer the questions before flipping to the next page, which contains the outcome as well as the answers and discussion.

CASE STUDY 1.   BIOMIMETIC ONLAY

This is a beautiful example of replacing a large amalgam with an indirect restoration (onlay or crown), a procedure that is often declined by insurance. Receiving a claim denial for this type of case is usually due to lack of correct documentation. Therefore, let's discuss this case and how to properly approach it and prepare the claim in order to achieve reimbursement for the patient's benefit.

Case Notes: 42 y/o patient presents with decay underneath a prior massive amalgam restoration. Patient has non-lingering sensitivity to cold stimulus, and pain to direct pressure.

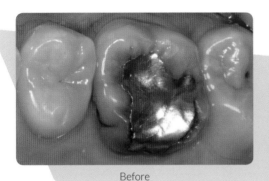 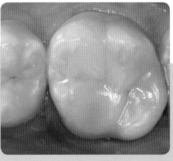

Before   After

Insurance Questions to Answer:

1. What is the most common treatment for this case?
2. What internal or insurance codes would you use?
3. Which pictures and x-rays would you want to prepare and include for the best chance of insurance reimbursement?
4. What narrative might you want to construct for this case for insurance?

The most common treatment for this type of case would be a buildup and crown. For this case, however, Dr. Sergie is highly trained in more conservative treatment methods (biomimetics) and was able to solve this problem with an onlay. Since most dentists would treat this as a crown, we will use that as the discussion for coding.

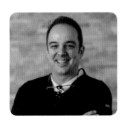

Dr. Aly Sergie maintains a restorative practice in Dallas, Texas, focusing on adhesive, cosmetic, and implant dentistry. He is known for making complex issues in dentistry easy to understand. The foundations of what he teaches is based on dental photography, adhesive dentistry, and treatment acceptance. You can find out more of this information at MondayMorningSolutions.dental and LearnDentalPhotography.com

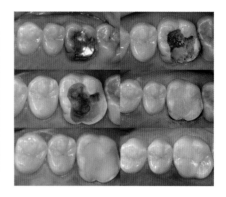

CODING RECOMMENDATIONS
D2950 – Core buildup
D2750 – Porcelain crown
D3110 – Direct pulp cap
S2700 – Internal code for custom staining
S2750 – Internal code for additional lab fee
for premium lab

Insurance Answers for Biomimetic Onlay Case

Before and After Photos to send

1. Photo after restoration removal with decay (left), photo showing fractures internal to both mesial and distal (right). You can also see the direct pulp exposure in this photo.

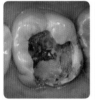 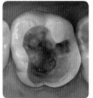

NOTE
The best time to take the pre-op PA that you will send to insurance for this case is at the point shown by the photos on the left (see Chapter 23 for discussion).

2. After Buildup Photo. An x-ray would not be required with a good photo instead. Ideally this photo would be post-prep as seen here on the right.

Case Narrative

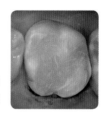

All crowns and buildups should be submitted with a narrative. A basic narrative to send for this case is below. You can refer to Chapter 23 for a full discussion on narratives for crowns and buildups.

"Patient presents with fractured and decayed tooth. Patient has cracked tooth syndrome based on symptoms of pain to biting pressure, confirmed with positive tooth sleuth results. Decay is present on MODL surfaces and internal fractures on the mesial and distal pulpal floors require occlusal coverage restoration. Direct carious pulpal exposure noted, requiring direct pulp cap as an additional service, long-term prognosis is excellent. Build up is required due to 80% of sound tooth structure missing after decay removal. Please refer to photos for decay, fractures, missing tooth structure, and after buildup documentation."

Summary

This is a common scenario seen daily in dental offices where there is an obvious clinical need for an indirect restoration. However, explaining to the insurance company why the indirect restoration treatment is necessary can be a challenge. Changing how you approach these cases can mean the difference between achieving reimbursement vs a headache. Remember, reimbursement fights are in the best interest of the patient, as anything not collected from insurance should and will be the patient's responsibility to pay.

CASE STUDY 2.   CADCAM CROWN REPLACEMENT

This is another beautiful case submitted by Dr. Sergie. What you see here is a pronounced situation where former restorations failed. The common challenge when submitting claims to correct previous dental work is getting all parts of the case reimbursed. Typically, the denial of this type of case will be due to lack of correct, clear documentation. Therefore, let's discuss how to best prepare a claim for this case in order to obtain full reimbursement for the patient's benefit.

Case Notes: 52 y/o patient presents with decay under prior CADCAM restorations on #29 and 30. Patient has non-lingering sensitivity to cold stimulus and notable sticky decay around the margins.

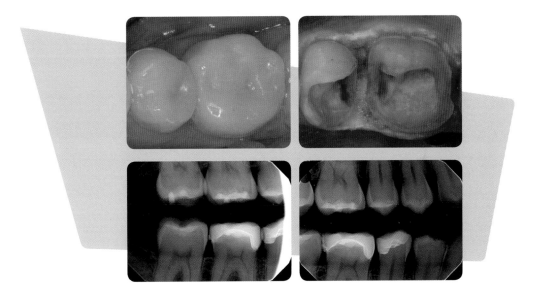

Insurance Questions to Answer:

1. What initial challenge do you see for this case getting reimbursed?
2. What codes would you file in the insurance claim? What internal office codes might you use?
3. Which pictures and x-rays would you want to attach to the claim to achieve the best chance for insurance reimbursement?
4. What narrative might you want to submit to ensure the reason for this case is clear for an insurance claims examiner?

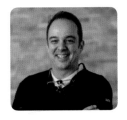

Dr. Aly Sergie maintains a restorative practice in Dallas, Texas, focusing on adhesive, cosmetic, and implant dentistry. He is known for making complex issues in dentistry easy to understand. The foundations of what he teaches is based on dental photography, adhesive dentistry, and treatment acceptance. You can find out more of this information at MondayMorningSolutions.dental and LearnDentalPhotography.com

Insurance Answers for CADCAM Crown Replacement Case

The initial challenge with cases like this is that the x-rays alone would often result in claim denials. The decay that we notice clinically does not always show up clearly on an x-ray.

Since some problems do not show up well on an x-ray, photos and narratives become of primary importance. But not any photo will work. Pre-op photos often may not show a good picture of the true problem.

Photos to Send

1. After restoration removal, with decay, showing missing tooth structure and need for a buildup that would not be evident on an x-ray.
2. The best x-rays to send are at this post-restoration removal stage.
3. After-buildup photo. An x-ray would not be required with a good photo instead.
4. See Chapter 23 for further discussion about which photos and x-rays are best to submit for crowns and buildups.

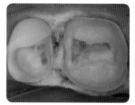 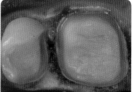

CODING RECOMMENDATIONS
D2950 – Core buildup
D2750 – Porcelain crown
D3120 – Indirect pulp cap
S2750 – Internal code for additional lab fee for premium lab
* The premolar buildup might get remapped to a D2949. Suggest estimating as zero coverage.

Case Narrative

All crowns and build ups should be submitted with a narrative. A basic narrative to send for this case is included below. You can refer to Chapter 25 for a full discussion on narratives for crowns and build ups.

"Patient presents with decay under distal of #29 prior onlay and mesial and distal of prior crown #30. Near pulpal exposure noted #30, requiring indirect pulp cap as an additional service, long-term prognosis is excellent for avoidance of RCT with this procedure. Buildup is required due to 65% of sound tooth structure missing after decay removal. Please refer to photos for decay, missing tooth structure, and after buildup documentation."

Summary

This is a common scenario seen in dental offices where there is an obvious clinical need for an indirect restoration, but with challenges in relaying that information to an insurance company thoroughly enough for reimbursement, especially with buildups. Remember, reimbursement fights are in the best interest of the patient, as anything not collected from insurance should and will be the patient's responsibility to pay. Ultimately, the office should collect the same amount in total for a case no matter how insurance responds.

CASE STUDY 3. **PALATAL VENEERS**

Cosmetic-type work is often declined by insurance and if in-network, may likely result in disallowances as well. Therefore, cosmetic cases should be undertaken with full advance knowledge of whether a patient has insurance or not. This is not because the office needs to bill differently but rather because there will be necessary additional paperwork for

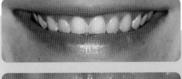
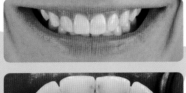
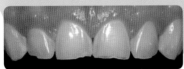
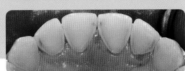

in-network patients to undergo these types of cases without insurance consideration.

In this case, a relatively young patient has sustained clear damage and decay resulting from bulimia. There are two concerns at play. The first is to repair the actual damage to the teeth. The second is to improve the outward appearance of the teeth. Potentially different treatments steps can be considered for this patient: (1) Fill any cavities sustained; (2) build up portions of teeth that have suffered damage; and (3) improve the cosmetic appeal. In this case, the dentist has opted to install a palatal veneer instead of the typical facial veneer because most of the damage was caused by acid erosion on the palatal surface. The patient is currently asymptomatic, and her main concern is cosmetic.

Insurance Questions to Answer:

1. How are cosmetic cases different with insurance?
2. Which codes would you file to insurance in this case? Any internal codes to think about?
3. What documentation would you want to submit for the best chance of insurance reimbursement?
4. Which waivers should be addressed?

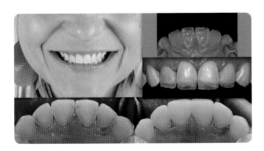

One of the most common challenges with anterior veneers is working with the occlusion. In this case, Dr. Sergie created palatal veneers to achieve a stronger and more uniform occlusion, allowing composite to guide the appearance of the final result. This is another great example of treatment that is outside the realm of basic insurance coding.

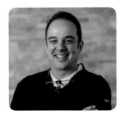

Dr. Aly Sergie maintains a restorative practice in Dallas, Texas, focusing on adhesive, cosmetic, and implant dentistry. He is known for making complex issues in dentistry easy to understand. The foundations of what he teaches is based on dental photography, adhesive dentistry, and treatment acceptance. You can find out more of this information at MondayMorningSolutions.dental and LearnDentalPhotography.com

Insurance Answers for Palatal Veneer Case

The common challenge with atypical cases is that ADA codes were designed to communicate procedures that insurance companies will potentially reimburse. Cosmetic cases are often not covered by insurance, and therefore fall outside the range of insurance reimbursement, coding, and fee capping. The additional challenge with this case is the coding for veneers and buildups do not match the services provided. D2962 is for labial veneers, and there is no code for palatal veneers. Core buildups are to support crowns—there is no code for a restoration to support a veneer.

> **CODING CONCERNS**
>
> D2962 – Porcelain labial veneer – laboratory
> *There is no code for a palatal veneer.
> D2950 – Core buildup
> *Core build ups are to support crowns, not veneers.

With the composite, the closest code is for a composite veneer D2960.

If you want some form of reimbursement for this case, you could file composite fillings for the anterior decay.

You will still need to use some type of coding to document in your ledgers. It would be appropriate to either use the closest ADA codes to what you are doing, or an internal bulk code for the total case. One could use the normal labial veneer code (D2962) as palatal veneers instead. Anterior composite coding would be the most appropriate as there is decay to remove and might bring in some insurance reimbursement. The increased length of tooth is a composite veneer. Upgrade codes would include additional costs for using cosmetic labs and multiple shades/stains for color matching.

> **POTENTIAL CODING FOR CASE**
>
> Insurance
>   D23XX – Composite fillings
> Internal
>   D2960 – Composite labial veneer – chairside
>   D2962 – Porcelain veneer – lab (palatal)
>   S2960 – Upgrade lab fee for premium lab
>   S2999 – Upgrade code for multiple/custom shade matching.

Documentation to Send

Fillings are typically auto-adjudicated; therefore, if you are only submitting insurance in this case for the composite fillings, no specific documentation should be required.

Waivers

The simplest way to handle this case is to put the cosmetic side of the case under a HIPAA waiver and remove insurance from the picture completely. See Chapter 18 for discussion of HIPAA waivers. When insurance is no longer an issue in this case, it can be treated basically as fee-for-service.

Summary

Most insurance policies contain exclusions clauses stating that they will not reimburse for cases of a cosmetic nature. While this is a concern for the patient, it should not be a major concern for the office. These policies are employer chosen, and it is rare for cosmetics to be covered by a third party. Use insurance for what it is designed to pay, and then run the rest as a non-insurance-based treatment. Any reimbursement in this case should be looked at as a huge win for the patient since the case and chief complaint are cosmetic in nature.

CASE STUDY 4. CROWN REPAIR

Cases can be difficult from an insurance view, but they can be difficult from a clinical view as well. This adult female patient presented with two adjacent crowns (#14, 15) with an open contact (gap) which was causing food to get packed between them. The traditional way to handle this would be to replace one of the crowns in order to close the gap.

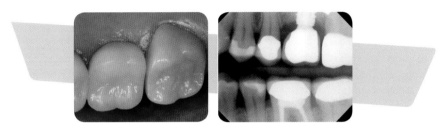

Instead, this case highlights an "outside the box" solution, which does raise some interesting ways to handle billing and insurance. Instead of replacing a crown, Dr. Sergie decided to repair the problem with a composite filling bonded to the crown. Many dentists would not treat this case in this manner due to the unpredictable nature of the process if not done perfectly.

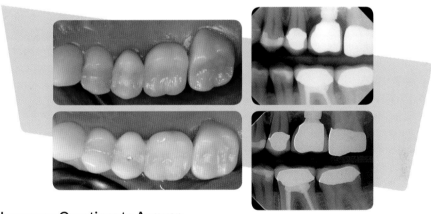

Insurance Questions to Answer:

1. How would you code this treatment?
2. Would insurance be involved?
3. Which documentation would you prepare to have the best chance of insurance reimbursement?
4. How might you discuss this treatment option with the insurance-driven patient?

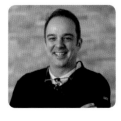

Dr. Aly Sergie maintains a restorative practice in Dallas, Texas, focusing on adhesive, cosmetic, and implant dentistry. He is known for making complex issues in dentistry easy to understand. The foundations of what he teaches is based on dental photography, adhesive dentistry, and treatment acceptance. You can find out more of this information at MondayMorningSolutions.dental and LearnDentalPhotography.com

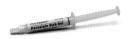

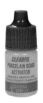

CODING RECOMMENDATIONS
D2980 – Crown repair
S2980 – Internal code for additional materials

Insurance Answers for Crown Repair Case

Supplies: This case required porcelain etchant, air abrasion, and porcelain bonding agents; most of which are not carried in a typical general dental office. Insurance will not reimburse for different methods of treatment, such as lasers or more expensive supplies. Therefore, these additional costs must be borne by the patient and charged separately.

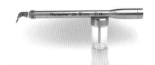

Documentation to Send

X-rays: While a bitewing is more diagnostic in this case, insurance often wants to see a PA with any crown-related procedure. It would be important to have both available.

Photos: The most important purpose for any photo is to help show what might not be as evident in an x-ray. In this case, it would be the open contact (gap). It can also be important to show the post-op repaired restoration as well.

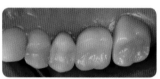

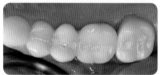

Narrative: The narrative is going to be the most important part of a case like this. On the initial view of the x-ray, many examiners might miss the problem presented as this case does not involve the decay/fracture problems typical to a crown case. The goal is to try to get insurance to see that by covering this crown repair, they are saving money instead of replacing a crown (the more common solution to this type of problem).

Waivers

An upgrade waiver for atypical materials/supplies would be ideal in this case. See Chapter 18 on upgrades.

Discussion with Patient

The goal in the treatment discussion with this patient about insurance should be less about coverage and more about overall savings. This case has a fair chance of not being reimbursed by insurance. However, the alternative is to replace a crown, which has even less chance of coverage because there's no fracture or decay and would cost the patient far more in the long run.

Crown repair codes can be hit or miss on coverage, so it would be important to advise the patient ahead of time that they might be responsible for the entire amount. Any reimbursement in this case should be looked at as a huge win for the patient.

POTENTIAL NARRATIVE:

"Patient presents with open contact #14/15 with food packing, periodontal pocketing, and potential for crown and/or implant loss. Crown repair necessary to close the contact gap, stop the food packing, and prevent more extensive decay and/or future treatment."

CASE STUDY 5.   **FRACTURED TOOTH**

Problems we see clinically do not always show up with an x-ray. This can present a challenge for insurance claims examiners as they rely heavily on x-ray attachments. The following case is a good example of where needed treatment for a fractured tooth might in fact be denied. Typically, the denial of this type of case is simply due to lack of clear documentation. Therefore, let's discuss this case and how to manage it within a realm of insurance to achieve reimbursement for the patient's benefit.

Case Notes: 32 y/o patient presents with chief complaint of "periodic pain on upper right when biting. Patient has no sensitivity to thermal stimulus but does have pain to direct pressure and release. Exam reveals premolar #5 fractured from mesial to distal.

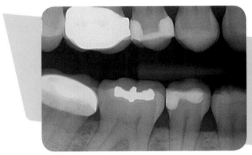 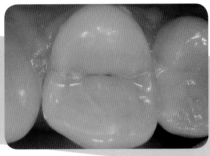

Insurance Questions to Answer:

1. Why is this an insurance challenge?
2. Which pictures and x-rays would you want to submit for the best chance of insurance reimbursement?
3. What narrative might you want to include with this case for insurance?

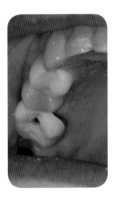

The case was successfully treated with a crown. The challenge comes in communicating to the insurance company in order to receive reimbursement.

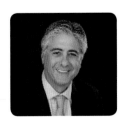

Dr. Sonny Spera owns and maintains fee-for-service practices, Progressive Dental, in New York and Pennsylvania. They have a fully integrated on-site dental lab with 2 CDTs. He focuses on digital dentistry with a passion for clinical diagnosis, restorative dentistry, practice management, team building, and growth. Dr Spera is a graduate of SUNY Buffalo Dental School. He is also a member of Academy of General Dentistry, International Association of Orthodontics, the American Academy of Dental Implant Association, and the Pierre Fauchard Academy.

Insurance Answers for Fractured Tooth Case

CODING

No coding challenges with this case, it is a simple D2740 – Porcelain Crown.

Photos and X-Rays to Send

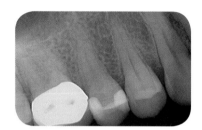

1. Bitewing x-rays serve no diagnostic or insurance value in this case. Any time a crown is done, a periapical (PA) is typically necessary to support the claim.
2. A photo showing the fractures from mesial and distal would be one of the most important attachments to include. Alternatively, or additionally, a photo showing internal fractures would help.

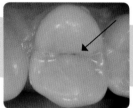
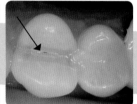
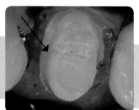

3. However, since the photo greatly depends on the quality of the image as well as the size, it can be very helpful to send a trans-illuminated photo, which highlights the fracture far better.

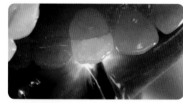

Case Narrative: All crowns but the most obvious crown due to fracture or decay should be submitted with a narrative. A basic narrative to send for this case is as follows:

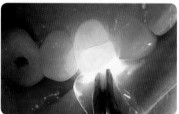

"Patient presents with a fracture completely through the tooth #5 from mesial marginal ridge to distal marginal ridge and across the pulpal floor (see photos provided). Patient has cracked tooth syndrome based on symptoms of pain to biting pressure, confirmed with positive tooth sleuth results. Crown required to stop breakage and prevent tooth loss."

You can refer to Chapter 23 for a full discussion on narratives for crowns and build ups.

Summary

This is a common scenario seen in dental offices of cases with obvious clinical needs for an indirect restoration, but where there are challenges relaying that information to an insurance company thoroughly enough for reimbursement. X-rays do not always show the problem, making photos and narratives an integral part of communications. Remember, reimbursement fights are in the best interest of the patient, as anything not collected from insurance should and will be the patient's responsibility to pay.

CASE STUDY 6.   ALL-ON-4

This is a beautiful case of a hybrid denture (All-on-4) from Dr. Christian Yaste. Complex cases can present challenges when submitting insurance claims. Almost any way you approach the claim, the result will be to max out the patient's policy benefits. Therefore, the most important understanding comes from how to code the case out, especially as an in-network provider, in order to make it feasible for an office to handle financially.

Case Notes: 32 y/o patient presents with multiple failing restorations and moderate periodontal disease. Main concerns were generalized sensitivity and esthetics. The patient was interested in an implant-based option due to a history of anterior trauma, early extensive decay, root canals not restored with crowns, rapid dental decline, and collapsed occlusion.

This case was started by acquiring diagnostic information such as CBCT, exam, photos, and preliminary impressions. The surgery was completed with a lab tech and dental anesthesiologist on site. A temporary restoration was seated initially. For try-in phases a milled model was used to simulate the expected outcome of the teeth for evaluation of function, occlusion, esthetics, and for patient approval. This case was finished over a period of several months with an implant retained zirconia hybrid restoration.

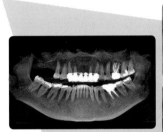
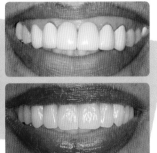
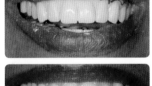
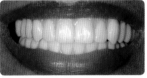

Insurance Questions to Answer:

1. Can an in-network office make this financially work?
2. What forms/waivers would you want to obtain from a patient?
3. What ADA codes would you file to insurance? Internal codes?
4. How might you present this to an insurance-based patient?

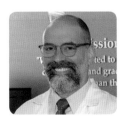

Dr. Christian Yaste graduated from the University of Michigan School of Dentistry in 1996 and then completed a two-year post graduate program in Oral Medicine at the Carolinas Medical Center in Charlotte, North Carolina Dr. Yaste is a founding partner at the Ballantyne Center for Dentistry and Charlotte Dental Implant Solutions, the only dental practice in 2019 to be ranked by Fortune Magazine in the "Top 35 places to work in healthcare in the US." The focus of his practice is helping adult patients who have complex and unique dental problems with an emphasis on sedation, cosmetic, and implant dentistry. Dr. Yaste is a clinician, mentor, educator, and has authored a book designed to help patients understand the changes in dentistry over the past two decades. He is passionate about using technology and finding cost effective solutions for dentists and patients.

Insurance Answers for All-on-4 Case
Can an In-Network Office Make This Work Financially?

Absolutely. This type of case is much easier to manage than traditional dentistry from an insurance view, seeing as most everything will be non-covered. See Chapter 17 for more details on non-covered services.

The waivers you will want to think about are either upgrade waivers, or HIPAA forms to not bill insurance for most of the case. The HIPAA option will remove the case almost completely from insurance entanglement, and typically make life much easier for the team and the patient. See Chapter 18 for discussions on upgrades and opt-out forms.

Patient Discussions

These hybrid cases are often all-or-nothing approaches. Unlike traditional dentistry, there is not really an option to remove parts of the plan. If you see the coding list on the right, this level of complexity can confuse even an experienced dental team member; what do you think the average patient will understand?

The offices who manage these cases often illustrate treatment with flat case fees to remove the complexity for all involved. One thought is to make sure that if you do need to itemize out a plan, ensure that the sum total of the individual items far exceeds the full case fee. Remove any ideas the patient might have that it is a menu to pick and choose from. See Chapter 22 for discussions on treatment planning and itemization.

TYPICAL CODING

D7210 – Surgical extractions
D6010 – Endosteal implants
D6190 – Surgical guide
D0367 – CBCT scan
D6114/D6115 – Hybrid dentures (teeth and acrylic only)
D6056 – Prefab abutments
D6051 – Temporary abutments
D6118/9 – Temporary dentures
D6055 – Titanium bar
D9xxx – Sedation
D73xx – Alveoloplasty
D7921 – PRF
Sxxxx – Temporary try-in denture
Sxxxx – Zirconia material upgrade
Sxxxx – On-site lab technician

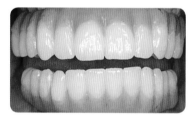

Treatment plans for cases like this are much better presented to the patient as full case fees. Itemizing out an insurance code list tends to only add confusion and a potential for patients to want to "pull things off the menu," which is not really an option. Coding should purely be used to help for insurance reimbursement, not for patient illustration or education.

Summary

Hybrid cases are becoming far more common in modern dentistry. Whether your office treats these types of cases or not, the understanding of how to code and submit these cases with insurance can be used on a variety of other types of general dentistry. Remember, reimbursement fights are in the best interest of the patient, as anything not collected from insurance should and will be the patient's responsibility to pay.

CASE STUDY 7.   COSMETIC VENEERS

Cosmetic work of most types is often declined by insurance, and if in-network, can generate disallowances as well. Cosmetic cases should be approached with full knowledge of whether a patient has insurance or not. This is not because the office needs to bill differently, but there will be necessary additional paperwork for in-network patients to fully understand their financial obligations for these types of cases and what insurance does and does not allow.

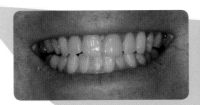 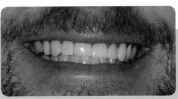

Case Notes: 41 y/o WM patient presents with history of multiple dental restorations of different color, uneven bite and smile, and lower crowding. Patient is asymptomatic and his main concern is cosmetic.

Insurance Questions to Answer:

1. How are cosmetic cases different with insurance?
2. What codes would you file to insurance? Internal?
3. What waivers should be addressed?

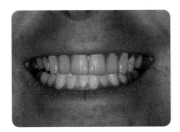

One of the most common challenges with anterior cosmetics can be occlusion and meeting the patient's esthetic goals. In this case, Dr. Danna provided a digital mock-up of the case to help with communicating goals. She also planned for some lower orthodontics to correct mild crowding concerns. This is another great example of treatment that is outside the realm of basic insurance coding.

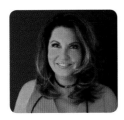

Dr. Jodi Danna graduated from Baylor College of Dentistry in 1995, completing her post-graduate program in Cosmetics and Geriatrics. Dr. Danna opened "The Danna Smile" in 2002. She holds Fellowships in the Academy of General Dentistry, the American College of Dentists, and the International College of Dentists. Dr. Danna was honored to be the 2017 Southwest Dental Conference Chairman and President and Boards Parliamentarian for the Dallas County Dental Society. In addition, she is the co-founder of Berman Instruments, providing high-quality, low-cost instruments for dentists.

Insurance Answers for Cosmetic Veneers Case

The common challenge with atypical cases is that ADA codes were designed to communicate procedures that insurance companies will potentially reimburse. In general, cosmetic cases are specifically not covered by insurance, and therefore fall outside the range of insurance reimbursement, coding, and fee capping. Unless there is decay or other non-cosmetic issues with the current restorations, one should expect this case to come with limited to no reimbursement. Some level of reimbursement may be achieved from the occlusal guard or removable ortho appliance if the patient's policy covers those services.

CODING

D2962 – Porcelain Veneers
D8210 – Removable Ortho Appliance
D9944 – Occlusal Guard – Hard, Full Arch
S9950 – In-Office Bleaching
S0150 – Digital Simulation Design
S2962 – Upgrade Lab Fee for cosmetic lab
S2999 – Upgrade Code for custom shade matching.

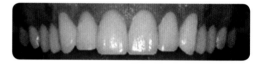

TREATMENT PLAN

Phase 1: Bleaching, Impressions for Lower Spring Retainer
Phase 2: Prep Veneers #5-12. Fabricate Provisionals.
Phase 3: Place Veneers, Impress for Occlusal Guard
Phase 4: Deliver Occlusal Guard

Upgrade codes might include additional costs for using cosmetic labs, digital simulation design, and custom color matching. Bleaching would also be an internal code. There is an ADA code for bleaching, but it is per arch, which is rarely done. ADA codes are also designed to communicate with insurance companies for potential reimbursement.

Since bleaching is never a covered service, there is no reason to use an ADA code. See Chapter 18 and 20 for discussions of upgrades and internal coding.

Waivers

The simplest way to handle this case is to separate the cosmetic side of the case, placing that portion under a HIPAA waiver to remove insurance from the picture completely. When insurance is no longer an issue in this case, it can be treated basically as fee-for-service. See Chapter 18 for discussion of HIPAA waivers.

Summary

Most insurance policies have exclusions documenting that they will not reimburse for cases of a cosmetic nature. While this may be a concern for the patient, it should not be a major concern for the office. These policies are employer chosen, and it is rare for cosmetics to be covered by a third party. This is no different than if you would purchase an auto liability policy that only has partial car replacement value. If you total your car, insurance will only pay for what the policy purchased designated, even if that is not enough to buy a replacement car.

Use insurance for what it is designed to pay, and then treat the rest as a non-insurance-based treatment. Any reimbursement in this case should be looked at as a huge win for the patient since the case and chief complaint are cosmetic in nature.

CASE STUDY 8. COSMETIC IMPLANT BRIDGE

Cosmetic type work often comes with challenges of being declined by insurance, and if in-network, a lot of disallowances as well. Cosmetic cases should be entered into with full knowledge of whether a patient has insurance or not. This is not because the office needs to bill differently, but there will be necessary additional paperwork for in-network patients to ensure clear financing for these types of cases.

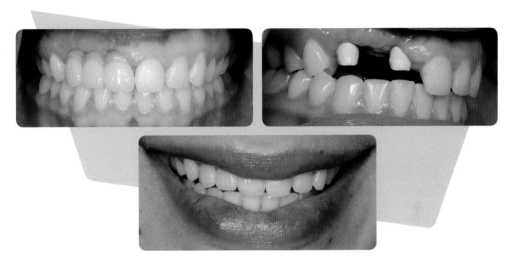

Case Notes: 24 y/o patient presents with history of trauma and missing teeth and bone on the upper right anterior.

Insurance Questions to Answer:

1. How are cosmetic cases different with insurance?
2. What codes would you file to insurance? Internal?
3. What waivers should be addressed?

One of the most common challenges with anterior cosmetics can be occlusion and meeting the patient's esthetic goals. In this case, Dr. Danna provided a digital mock-up of the case to help with communicating goals. She also planned for some lower orthodontics to correct mild crowding concerns. This is another great example of treatment that is outside the realm of basic insurance coding.

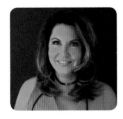

Dr. Jodi Danna graduated from Baylor College of Dentistry in 1995, completing her post-graduate program in Cosmetics and Geriatrics. Dr. Danna opened "The Danna Smile" in 2002. She holds Fellowships in the Academy of General Dentistry, the American College of Dentists and the International College of Dentists. Dr. Danna was honored to be the 2017 Southwest Dental Conference Chairman and President and Boards Parliamentarian for the Dallas County Dental Society. In addition, she is the co-founder of Berman Instruments, providing high quality, low-cost instruments for dentists.

Insurance Answers for Cosmetic Implant Bridge Case

The common challenge with atypical cases is that ADA codes were designed to communicate procedures that insurance companies will potentially reimburse. Typically, cosmetic cases are specifically not covered by insurance, and therefore fall outside the range of insurance reimbursement, coding, and fee capping. Unless there is decay or other non-cosmetic issues with the current restorations, one should expect this case to come with limited to no reimbursement. Limited reimbursement may come from the occlusal guard or removable ortho appliance if the patient's policy covers those services.

Upgrade codes might include additional costs for using cosmetic labs, digital simulation design, and custom color matching. Bleaching would also be an internal code. There is an ADA code for bleaching, but it is per arch, which is rarely done. ADA codes are also designed to communicate with insurance companies for reimbursement. Since bleaching isn't ever a covered service, there is no reason to use an ADA code. See Chapter 18 and 20 for discussions of upgrades and internal coding.

> **CODING SUGGESTIONS**
> D2962 – Porcelain Veneers
> D8210 – Removable Ortho Appliance
> D9944 – Occlusal Guard – Hard, Full Arch
> S9950 – In-Office Bleaching
> S0150 – Digital Simulation Design
> S2962 – Upgrade Lab Fee for cosmetic lab
> S2999 – Upgrade Code for custom shade matching.

> **TREATMENT PLAN**
> Phase 1: Bleaching, impressions for lower spring retainer
> Phase 2: Prep veneers #5–12, fabricate provisionals
> Phase 3: Place veneers, impress for occlusal guard
> Phase 4: Deliver occlusal guard

Waivers

The simplest way to handle this case is to place the cosmetic side of the case under a HIPAA waiver and remove insurance from the picture completely. See Chapter 18 for discussion of HIPAA waivers. When insurance is no longer an issue in this case, it can be treated basically as a Fee-For-Service case.

Summary

Most insurance policies have exclusions that they will not reimburse for cases of a cosmetic nature. While this is a concern for the patient, it should not be a major concern for the office. These policies are employer chosen, and it is rare for cosmetics to be covered by a third party. Use insurance for what it is designed to pay, and then approach the rest as a non-insurance-based treatment. Any reimbursement in this case should be looked at as a huge win for the patient since the case and chief complaint are cosmetic in nature.

CASE STUDY 9.   SINGLE IMPLANT

Implants are becoming more commonly treated within a general practice setting. The predictability and longevity of implants is a key driving force toward dentists switching from trying to save questionable teeth to installing more predictable implants instead. This is a common implant case that can highlight several concerns with insurance and reimbursement.

Correct documentation and coding are vital to successfully obtaining approval for insurance reimbursement. Understanding how insurance works with implants involves more than just knowing the basics of policy coverage. Therefore, let's discuss this case and how to manage it within a realm of insurance to provide the patient the most accurate estimate.

Case Notes: 52 y/o WM patient presents with decay under prior crown. When removed, the tooth was broken below the gumline. Due to the poor long-term prognosis of trying to save the tooth, the patient elected to have implant replacement.

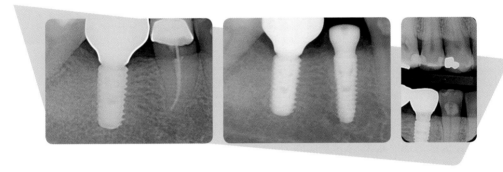

Insurance Questions to Answer:

1. Are implants covered for all patients?
2. What codes would you file to insurance? Internal?
3. Which pictures and x-rays would you want to submit for the best chance of insurance reimbursement?
4. What other insurance reimbursement concerns might you need to think about?

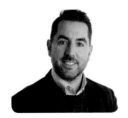

Dr. Paul Goodman is a practicing general dentist and the managing partner of a group practice with two locations, along with his brother, Jeffrey, in Mercer County, New Jersey. In 2017, Dr. Goodman founded Dental Nachos. Dental Nachos is dedicated to increasing the success and decreasing the stress of dentists and teams! Dr. Goodman is also a practice broker, speaker, and coach for dentists. After graduating from the University of Pennsylvania School of Dental Medicine in 2002, Dr. Goodman pursued additional training at Albert Einstein Medical Center in Philadelphia. During his general practice residency and hospital fellowship at Albert Einstein Medical Center, Dr. Goodman had the fortunate opportunity to learn how to place and restore dental implants. Dr. Goodman has a passion for teaching, speaking, and giving back to the dental community. Dr. Goodman can be reached at drnacho@dentalnachos.com or by visiting www.dentalnachos.com.

Insurance Answers
for Single Implant Case

Implants are not covered for all patients. Typically implant coverage is an add-on that employers can choose to offer or not. As such, many policies do not include coverage for implants at all. If there is no implant coverage, there may be no alternative/downgraded benefit coverage (of a partial) either should the patient elect to proceed with an implant.

TREATMENT CASE

D7210 – Extraction-surgical/erupt tooth
D7953 – Bone graft socket
D0383 – CT image, both jaws
D6190 – Implant guide
D6010 – Surg place implant: endosteal
D6011 – Second stage implant surgery
D6057 – Custom abutment-incl placement
D6058 – Abutment supported Pporc/cer cr.
D3 – Insert crown

This can be beneficial to the office in most states due to how non-covered services are handled. This removes the restrictions that the insurance company places on the quality of care that can be delivered. See Chapter 17 for more details about non-covered benefits.

Coding

You can see the chart on the right has the codes that were filed in this specific case. Potentially one could also have coded for a membrane as well if one was used. The D3 Insert crown code is an example of an internal code for tracking purposes that would not be submitted to insurance.

Photos and X-Rays

Photos are not usually requested or required for claims involving treatment for extractions, bone grafts, and implants. However, occasionally they are, which is why it is good to always document these thoroughly, regardless of specific insurance requirements.

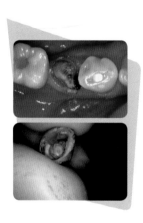

X-rays are highly important and often the only documentation the insurance company requests to see. Some policies and companies will cover implants with minimal required data. However, enough companies require more specific information that it is prudent to always have good photographic documentation available as well, if needed. You cannot obtain pre-op information that was missed after treatment is started.

The reason for this documentation necessity is what is most important to understand about implant treatment. Many policies are written with LEAT clauses (see Chapter 6). Partials are considered a LEAT in a case where a patient is missing a tooth on both sides of the mouth in the same arch (top or bottom). This is why many insurance companies require a pano or FMX to evaluate a claim for an implant. They are wanting to see whether the policy would need to pay for the implant or the lower-cost, removable partial denture.

Many insurance policies also have a missing tooth clause (MTC, Chapter 6). This means if the tooth was removed before the insurance policy took effect, the replacement of the tooth (implant in this case), would not be covered.

The best practice with implant treatment is to always get an FMX or pano before the removal of the tooth. This will give you the best chance of obtaining insurance reimbursement for your patient.

CASE STUDY 10. HEMI-SECTION

Occasionally dentists are provided with cases that are outside the ordinary and which require more complex treatment. These cases can be both interesting and gratifying to treat, providing great results for patients. However, they can also become complex to handle within an insurance-driven world.

Here is such a case where the treatment provided was a hemi-section, which can be difficult to accomplish. Correct documentation and coding are vital for successfully obtaining approval for insurance reimbursement.

Case Notes: 32 y/o patient presents with non-restorable external cervical invasive resorption under the bone on the mesial of #30. In order to save the tooth in a patient so young, a hemi-section was performed. A hemi-section is when half of the tooth and root is removed in order to save the remaining half. The tooth was then restored with a bridge to maintain a balance with normal chewing pressures.

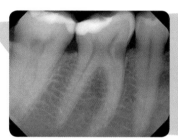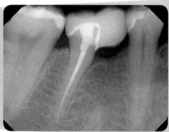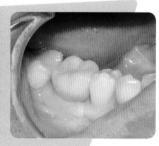

Insurance Questions to Answer:

1. What codes would you file to insurance?
2. Would you expect insurance to cover every code?
3. Which pictures and x-rays would you want to have the best chance of insurance reimbursement?
4. What important points should be discussed with the patient regarding insurance with this type of treatment option?

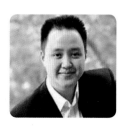

Dr. Raymond Zhu completed a Bachelor of Science Degree at the University of Toronto and received his Bachelor of Science Degree in Dentistry, and his Doctor of Medical Dentistry degree from the University of Manitoba. At both universities he was on the Dean's Honor List, recognizing him as one of the top students in his class. In addition to numerous awards, Dr. Zhu received the distinguished University Gold Medal for graduating with the highest standing in Dentistry. Dr. Zhu began his career in private practice in Winnipeg, Manitoba. In addition to private practice, he was also a part-time clinical instructor at the Faculty of Dentistry, where he has taught first-, second-, and third-year dental students in the disciplines of Crown and Bridge, Root Canal therapy, and Dental Anatomy and Occlusion. He is currently in full-time private practice.

Insurance Answers for Hemi-Section Case

Coding

The final restoration is and is not a bridge. It is a bridge in that it spans a gap with a missing tooth root but does not span a gap with a complete missing tooth. It would be appropriate to treat this as a three-unit bridge, a two-unit bridge (two abutments, no pontic), or as a single crown with a wing (as seen in this case). A three-unit bridge is likely to cause insurance reimbursement concerns, as there is no tooth normally between #29 and 30. In the case of a two-unit bridge, it is possible that insurance would pay for the crown on #30 but not #29 since there is nothing wrong with #29.

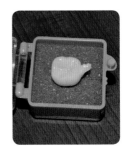

Photos and X-Rays

The more uncommon, difficult, or expensive the procedure, the more documentation is likely to be needed to correctly communicate with the insurance company. You can expect this type of case to be denied on the first round until you can get it in front of an actual dentist reviewer to evaluate the case. Claims examiners are not typically trained to handle cases that fall outside the ordinary. This usually requires an appeal of the denial.

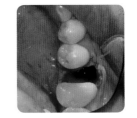

Both x-rays and photos are highly important to include in order to show not only what was done, but also to show the successful outcome. Many insurance policies are written such that treatment with a questionable prognosis are not covered. Therefore, in more extraordinary cases, it is important to show final images that depict a high chance for long-term success.

You will also want to be aware of any LEAT clauses where insurance might pay for a partial instead of a bridge (see Chapter 6). If this is the case, then a pano or FMX should also be attached.

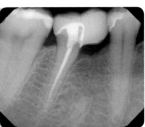

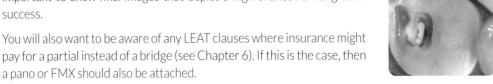

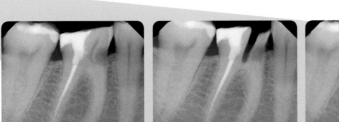

CASE STUDY 11. **EXTRACTION AND GRAFTING**

Case pictures of restorations often get the most "oohs and aahs" in dentistry, but even basic surgery is highly important in the day-to-day life of a dental office. Surgical cases are generally more straightforward when dealing with insurance. What follows is a well-documented extraction and grafting case by Dr. Napoletano. This particular example makes a great starter case study for testing your insurance knowledge.

Case Notes: Patient presents with a buccal abscess, non-restorable. The patient expresses interest in replacing the tooth with an implant, so the chosen treatment is an extraction and socket preservation graft for future implant placement.

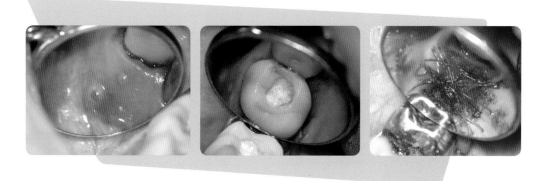

Insurance Questions to Answer:

1. What codes would you file to insurance?
2. Which pictures and x-rays would you want to include for the insurance claim?
3. What narrative might you want to develop for this case for insurance purposes?
4. Any reimbursement concerns to think about?

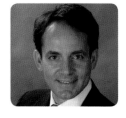

Donato (Dino) Napoletano, DMD, is a restorative dentist at Donato Dental in Middletown, New York, where he routinely utilizes technologies such as Dental Operating Microscopes, CEREC, and multiple laser wavelengths in the diagnosis and treatment of caries and periodontal disease. He is also a technology integration consultant and director of continuing education at Donato Dental Systems, LLC, dedicated to helping dentists evaluate, select, and integrate various technologies in a systematic and time-efficient manner. Donato (Dino) Napoletano, DMD, graduated from Boston University School of Dental Medicine in 1987 and has been in private practice in his hometown of Middletown, NewYork, since 1988. He also helps dentists across the country integrate various technologies to their practice.

Insurance Answers for Extraction and Graft Case Coding

The recommended coding is on the right. One common mistake made by offices is the bone graft code itself. Typically, D7953 is only a covered code when patients have implant coverage. This is why when getting breakdowns teams will find D7953 not covered but are told by the insurance company that D4263 – bone replacement graft is covered. The problem is that D4263 is a periodontal code that is only meant for grafting around a natural tooth. This would be an inappropriate code to use after an extraction. D4263 will likely be automatically denied when done with an extraction. Even if it does get paid initially, it will be demanded as a refund later for incorrect reimbursement. Do not fall into this common trap. If D7953 is not covered by the insurance policy, then the patient will need to pay out of pocket without insurance help; do not switch codes.

CODING RECOMMENDATIONS

D7140/D7210 – Extraction
D7953 – Bone replacement graft
for ridge preservation
D4266/D4267 – Membrane

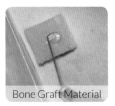
Bone Graft Material
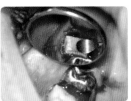

The other coding/insurance challenge is with membranes. The D4266/D4267 code is for a resorbable/non-resorbable membrane. This code does frequently get denied when completed on the same day as D7953. The denial is in part due to the fact that the membrane codes are actually perio codes and sometimes are seen as only covered when done in conjunction with a natural tooth.

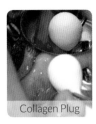
Collagen Plug

Similar to the bone graft, if you place a membrane for socket preservation after an extraction, it is highly likely the patient will need to pay out of pocket for that membrane. An alternative option would be to use a bone plug, which would not need a covering at all. Or to use a collagen plug or collagen tape instead of the membrane. This will help keep the cost down for both the office and patient.

Photos and X-Rays

The primary x-ray needed for an extraction would be a PA or pano. With the graft code, you might get a request for a pano due to the LEAT clause (see Chapter 6). If an insurance company determines it will not reimburse for an implant in the future, it will likely not reimburse for the bone graft either. Typically, photos are not necessary for insurance reimbursement for extractions and bone grafts. The patient either has coverage or does not.

Narratives

Like photos, narratives are not usually necessary for a bone graft, either they are covered, or they aren't. If you completed a surgical extraction, you might need a narrative to avoid receiving a "down-code" to simple extraction (see Chapter 20).

Reimbursement Concerns

The main reimbursement concerns have been addressed, as they all revolve around whether the insurance policy has implant coverage or not. It is important to let the patient know ahead of time what their expected co-pay will be to avoid unnecessary headaches.

CASE STUDY 12.   BUILDUP AND CROWN

Buildups and crowns, though common procedures for a dental office, also tend to generate a fairly high level of concerns and denials from insurance carriers. Since crowns are completed almost daily, this is one of the most important procedures for the dentist and team to document carefully for best chance of claim approval. Chapter 23 delves into this in depth, but this is such a beautifully documented case by Dr. Napoletano that we included it within the case studies.

Case Notes: Patient presents with a broken crown with decay around the margins.

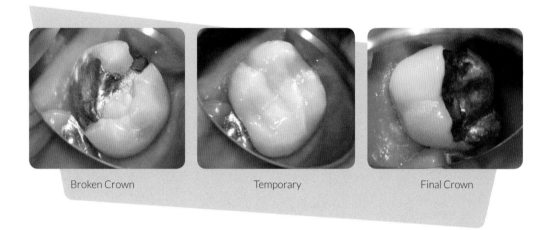

Broken Crown   Temporary   Final Crown

Insurance Questions to Answer:

1. What are the three most common items insurance wants to see to approve a buildup?
2. Which pictures and x-rays would you want to capture and include?
3. Which of the pictures shown below would be best to send, if only one?
4. What narrative might you want to document for this case for insurance?

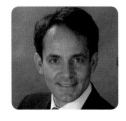

Donato (Dino) Napoletano, DMD, is a restorative dentist at Donato Dental in Middletown, New York, where he routinely utilizes technologies such as Dental Operating Microscopes, CEREC, and multiple laser wavelengths in the diagnosis and treatment of caries and periodontal disease. He is also a technology integration consultant and director of continuing education at Donato Dental Systems, LLC, dedicated to helping dentists evaluate, select, and integrate various technologies in a systematic and time-efficient manner. Donato (Dino) Napoletano, DMD, graduated from Boston University School of Dental Medicine in 1987 and has been in private practice in his hometown of Middletown, New York, since 1988. He also helps dentists across the country integrate various technologies to their practice.

Insurance Answers
for Buildup and Crown Case

Coding

Coding should not be a concern. The only complexity is making sure the crown code used
matches the material provided. It is important
to note that many insurance policies only cover
a lower-cost crown material (base metal or all metal). This is a downgrade,
and the patient would be responsible for the total of the network fee. See
Chapter 6 for more details on downgrades.

**MOST COMMON BUILDUP
REQUIREMENTS**
- \> 65% of missing tooth structure
- < 2 mm ferrule height
- At least 1 cusp missing

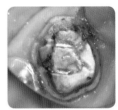

X-Rays

While most dentists want to see a pre-op BW x-ray for a crown, often insurance requires a pre-op PA. This is mostly because insurance policies
are written to reimburse crowns only for teeth with a good long-term
prognosis. They are looking at the root surface and bone to make sure the
tooth (and subsequent crown) has a high expected life span. If the decay
does not show up well on the PA, it is recommended to also submit a good
bitewing to show the decay.

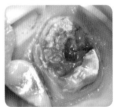

Post-op PAs are often required as well to show the original problem was
fixed.

Many insurance companies ask for an x-ray of the buildup. A photo can be
substituted instead.

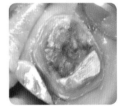

Photos

The most important two photos to submit for buildups are mid-op, before,
and after the BU is done (shown on the right). The before picture ideally should be as indicative of problems as possible (before decay removal
and/or showing internal fractures). The photo on the top right is the best
of the three from the previous page as it is clean of cement but still shows
the decay and staining.

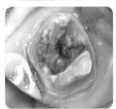

Narratives

Clear narratives are also important to include with the claim for buildups
and crowns. The main points you want to address are (see Chapter 23 for
full narrative breakdown):

- What is the problem (decay, fracture, pain, etc.)?
- How severe is the problem?
- What do you see that does not show up well on the x-ray
  and/or photo?
- Which of the most common buildup requirements does
  this case satisfy?

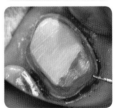

CASE STUDY 13.   LANAP

Periodontal procedures make up some of the most common procedures in any office. It is important to know how insurance policies will respond to perio cases, both in what codes may or may not be covered, as well as additional services that will not be recognized. This is a beautifully documented case of periodontal surgery by Dr. Napoletano that was treated with LANAP. LANAP, which stands for Laser-Assisted New Attachment Procedure, is a process where a laser is used to clean and disinfect infected tissue far better than traditional methods.

Case Notes: Patient presents with generalized severe periodontal disease and teeth in poor occlusion. Mobility and pus drainage were noted in multiple locations. Prognosis with traditional therapies would be guarded. After periodontal therapy, the patient was placed into orthodontia to correct the malocclusion. Below you can see the before and after photos, x-rays, and perio charts.

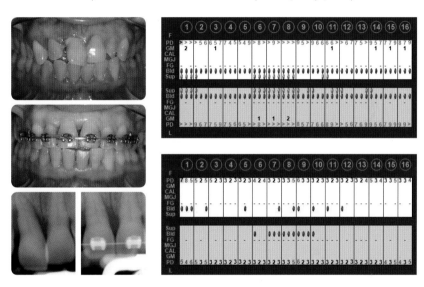

Insurance Questions to Answer:

1. Can you bill more for a procedure that is treated with a laser?
2. Which pictures and x-rays would you want to capture?
3. What information is missing from the perio charts that is necessary to include with insurance?

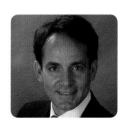

Donato (Dino) Napoletano, DMD, is a restorative dentist at Donato Dental in Middletown, New York, where he routinely utilizes technologies such as Dental Operating Microscopes, CEREC, and multiple laser wavelengths in the diagnosis and treatment of caries and periodontal disease. He is also a technology integration consultant and director of continuing education at Donato Dental Systems, LLC, dedicated to helping dentists evaluate, select, and integrate various technologies in a systematic and time-efficient manner. Donato (Dino) Napoletano, DMD, graduated from Boston University School of Dental Medicine in 1987 and has been in private practice in his hometown of Middletown, NewYork, since 1988. He also helps dentists across the country integrate various technologies to their practice.

Insurance Answers for LANAP Case

Coding

Periodontal surgery alone should not be a challenge with a case like this. Insurance will either re-imburse for this surgery or it won't. Many times, a policy will also hit the yearly maximum before finishing the case, leaving dental insurance as only a small coupon that can be applied for treatment.

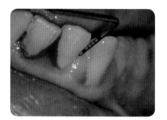

MAIN CODING CHALLENGE

Lasers are far more expensive to purchase and use, but codes are not descriptive of the method of treatment.

Insurance will not reimburse or authorize more for treatments performed with a laser.

The challenge comes because lasers are far more expensive to purchase and use than traditional methods of surgery. However, dental codes are not descriptive of the method of treatment. This means that if there are two methods for the same procedure, even though one may cost far more, in-surance will reimburse the same amount for either. For an out-of-network office, this choice affects the patent in terms of what they must pay. For an in-network office, office teams need to understand internal coding and how to charge for upgrades if you want to adequately recoup costs for your time and service. The office can charge an upgrade fee for use of a laser if optional (see Chapter 18 for upgrade charges).

Photos and Narratives

Similar to most other periodontal services, surgical cases are much more likely to be approved by insurance when you provide a great set of full mouth x-rays, quadrant photos of probes in position with bleeding, and periodontal charts. The most important piece of information from a perio chart is clinical attachment loss (CAL), which is not presented on the first page. See Chapter 23 for a full discussion.

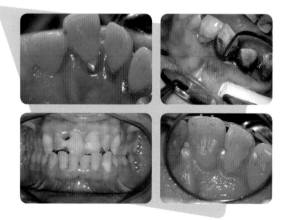

Summary

This case is a great example of an amazing service that is provided to the patient, yet at the same time, one that insurance will often not adequately cover. The challenge is more about understanding up front what insur-ance will and will not reimburse.

Then the office needs to make the decision on what steps they are going to take in re-sponse.

CASE STUDY 14.   COMBINATION IMPLANT AND VENEERS

The cases where dentists can achieve the greatest impact for our patients are often the more complex. When you combine emergency care with cosmetics, you can significantly change someone's smile and outlook on life. As mentioned in previous cases, cosmetic work of most types is often declined by insurance and if in-network, can generate disallowances as well. Therefore, cosmetic cases should be approached with full knowledge of whether a patient has insurance or not. This is not because the office needs to bill differently, but there will be necessary additional paperwork for in-network patients to fully understand their financial obligations for these types of cases and what insurance does and does not cover.

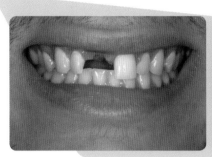 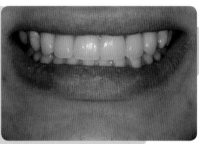

Case Notes: Young adult patient presents with broken front tooth due to a sports accident. He has a secondary concern of wanting to brighten, widen, and improve his overall smile. Case was completed with an implant on #8, veneers from #6–11, and buccal composite bonding on #4, 5, 12, 13.

Insurance Questions to Answer:

1. How are emergency/cosmetic cases different with insurance?
2. What part(s) of this case could be considered by insurance?
3. What codes would you file to insurance?
4. What waivers should be addressed?

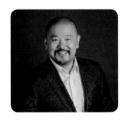 Jerry Hu, DDS, DABDSM, DACSDD, MICOI, FICOI, AFAAID, FIAPA, LVIF, FIADFE, travels the world to educate, research, and work on his numerous patent/IPs in dentistry. He is the founder of O2&U, which is a dental sleep medicine company based in Melbourne, Australia. He has taught seminars both hands-on and lectures all over North America and Asia in cosmetic, implant. and dental sleep medicine. He has been published in many peer-reviewed journals, such as AACD's *JCD*, including cover, as well as AGD's *General Dentistry*, AADSM's *JDSM*, and even *Aegis Inside Dentistry*, *DSP*, *Dental Economics*, and *Dentistry Today*. In 2019, he made the list of most recognized lecturers in dentistry for *Dentistry Today*. He also teaches weekly clinical pearls on Facebook's Dental Clinical Pearls forum. He has won many national competitions and awards in cosmetic dentistry, including MACSTUDIO nationwide model search and IAPA's Aesthetic Eye.

Insurance Answers for Implant and Veneers Case

The common challenge with atypical cases is that ADA codes were designed to communicate procedures that insurance companies will potentially reimburse. Cosmetic cases often are specifically not covered by insurance and therefore fall outside the range of insurance reimbursement, coding, and fee capping. Unless there is decay or other non-cosmetic issues with the current restorations, one should expect this case to come with limited to no reimbursement. Potential reimbursement may be achieved from tooth #8 due to trauma and the occlusal guard or any removable ortho appliance if the patient's policy covers those services.

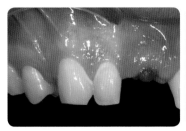 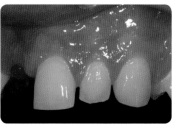

Internal upgrade codes might include additional costs for using cosmetic labs, digital simulation design, and custom color matching. Bleaching would also be an internal code. There is an ADA code for bleaching, but it is per arch, which is rarely done. ADA codes are also designed to communicate with insurance companies for potential reimbursement. Since bleaching is never a covered service, there is no reason to use an ADA code. See Chapters 18 and 20 for discussions of upgrades and internal coding.

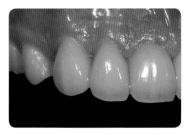 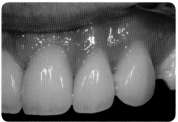

Waivers

The simplest way to handle this case is to separate the cosmetic side of the case, placing that portion under a HIPAA waiver to remove insurance from the picture completely. When insurance is no longer an issue in this case, it can be treated basically as a fee-for-service case. See Chapter 18 for discussion of HIPAA waivers.

Summary

Most insurance policies have exclusions documenting that they will not reimburse for cases of a cosmetic nature. As with a previous case, this may be a concern for the patient, it should not be a major concern for the office. These policies are employer chosen, and it is rare for cosmetics to be covered by a third party. This is no different than if you would purchase an auto liability policy that only has partial car replacement value. If you total your car, insurance will only pay for what the policy purchased designated, even if that is not enough to buy a replacement car.

Use insurance for what it is designed to pay, and then treat the rest as a non-insurance-based treatment. Any reimbursement outside the broken tooth in this case should be looked at as a huge win for the patient since the rest of the case and chief complaint are cosmetic in nature.

CASE STUDY 15. EMERGENCY IMPLANT CROWN

As implants become more common, so do the potential emergencies revolving around their treatment. In emergency situations, dentists understandably focus on taking care of the patient with minimal consideration of the insurance and billing side. Unfortunately, a lack of consideration of the financial implications can lead to burnout of providers, as they can feel inadequately reimbursed for their time. As a result, there are offices who simply turn away emergency treatment, which is not good for the patients.

Better understanding of coding, billing, and insurance can help alleviate the challenges involved with emergency care and provide the dentist with adequate compensation for what can often be a priceless service to the patient.

Case Notes: Patient presented with an implant placed by another provider. The patient shattered his flipper and was about to leave the country for several weeks. He needed an immediate solution and was seen on an emergency basis. The tissue around the implant was not yet in a good condition and the natural coloration of the teeth provided a difficult problem to overcome in matching teeth.

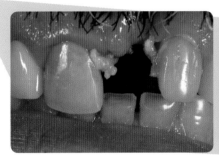 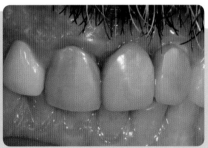

Insurance Questions to Answer:

1. What codes would you think about for this case?
2. Which of those codes would be potentially reimbursed by insurance?
3. Any necessary pictures or x-rays that you should think about obtaining?
4. What other insurance reimbursement concerns might you need to think about?

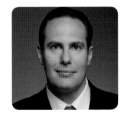

Dr. Arthur Volker graduated from the Columbia University School of Dental and Oral Surgery. Dr. Volker is a Diplomate of the World Congress of Minimally Invasive Dentistry and is a Fellow of the Academy of General Dentistry and the American College of Dentists. He was a clinical attending at the Coler-Goldwater Specialty Hospital and Nursing Facility on Roosevelt Island, and is in private practice in New York, with an emphasis on digital and minimally invasive dentistry. Dr. Volker has published articles and lectures nationally and internationally on such topics as cosmetic dentistry, minimally invasive dentistry, dental materials, and dental implants.

Insurance Answers for Emergency Implant Crown Case

Insurance is around to help with long-term solutions and is not often in the business of paying for temporary work. This means that most temporary solutions are non-covered services. The downside for patients is that this means there is no assistance for when they face an emergency situation and only want or can have a temporary solution. The benefit to the office is this means insurance rarely is involved with either the billing or fee setting side of these cases. This removes the restrictions that the insurance company places on the quality of care that can be delivered. This is why dentists and teams often should encourage patients to not delay treatment so they can avoid the emergencies.

> **CODING RECOMMENDATIONS**
> D0140 – Limited exam
> D0220 – 1st PA x-ray
> D6051 – Interim abutment
> D6085 – Provisional implant crown
> D9440 – Office visit after hours

Coding

The recommended coding for this case is seen on the upper right. Only the exam and x-ray are possible for insurance to cover, making most of this type of visit a fee-for-service arrangement. See Chapter 17 for more details on non-covered services.

Photos and X-Rays

Photos and x-rays are not usually requested by an insurance carrier to reimburse for exams and x-rays. Taking them would be purely for documentation purposes for the dentist and clinical chart.

Reimbursement

One point to think about with afterhours care is that insurance companies cannot be reached to verify coverage or benefits. In addition, during an emergency, the dentist only brings a single team member. Their focus should be purely on handling the emergency and not worrying about insurance coverage. Cases like this are ideally paid for 100% by the patient, leaving insurance to reimburse the patient later. An office can choose to either accept assignment of benefits or pass AOB on to the patient.

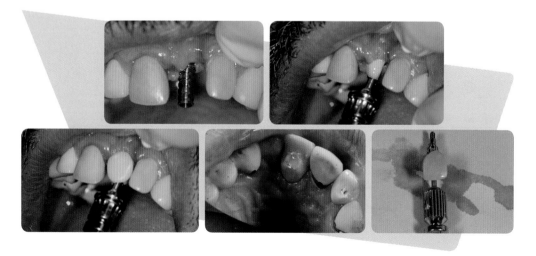

CASE STUDY 16.   RESIN VENEERS

Composite (resin) can be used for a variety of procedures. Dental teams most often think about it for use as a filling material. However, it can also be used for several other applications, in this case, for cosmetic veneers.

Case Notes: Patient presented with "black triangles" after orthodontic treatment. Black triangles refer to the dark spaces seen between teeth that either have too much of a triangle shape or have too much gum recession. These black triangles can be a cosmetic challenge, as they tend to draw the eye directly to the spot. The procedure to fix these is commonly called "bonding" by patients. However, the procedure is often miscoded by dental teams.

This beautiful case, presented by Dr. Volker, highlights an area of dentistry that can make a huge difference for patients. The location and blending of resin in these cases can be a challenge for many dentists. For in-network dentists, it is important to understand correct billing for this technique in order to make them worthwhile to learn to do.

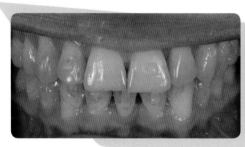 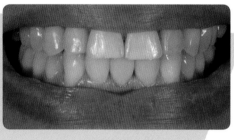

Insurance Questions to Answer:

1. What code would you think about for this case?
2. Would this be potentially reimbursed by insurance?
3. Any necessary pictures or x-rays that you should think about obtaining?
4. What other insurance concerns might you need to think about?

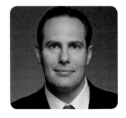

Dr. Volker graduated from the Columbia University School of Dental and Oral Surgery. Dr. Volker is a Diplomate of the World Congress of Minimally Invasive Dentistry and is a Fellow of the Academy of General Dentistry and the American College of Dentists. He was a clinical attending at the Coler-Goldwater Specialty Hospital and Nursing Facility on Roosevelt Island, and is in private practice in New York, with an emphasis on digital and minimally invasive dentistry. Dr. Volker has published articles and lectures nationally and internationally on such topics as cosmetic dentistry, minimally invasive dentistry, dental materials, and dental implants.

Insurance Answers for Resin Veneers Case

Fillings versus Veneers

A filling is typically a replacement of tooth structure that fits within the original tooth; it "fills" a defect. In trauma cases, it can sometimes be used slightly outside of the borders of natural structure. However, at some point, it becomes more outside of the boundaries of the tooth and is no longer adaquate to refer to it as a "filling."

This is where resin veneers take over. Porcelain is most commonly thought of when the term veneer comes up. However, veneers can also be resin based (filling material). A veneer is a restoration that covers the outer section of a tooth. It does not fill a tooth; it expands and/or reshapes the tooth.

Coding

It would be inappropriate to code the service provided in this case as a D2335 composite filling. As mentioned, this treatment goes well beyond the idea of "filling" a defect in the tooth.

The D2960 - direct placement resin veneer is the correct code to use. This code is almost always seen as cosmetic by insurance companies, therefore they classify it a non-covered service and is no longer applicable to insurance discounted fees in most states. See Chapter 17 for more details on non-covered services.

Photos and X-Rays

Photos and x-rays are not typically requested for cosmetic services, as claims are often denied outright. Taking them would be purely for documentation purposes for the dentist and clinical chart.

Narrative

It is always important to be honest with the insurance company to avoid any hint of fraud. When dealing with a cosmetic case, it is advised to write a note or narrative to the insurance company that the treatment is cosmetic in nature. It would also be advisable to let the patient know that this service would not likely be reimbursed so they can prepare to pay for the entire service fee.

CODING CONCERNS

D2335 – Anterior 4+ surface composite filling

vs

*D2960 – Resin veneer - direct

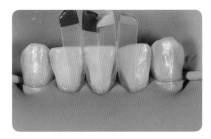

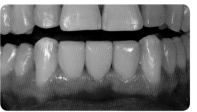

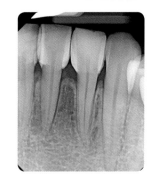

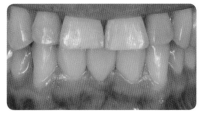

Glossary

When learning any new concept, it is vitally important to understand the language and terminology used in that arena. If you are new to dental insurance, it might be a good idea to read through this section more than once. If you have been working with insurance for a while, a quick read might still be a good refresher.

American Dental Association (ADA). The ADA is responsible for creating and maintaining the dental codes used with insurance billing. They also recommend the guidelines that go with that process. It is important to understand the ADA is a trade organization and not a regulatory body. This means they do not set laws that must be enforced; they can only recommend changes to the industry.

Appeal. When dental services are performed for an insured individual, and subsequently a claim is submitted for payment, the insurance company will review the claim in detail. If the claim is not adequately substantiated in their eyes, the claim may be denied. If the insured or dentist/dental provider does not agree with the denial, the claim may be resubmitted for a second review. The process for resubmitting the claim to change the outcome/decision is considered an "appeal" for further consideration.

This is different than reprocessing a claim. You only have two chances to appeal.

Assignment of Benefits (AOB). Insurance companies will assign benefits to either the patient or the office. Whoever is assigned the benefit is where the reimbursement check is sent. Most insurance companies allow AOB to go to either the provider or the policyholder based on what is designated in the claim. A few companies, such as Delta Dental, will typically only send AOB to the policyholder when the provider is out of network.

Benefit Year. The 12-month period a member's dental plan covers. The plan year is not always a calendar year; it depends upon the company. It could also be based on a fiscal year (e.g., April–March, Oct–Sept, or July–June).

Benefits. Dental benefits are the specific treatments and services that a dental insurance policy agrees to cover. There are seven basic areas of dental care that can be included in a typical plan.

1. preventive care, i.e., cleaning, routine office visits
2. restorative care, i.e., fillings and crowns
3. endodontics, i.e., root canals
4. oral surgery: tooth removal and minor surgical procedures such as tissue biopsy and drainage of minor oral infections
5. orthodontics: retainers, braces, etc.
6. periodontics: scaling, root planing, and management of acute infections or lesions
7. prosthodontics: dentures and bridges

These seven types of procedures can be divided into three broad areas of coverage, that is, preventive, basic, and major. You can see a thorough analysis in Chapter 6.

Breakdown. A dental insurance breakdown is an itemized illustration of what insurance companies will pay for specific procedures. Offices create breakdowns so that an estimate can be made for the patient's treatment plan. Every insurance policy is unique, which makes breakdowns one of the most important tools in the office if you are going to be accepting assignment of insurance benefits. Even if you collect all money up front, patients will want to understand/request information as to how their insurance carrier might reimburse them for their treatment plan.

Breakdowns may come directly from an insurance company in the way of a fax, online list, or automatic phone system. However, the most common way of obtaining a detailed breakdown of policy coverage is by speaking to an insurance representative on the phone.

Cafeteria Plan. A cafeteria plan gets its name from a cafeteria but has nothing to do with food. Just as individuals make food selections in a cafeteria, employees can select the benefits of their choice from a pool of options offered by their employers. One big reason why health insurance is offered through employers is so the employee can purchase them with pre-tax money out of their paycheck. A cafeteria plan provides the opportunity for employees to select from a menu of benefits, choosing the benefits they decide are tailored to their personal needs. The benefit to the employer is lowered payroll taxes for both the employee and employer.

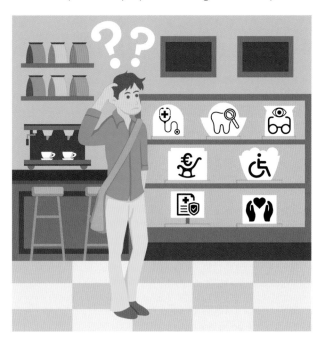

Cafeteria plan selections include insurance options, such as health savings accounts (HSAs), life insurance, disability insurance, and of course medical and dental insurance.

Claim. A formal request to an insurance company to cover all or part of the cost of a dental procedure. Claims are reviewed by the insurance company and are either approved, returned for more information, or denied. When approved, payment of the claim can be made directly to the dental office or, if the patient pays the dentist up front, then the insurance company can reimburse the insured.

Claims Bundling. Systematic combination of unique dental services by insurance companies in order to reduce the benefit to the patient/subscriber.

Claims Examiner (Agent). The insurance company employee who handles claims and determines whether the treatment meets the policy guidelines for reimbursement. They are often not dentists and are only minimally trained in dentistry.

"Clean Claim". A claim with all fields completed and that complies with the payer's published filing requirements. According to most state laws, clean claims must be paid in 30/60 days. This is why it is so important for the team to send claims out correctly the first time. The law often does not have restrictions on claims that are not clean or accurate.

Clearinghouse. A middle-man entity that translates electronic claims information submitted from dental offices into usable information for each insurance company.

Coordination of Benefits. This is the process by which a secondary insurer coordinates payment for a claim after the primary insurer has determined payment. There are a few different ways that insurance companies could possibly coordinate benefits, which can result in anything from zero payment to coverage up to a dental office's full fee. This complexity often leads to a lot of challenges for the dental team. See Chapter 9 for more details.

Contracted Dentist. A dentist is considered contracted or in-network when the dentist and insurance company agree to a reduced fee that's lower than the office's full fee or "retail" price. When a patient chooses services from a contracted, in-network provider, their resulting fee is lower than if they went to a dentist who was out of network or non-contracted. The contracted dentist also agrees to a set of rules that must be followed to work with that company.

Deductible. The amount of money that the policyholder is required to pay up front to the provider before dental policy benefits are considered or approved. The deductible is usually an annual amount, often ranging between $50 and $100. A policy may require one deductible to cover the entire family, or it could require a deductible for each member of the family. The deductible does not need to be paid until the patient has dental procedures done that are subject to the deductible and a claim is submitted. Commonly, procedures that are covered at 100% do not invoke the deductible.

For example, if the patient comes in for a treatment costing $100, and the deductible for their policy is $100, then the patient must pay the first $100 directly to the dentist. The next visit to the dentist in the same coverage year will then qualify for payment or reimbursement by the insurance company according to the terms of the policy. Even when a patient's deductible has not yet been met and they owe the dentist the deductible amount, a claim for those services must still be filed with the insurance company. Filing with the insurance company is to make them aware that services have been rendered and the deductible amount has been satisfied by the patient.

Denial. This is a potential response by an insurance company to a claim that means the insurance company will not reimburse for a specific procedure, but the office can proceed to collect the fee from the patient.

Dental Plan. A dental plan is quite simply a specific insurance product that is purchased by an employer as a benefit to be offered to their employees or by an individual for themselves. There are many different types of dental plans, including Preferred Provider Organizations (PPO), Dental Health Maintenance Organizations (DHMO), and Direct Reimbursement.

Dependents. Any family member who may be covered under a dental insurance policy in addition to the policyholder (insured). Usually it includes spouse and/or children living with the insured.

Disallow. This is a potential response by an insurance company to a claim. A disallow means the insurance company will not reimburse for a requested procedure and also determines that the in-network dental office should not charge for the procedure either. This is one of those rules that may be included in an in-network contract the dentist signs, a clause which can often be more onerous than the reduced fee schedule. It is important to understand the ADA is firmly against the use of disallowing costs.

Dual Coverage. Dual coverage means a patient is covered by multiple insurance companies that may provide reimbursement. This typically does not mean double coverage though. Secondary insurance policies usually do not pay as much as primary.

> **Q: My patient has dual coverage; does this mean they get four cleanings per year?**
> A: Generally, no.

Explanation of Benefits (EOB). Once a claim has been reviewed and approved or denied for payment, both the dental office and the policyholder will receive a notice from the insurance company explaining in detail what treatment was approved, what amount was paid (or denied) to the dentist, and what amount may still be owed by the insured. This document is referred to as an EOB. EOBs are not standardized by the ADA; each insurance company has a different layout for their EOBs. It is important to learn how to read these statements and understand what information they are trying to convey back to you. See Chapter 10 for a walkthrough of some common layouts and how to understand them.

Explosion Code (Macros): Many dental codes are commonly used together to describe a given procedure. For efficiency, an explosion code (aka macro) is the term for one button in a dental software system which will in turn input multiple codes at once into a patient's chart. For example, an Explosion Crown Code enters an x-ray, build up, crown, and seat code at the same time.

Fee for Service (FFS). A provider that treats patients without signing any contracts or agreeing to follow any specific fee schedule and then collects payment from patients directly when a service is provided. If they file claims on behalf of a patient, assignment of benefits is sent to the patient.

Frequency Limitation. The time period after which insurance will reimburse for services again. Example: many insurance policies have a six-month frequency limit for exams, meaning they will not reimburse for another exam conducted after five months due to frequency limitations but will reimburse after six months have passed since the last exam.

Group Coverage. Group dental plans provide insurance not to an individual but to an entire group. For example, a dental insurance provider may provide dental coverage to an employer for his or her employees. Dental insurance providers tend to prefer to offer group insurance because group insurance offers the most profitable form of dental insurance for insurance companies. Many individuals also like group insurance because it offers the most cost-effective, flexible, and comprehensive type of dental insurance.

Inclusive (Bundled) Services. Dental services that are bundled together by insurance companies as part of another unique service.

In-Network. This term refers to a provider who has signed a contract with an insurance company to follow a specific fee schedule, along with a set of rules determined by the insurance company. In exchange, the insurance company will list the provider online for more visibility to patients.

Insured. An insured is any individual who is covered under a specific insurance policy. An insured may be your patient, a spouse, or family member of the patient.

Non-Duplication of Benefits. This is a common clause with coordination of benefits that means the secondary insurer will reimburse nothing if the primary insurer pays equal to the secondary payment benefit or greater. See Chapter 9 for more details.

Out-of-Network (OON). A provider that treats patients without signing an insurance contract or agreeing to follow any specific fee schedule but still files claims for patients and waits for reimbursement. The reimbursement amount for an out-of-network provider is usually higher than the amount for an in-network-provider.

Policy. A dental insurance policy is a formal contract between two parties. Most often the policy is in effect for one year, when it must then be renewed. One party, the "insured," is the individual who may need dental treatment during the course of the contract year. The other party is the insurance carrier, who agrees to provide payment for dental service rendered according to the agreed-upon parameters of the policy contract. A policy is usually unique to the employer or group, meaning each patient will likely have a different set of coverage than another's.

Policyholder. The individual whose dental health is covered under the terms of the policy or insurance contract. Many times, the policyholder will be the patient you are seeing, but parents or spouses could also be the policyholder instead.

Pre-authorization (Pre-Auth). A pre-authorization provides written advance approval for the planned services, which is generally valid for 60 days. Certain types of services require advance approval, or pre-authorization. This pre-authorization for specified procedures is important, and the failure to obtain it may result in denial of the claim. Pre-authorizations are common with medical policies and are almost non-existent in dental policies. Dental policies use pre-determinations instead.

Predetermination (Pre-D). A predetermination provides written coverage details for the planned services, which is generally valid for that benefit year. Pre-Ds do not guarantee payment like Pre-Auths.

While not common, certain types of services may require advance predetermination. This pre-D for specified procedures is important, and failure to obtain it when required may result in denial of the claim.

Premium. The premium is the amount of money that the employer and policyholder pay monthly (or bi-weekly) in order to have insurance coverage. Most often that premium is made through payroll deduction out of the employee paycheck. The employer then sends the premium payments on behalf of their employees in bulk to their insurance company.

Progressive Plan. This is a term used for an insurance policy that increases in benefits for every year the subscriber is a part of the plan. Example: annual maximum for the plan for year one, two, and three are $1000, $1250, and $1500, respectively.

Prompt Payment Laws. These laws are passed by all states. They require insurance companies to pay "clean claims" within a certain time period. Prompt Payment Laws do not generally apply to self-funded (ERISA) plans. However, some PPO self-funded contracts will spell out a prompt payment policy.

Reprocessing/Reconsideration. Insurance companies will often ask for additional information to process a claim. When you provide this new information and resubmit the claim, it is called reprocessing. This is different than an appeal because there may not be a decision to appeal yet. It is often better to ask for a claim to be reprocessed in order not to use up one of your appeal chances.

Reference Numbers. When you call an insurance company for information, such as to get a breakdown, the call will be recorded. This recording is given a reference number. It is important to save these reference numbers for use later. If you are given incorrect information during a call, using the reference number and recorded call can persuade an insurance company to abide by the information that they provided (even if it was shown to be incorrect later).

Rollover. An insurance policy will usually have a yearly maximum. If the policyholder does not use all of the money in a given plan year, any remainder will disappear. Occasionally policies will include a rollover clause, which means part or all of that unused maximum will be useable the following year. Typically, this rollover of benefits is only for one year. For example if a policy has a rollover clause and the patient does not use their insurance for three years, they will only have two years of maximum funds to use.

Self-Funded Plan. Insurance plan where the employer takes all financial risk themselves but hires an insurance company to provide networks, call centers, and administrative support. This is different from traditional insurance (fully insured) where the insurance company handles everything, including the financial risk.

Subscriber. This term refers to the individual whose dental health is covered under the terms of the policy or insurance contract. Many times, the subscriber will be the patient you are seeing, but in other cases, you'll find parents or spouses might be the subscriber instead.

Verification. Verification is the process of double-checking whether the patient has active dental insurance coverage. This is often done by fax or phone but can occasionally be retrieved from online platforms with some insurance companies.

Acknowledgments

I began the process of writing this book in early 2020. Covid-19 hit the scene while I was still in the early stages of drafting the material. Like other businesses, my dental practice was closed for several months, which truthfully allowed me more time than anticipated to write. The timing was certainly a gift, as I did not appreciate just how much time would be required to cover the vast topic of dental insurance. Nor did I appreciate how many people would end up helping me get to the finish line.

Writing a book of any kind starts out as a concept, then a first outline, and slowly takes shape through many writings and rewritings over a long period of time. My first book was under 150 pages. At the time, it was a daunting project. My second book, the insurance text you now have in your hands, is over 300 pages and significantly more technical in content. While dental insurance is certainly one of my most favorite topics, the process of creating a teaching/reference manual of this size and scope cannot be accomplished without the help of many talented and dedicated people.

Working full time, and with two small children at home, there is little time left over to accomplish something so significant as writing a textbook. It certainly cannot be done without carving out time and space in our household to concentrate. I am blessed with a wonderful, supportive wife, Susan, who manages to carve out quiet time both for me to write, for her to provide great input, and create magical family time. Thank you, Susan; you are indeed a phenomenal life partner.

Special thanks to Rebecca Campbell, my mother, who serves as my "behind the scenes" writing partner and preliminary editor. Your expertise gained from a career in human resources within the insurance industry as well as your diplomatic instincts and communication skills were particularly valuable through the entire conception, outline, rough draft, and polishing phases of this 300-plus-page, technically detailed insurance manual. I am indeed grateful for our close and ongoing collaboration.

A thank you to Mark Ferber for your strategic insight and industry connections. You introduced me to the right resources to get this book off the ground, kept me moving forward with "mini-deadlines," as well as providing great feedback, ideas for content, and timely coaching along the way. I am not sure this book would have existed without your guidance and professional expertise.

To the entire team at Edra Publishing, thank you for helping me navigate the entire publishing process, answering questions, providing structure and feedback. You made this process easier than ever and made me appreciate why working with a publisher instead of self-publishing can be so much better!

In memory of my faithful, furry buddy Maxillary (Max), who was curled up in my lap for most of the time I was writing this textbook. You helped keep me company to finish writing but were sadly unable to see this book get published. Thank you for your constant presence and companionship over the last 14 years.

Thank you to all the amazing people who took time to read through a full rough draft of this textbook to give some great feedback! In particular, Minnie Garcia has been treatment coordinator at our dental practice for years and has accumulated a wealth of knowledge and experience in both dental and medical insurance.

Kinzie Broxon, who I also have the pleasure of calling a friend, has been a great resource. Her experience in dental insurance through her company, Dentalogic, has helped answer some tough, deep questions within the industry. Dr. Amanda Matsuhara, whom I have only had the pleasure of knowing for a short time, has some amazing insight into people and is the only other person I know to name a pet after dentistry!

There are so many people who touch our lives in various ways that it is impossible to acknowledge them all. Thank you to everyone who offers their time and talent to assist others improve and realize their dreams. The more we build each other up, the better our profession and society becomes.

Finally, a thank you to all the outstanding clinical dentists who submitted content for the case studies. This section is both a testament to what can be accomplished in dentistry as well as a great visual for learning through scenarios we see with insurance every day.

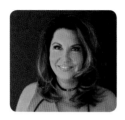

Dr. Jodi Danna graduated from Baylor College of Dentistry in 1995, completing her postgraduate program in cosmetics and geriatrics. Dr. Danna opened "The Danna Smile" in 2002. She holds fellowships in the Academy of General Dentistry, the American College of Dentists, and the International College of Dentists. Dr. Danna was honored to be the 2017 Southwest Dental Conference Chairman and President and Board's Parliamentarian for the Dallas County Dental Society. In addition, she is the co-founder of Berman Instruments, providing high-quality, low-cost instruments for dentists.

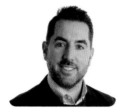

Dr. Paul Goodman is a practicing general dentist and the managing partner of a group practice with two locations, along with his brother, Jeffrey, in Mercer County, New Jersey. In 2017, Dr. Goodman founded Dental Nachos. Dental Nachos is dedicated to increasing the success and decreasing the stress of dentists and teams! Dr. Goodman is also a practice broker, speaker, and coach for dentists.

After graduating from the University of Pennsylvania School of Dental Medicine in 2002, Dr. Goodman pursued additional training at the Einstein Medical Center Philadelphia. During his general practice residency and hospital fellowship at Einstein Medical Center, Dr. Goodman had the fortunate opportunity to learn how to place and restore dental implants. Dr. Goodman has a passion for teaching, speaking, and giving back to the dental community.

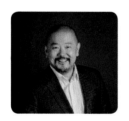

Jerry Hu, DDS, DABDSM, DACSDD, MICOI, FICOI, AFAAID, FIAPA, LVIF, FIADFE, travels the world to educate, research, and work on his numerous patent/IPs in dentistry. He is the founder of O2&U, which is a dental sleep medicine company based in Melbourne, Australia. He has taught seminars both hands-on and lectures all over North America and Asia in cosmetic, implant, and dental sleep medicine. He has been published in many peer-reviewed journals, such as AACD's *JCD*, including cover, as well as AGD's *General Dentistry*, AADSM's JDSM, and even *Aegis Inside Dentistry, DSP, Dental Economics*, and *Dentistry Today*. In 2019, he made the list of most recognized lecturers in dentistry for *Dentistry Today*. He also teaches weekly clinical pearls on Facebook's Dental Clinical Pearls forum. He has won many national competitions and awards in cosmetic dentistry, including MACSTUDIO nationwide model search and IAPA's Aesthetic Eye.

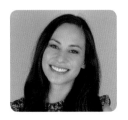

Dr. Amanda Matsuhara graduated from the University of the Pacific Arthur A. Dugoni School of Dentistry in 2019 and currently practices in San Francisco, both in private practice and at a community health clinic. Dr. Matsuhara has a passion for endodontics. Without many endodontists accepting Denti-Cal in San Francisco, she has made it her goal to make endodontic treatment more accessible.

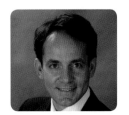

Donato (Dino) Napoletano, DMD, is a restorative dentist at Donato Dental in Middletown, New York, where he routinely utilizes technologies such as Dental Operating Microscopes, CEREC, and multiple laser wavelengths in the diagnosis and treatment of caries and periodontal disease. He is also a technology integration consultant and director of continuing education at Donato Dental Systems, LLC, dedicated to helping dentists evaluate, select, and integrate various technologies in a systematic and time-efficient manner.

Dr. Napoletano graduated from Boston University School of Dental Medicine in 1987 and has been in private practice in his hometown of Middletown, New York, since 1988. He also helps dentists across the country integrate various technologies to their practice.

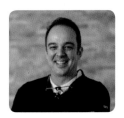

Dr. Aly Sergie maintains a restorative practice in Dallas, Texas, focusing on adhesive, cosmetic, and implant dentistry. He is known for making complex issues in dentistry easy to understand. The foundations of what he teaches are based on dental photography, adhesive dentistry, and treatment acceptance, which he teaches through Monday Morning Solutions and Learn Dental Photography.

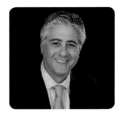

Dr. Sonny Spera owns and maintains five "Fee for Service" practices, Progressive Dental, in New York and Pennsylvania. They have a fully integrated on-site dental lab with two CDTs. He focuses on digital dentistry with a passion for clinical diagnosis, restorative dentistry, practice management, team building, and growth. Dr. Spera is a graduate of SUNY Buffalo Dental School. He is also a member of Academy of General Dentistry, International Association of Orthodontics, the American Academy of Dental Implant Association, and the Pierre Fauchard Academy.

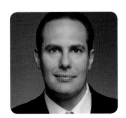

Dr. Arthur Volker graduated from the Columbia University School of Dental and Oral Surgery. Dr. Volker is a Diplomate of the World Congress of Minimally Invasive Dentistry and is a fellow of the Academy of General Dentistry and the American College of Dentists. He was a clinical attending at the Coler-Goldwater Specialty Hospital and Nursing Facility on Roosevelt Island and is in private practice in New York, with an emphasis on digital and minimally invasive dentistry. Dr. Volker has published articles and lectures nationally and internationally on such topics as cosmetic dentistry, minimally invasive dentistry, dental materials, and dental implants.

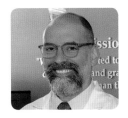

Dr. Christian Yaste graduated from the University of Michigan School of Dentistry in 1996 and then completed a two-year postgraduate program in oral medicine at the Carolinas Medical Center in Charlotte, North Carolina. Dr. Yaste is a founding partner at the Ballantyne Center for Dentistry and Charlotte Dental Implant Solutions, the only dental practice in 2019 to be ranked by Fortune Magazine in the "Top 35 places to work in healthcare in the US." The focus of his practice is helping adult patients who have complex and unique dental problems with an emphasis on sedation, cosmetic, and implant dentistry. Dr. Yaste is a clinician, mentor, educator, and has authored a book designed to help patients understand the changes in dentistry over the past two decades. He is passionate about using technology and finding cost-effective solutions for dentists and patients.

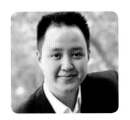

Dr. Raymond Zhu completed a bachelor of science degree at the University of Toronto and received his bachelor of science degree in dentistry and his doctor of medical dentistry degree from the University of Manitoba.

At both universities he was on the Dean's Honor List, recognizing him as one of the top students in his class. In addition to numerous awards, Dr. Zhu received the distinguished University Gold Medal for graduating with the highest standing in Dentistry.

Dr. Zhu began his career in private practice in Winnipeg, Manitoba. In addition to private practice, he was also a part-time clinical instructor at the Faculty of Dentistry, where he has taught first-, second-, and third-year dental students in the disciplines of crown and bridge, root canal therapy, and dental anatomy and occlusion. He is currently in full-time private practice in Maple, Ontario, devoted to comprehensive dentistry. He is a fellow and master of the International Congress of Oral Implantologists. He is also an affiliate clinician with RipeGlobal, one of the world's largest online dental networks.

About the Author

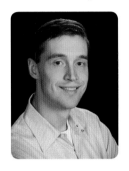

Dr. Travis Campbell, has been a practicing dentist since 2009, after graduating from Baylor University in Waco, Texas and then Baylor College of Dentistry in Dallas, Texas.

Yes, Dr. Campbell is a born and bred Texan, and proud of it! But even more notable… dentistry simply runs through his veins. He announced he "wanted to be a dentist" after his first dental visit at the age of three, and never once changed his goal. Today, dentistry remains a passion. He still loves the clinical side of treating patients, yet early on he developed a similar passion for the business end of running a practice. In fact, before he graduated from dental school, he built a vision and business plan for 380 Family Dentistry in Prosper, Texas. At the time, Prosper was a very tiny community well north of Dallas. There were cattle living across the highway from that first office!

Over the ensuing years, he has built that single dentist practice to its current position as one of the top one percent in the country. Through his experiences, he cultivated a personal "mission" to help other dentists avoid the typical pitfalls to become highly successful business owners.

Dr. Campbell is an author, trainer, speaker at dental conferences, a contributor to various online dental communities, and dental coach/consultant. He has been dubbed "The Practice Whisperer", which became the title of his first book released in 2019. Ever an entrepreneur, Dr. Campbell purchased a second dental practice, in Garland, Texas in the fall of 2019.

Having gained a reputation as an expert in the complex area of dental insurance, Dr. Campbell's new "moniker" is "The Dental Insurance Guy!" From understanding insurance to developing strategies to accelerate practice growth, Dr. Campbell delivers practical, actionable content that dentists and team members can use immediately. He dispels many of the myths and misinformation around today's dental insurance policies and explains how to navigate the complexities of being an exceptional dentist, business owner, and leader while still having a life outside of work.

Dr. Campbell lives in Prosper, Texas with his wife and two young children.

You can find more insurance related content, CE courses, articles, live Q&As, and much more by Dr. Campbell at www.TheDentalInsuranceGuy.com